Debarim Publishing
21566 Main St., Howe, OK 74940
www.debarimpublishing.com

Paperback ISBN-13: 979-8-9932402-5-1

COPYRIGHT PERMISSIONS

Excerpt(s) from *The Essential Home-Ground Flour Book* by Sue Becker, copyright © 2016. Used with permission of Robert J. Dees, president, Robert Rose, Inc., publisher.

Excerpt(s) from *Biological Ionization as Applied to Human Nutrition* by Alexander F. Beddoe, copyright © 1984-2008. Used with permission of Bruce Dickson, Publisher, Beddoe Books and Advanced Ideals.

Excerpts taken from *Merck Manual of Medical Information Home Edition* copyright © 1997 by Robert Berkow et al. Used with permission of Merck Research Laboratories, The Manuals Permission. www.merckmanuals.com

Excerpt(s) from *HANDS OF LIGHT* by Barbara Ann Brennan, copyright © 1987 by Barbara A. Brennan, Used with permission of Bantam Books, an imprint of Random House, a division of Penguin Random House LLC. All rights reserved.

Excerpt(s) from *Build a Better You* by Richard Brouse, D.C, copyright © 2001 by Dr. Richard Brouse. Used with permission of Dr. Richard Brouse.

Excerpts taken from *What Would Jesus Eat?* by Don Colbert, M.D., copyright © 2002 by Don Colbert. Used with permission of Harper Collins Christian Publishing. www.harpercollinschristian.com.

Excerpt(s) taken from *Design and Origin of Man* by Stuart Burgess. Copyright 2004. Used with permission of Day One Publications. www.dayone.co.uk

Excerpts from *What the Bible Says about Healthy Living* by Rex Russell, MD., copyright © 1996, 2006. Used with permission of Revell, a division of Baker Publishing.

Excerpt(s) from *Health in the 21st Century-Will Doctors Survive?* by Francisco Contreras, M.D., copyright © 1997. Used with permission by Dr. Francisco Contrera, Oasis of Hope Hospital, Tijuana, B.C. Mexico.

Excerpt(s) from *Restoring the Creation Mandate* by Roger L. DeHaan, V.O.M., copyright ©2007. Used with permission by Dr. Roger DeHaan.

Excerpt(s) from "God Said Man Said" podcasts #00991, "Corona Virus: You Won't Believe it!" and #01004, "Diet, Hygiene, Quarantine, and Hell to Pay," by Pastor Dave Paulovich and God Said Man Said Team used with permission. www.godsaidmansaid.com.

Excerpt(s) from *The Hebrew Yeshua vs The Greek Jesus*, by Dr. Nehemia Gordon, copyright © 2006. Used with permission by Nehemia Gordon, Ph.D. Excerpt(s) from "The Hebrew Yeshua vs The Greek Jesus," DVD by Dr. Nehemia Gordon. Used with permission by Nehemia Gordon, Ph.D.

Dietary Laws and *Torah*: Are They Relevant Today?

Cheryl M. Sutterby, DNOM

"Dear friend, I am praying that everything prosper with you and that you be in good health, as I know you are prospering spiritually."

3 *Yochanan* (John) 2

MEDICAL & HEALTH DISCLAIMER

Cheryl M. Sutterby is not a medical doctor and will not be providing any medical diagnostic procedures, treatment, or any other practices in the industry of allopathic medicine. This treatise is for educational purposes only. No medical claims are being made, and this book is not meant to diagnose or treat any condition or take the place of medical care.

This book is intended for educational purposes only. It is not intended to provide medical advice or to take the place of medical advice and treatment from your personal physician. Readers are advised to consult their own doctors or other qualified health professionals regarding the treatment of their medical problems. Neither the publisher nor the author takes responsibility for any possible consequences from any treatment, actions, or application of medicine, supplement, herb, or preparation to any person reading or following the information in this book. If readers are taking prescription medications, they should consult with their physicians and not take themselves off of medicines to start supplementation without the proper supervision of a physician.

PERSONAL ACKNOWLEDGMENTS

I am so thankful to *Yehovah Elohim,* God of Creation, for His wisdom, knowledge, understanding, and leading in preparing this dissertation that has become a book! Thank you for opening my spirit and mind to follow your lead.

I am thankful for my husband, Bruce Sutterby, for his patience, encouragement, and support as I have endeavored on the doctoral journey that led to this book. Without his suggestion that it become a book, it might never have been.

PROFESSIONAL ACKNOWLEDGMENTS

I thank my IIOM Doctoral degree mentors, Dr. Elisa Sharps and Dr. Jim Sharps, for their encouragement, academic support, and expertise.

Also, I would like to thank all the various pastors, teachers, and authors who have provided their life's work to help on this journey to the Creator and King of the Universe, *Yehovah Elohim*! I am so grateful for their books, articles, DVD's, podcasts, and more.

I am especially thankful for Lisa Rubin, of *Messianic Jewish Publishers,* for the permission to use scriptures and notes from *The Complete Jewish Study Bible: Insights for Jews and Christians*. This translation by David Stern definitely illuminates the Hebrew culture of God's Word.

Thank you also to Sarah Williams, of Debarim Publishing, whose encouragement and suggestions helped me move into this new journey of writing and publishing a book as a gift to Yah! Thank you!

TABLE OF CONTENTS

INTRODUCTION

Dietary Laws and *Torah*: Are They Relevant Today?

The focus of this book is to point out the relevance of the Hebrew *Torah* and the teachings of *Yeshua* Jesus and His followers in the life and lifestyle of those of us who follow Him. Although we will look at an overview of *Torah*, we will focus mainly on the importance of the *Torah* teachings that apply to an individual's health and lifestyle.

Chapter One –*Creation, Torah, and Our Health.* Section One of this book describes Creation, the health aspects of Creation, and the relevance of the *Torah*. It is a look at the message of *Torah* in the focus of health messages instituted in Creation and throughout Biblical history by our Creator.

Chapter Two – *Did Jesus (Yeshua) Do Away with Torah, including Dietary Laws?* This section of the book takes a look at various scriptures of the Words of Jesus in both Hebrew and Greek, establishing what Jesus taught based on the Hebrew culture and writings. Could there possibly be mistranslations, or at least misunderstandings, based on the two very different cultures? We will take a special look at *Matthew* 15, *Matthew* 23, and *Mark* 7.

Chapter Three – *Three Witnesses, Is Pork on the Menu?* In this section, we take a look at scriptures speaking about Peter (*Kefa*), Paul (*Sha'ul*), and James (*Ya'akov*) to reveal whether or not *Torah* was disregarded in their lives after Jesus' resurrection. Did they give their approval to God's Messianic congregations to serve and eat what *Torah* called 'unclean' animals?

Chapter Four – *Why "Unclean" – Pigs or People?* This section looks at the details of 'Clean' and 'Unclean' and the job description of those animals deemed 'unclean'. Some scriptures cause a bit of confusion, but they may not have anything to do with food at all. An example is what does it mean "You are not to boil a young animal in its mother's milk." *Exodus* 23:19, 34:26, and *Deuteronomy* 14:21. We shall find out!

Chapter Five– *Disease, Pharmaceuticals and Medicine, Clean or Unclean?* – How does God's Word in *Torah* affect medicines and pharmaceuticals we may be ingesting? Is science leading us in an unhealthy direction, causing more disease? Where are these diseases coming from anyhow? How do so many of them originate? Is this all related?

Chapter Six – *Awesomely and Wonderfully Made* – Let's look at how our bodies function and how science has assessed humankind's function over the years. We shall see just how fabulous we are! Our divine Creator blessed us greatly.

Chapter Seven – *Clean and Bountiful Foods for Health and Healing* – This section is an overview of the bounty of "clean" foods approved by our Creator for our health and enjoyment.

Summary, Conclusion, and Recommendations - This is the final section of this book. It contains a summary, conclusions, and recommendations for embracing the healthy lifestyle provided to us from the Beginning!

PREFACE

A question I have always pondered is whether or not Jesus upheld the *Torah,* or did he do away with it, as many people think? If He did away with it, perhaps it has no place in our lives today. As we look into these issues, we will adventure through the *Bible,* looking from Creation to beyond the Resurrection of the Messiah, seeking the answer.

The main Biblical teaching that affects health and healing the most is the teaching on 'clean' and 'unclean', especially regarding foods that today are referred to as '*Dietary Laws'*. And another question to consider is what should be considered *food* for human beings? In our world today, almost anything can be put in the mouth and eaten, but was that always the case, and should it be today?

In this treatise, I make the case that God's plan for our health and food was designed and instituted from the very beginning of His Creation and is still important today. I will look at the coordinated plan of Creation and the timing of each new 'kind' as life began to dance on the planet. God's original plan seems to have given us the gift of what we call '*Original Medicine'*.

Original Medicine was unveiled through each step of the Creation process as every new design blossomed from the gift of the previous creation. Needed benefits were provided for all living creatures and His image bearers. God, through *His Word,* spoke all into existence, and the world began!

As we learn from the *Book of John* (*Yochanan*) [1:1] "In the beginning was the Word, and the Word was with God, and the Word was God. [2] He was with God in the beginning. [3] All things came to be through him, and without him nothing made had being. [4] In him was life, and life was the light of mankind. [5] The light shines in the darkness, and the darkness has not suppressed it."[1 (page 1519)]

Yeshua Jesus has always been and will always be *The Word.*

Before the world began, God, Our Father, prepared a plan that included guidelines for His children's every need and facet of life. His desire was for our abundant life, close communion, and relationship with Him. As the *Great Physician,* He included in these guidelines eight areas of *Original Medicine*. We will look at these eight as we follow Creation. They are as follows:

- Fresh, pure air
- Pure, unadulterated water
- The sun's healing energy
- Live, natural foods – Fruit, Herbs, Vegetables
- Regular exercise
- Rest
- Moderation
- Belief and trust in the Divine Power [2]

God has always been interested in the health and well-being of all His creations, especially His *Image Bearers*, Humankind. Our Creation Mandate is located in *Genesis* [1:27] "So, God created humankind in his own image; in the image of God, he created him: Male and female he created them.

28 God blessed them: God said to them, 'Be fruitful, multiply, fill the earth, and subdue it. Rule over the fish in the sea, the birds in the air, and every living creature that crawls on the earth.'

29 Then God said, 'Here! Throughout the whole earth I am giving you as food every seed-bearing plant and every tree with seed-bearing fruit."[1 (page 4)]

From the beginning, Our Father provided not only our food, but everything we would need. And as the Inventor, Designer, and Creator of all, He provided instructions and guidelines for living in His newly Created World on His Created Planet. All Creation knew its purpose, and all knew what was expected of them.

Torah, a word used over the generations of Hebrew people to describe the teachings of God, was translated in Greek as '*nomos*', which has been rendered 'Law' in English.[1 (page 1852)] The *Torah* consists of the *Five Books of Moses*, called *The Pentateuch*, and includes the books of *Genesis*, *Exodus*, *Leviticus*, *Numbers*, and *Deuteronomy*.[1 (page 1852)] *Torah* is a significant body of work that was given to Moses during his 40-day tenure on *Mt. Sinai*. It incorporates so much more than the *Ten Commandments*. The *Torah* includes instructions and teachings on everything needed to be a healthy and civilized people that are set apart in holiness for their Creator, the God of Heaven and Earth.

So, the question is, are these writings and laws still relevant today, or were they done away with by *Jesus* during His time on earth?

Hanging on the balance of this knowledge is the relevance, or lack thereof, of all teachings provided from the beginning of time for God's people. As we will find out, these laws were known and important long before Noah and continued in some way until Moses obtained them in writing for all to benefit.

If *Jesus* considered the teachings of *Torah* information valuable for people seeking to be God's people, we should take a deeper look. If not, then we are back to where we started and on our own.

I hope this journey will be a blessing and confirmation of the extreme love and dedication of a gracious, loving Father to all His children.

CHAPTER ONE

CREATION, *TORAH,* AND OUR HEALTH

Where to begin? Without understanding God's overarching love for His Creation and His desire to commune eternally with His holy people, we cannot even begin to grasp all that He has given to us and planned for us.

A few hymns and songs come to mind when I think about the glorious details of creation and our Father's design. An old hymn of the church, written in 1901 by *Maltbie D. Babcok*, titled "*This is My Father's World,*" was one I learned in childhood and always brings my heart to worship. When I think of it, I break into song! This absolutely is our Father's World!

"*All Creatures of Our God and King*", written by *Francis of Assisi* in 1225, has been glorifying the Father and His Creation for hundreds of years. What joy and comfort the old hymns of the church can add to a worshipful look at *Yehovah* God of Creation!

A more recent song, "*So Will I*", written by *Joel Houston, Benjamin Hastings*, and *Michael Fatkin* in 2017, and performed by Hillsong, the worship group from Hillsong Ministries in Australia, can help us experience the amazing gift we have been given to be alive on God's earth. We are here at His invitation, and we can join Him in this eternal blessing. I hope you will have the opportunity to listen to this beautiful song and envision the expanse of eternity. [7]

In *The Book of Jubilees —The Little Genesis, The Apocalypse of Moses* in *The Apocrypha* compiled by *Joseph B. Lumpkin*, it is written "the angel of the presence (of the Lord) spoke with Moses according to the Word of the Lord, saying 'write the complete history of the creation, how in six days the Lord God finished all His works and all that He created, and kept Sabbath on the seventh day and made it holy for all ages and appointed it as a sign for all His works.'" The angel describes all that was created each day, culminating on the sixth day with His (God's) ultimate creation, humankind. Humankind are His image-bearers on the earth. [1 (Page 481)]

'*Adam*' means man-person, or human. The meaning of the word in Hebrew is 'red'. Hebrew *word puns* are a common practice in the Hebrew language, and one such used here is the name '*Adam,*' which is much like the word '*a-da-**mah***,' meaning earth. We are made of the elements of the earth, the water, and the air. [2 (Page 1814)]

From the beginning, God desired humankind to be in relationship and close communion with Him. We were to be holy, devoted people, set apart for Him. As His image-bearers, we share with Him spiritually. He breathed His Spirit life into the man-person and gave him a life set apart from all other created beings.

Two scriptures that speak to our unique form are *Genesis* 2:7 and *Genesis* 3:19b. *Genesis* 2:7 says, " Then, *ADONAI*, God, formed a person (Heb. *adam*) from the dust of the ground (Heb. *adamah*) and breathed into his nostrils the breath of life, so that he became a living being." The God of the Universe breathed His Spirit into us! Genesis 3:19b "for you were taken out of it (the ground); you are dust, and you will return to dust." [2 (pages 5 and 7)] Our bodies are lifeless shells until God shares His Spirit and breathes His Breath of Life in us. And through the finished work of Yeshua, we have eternal life even while here on earth!

Before I go any further, let me explain a bit about how I came to this topic. I have always been curious about ideas and concepts that didn't seem to fit together. I wondered why we were taught that scripture was written in *Greek*, *Latin*, or *English*, with no concern as to what the original language might have been. If the *Bible* story was primarily about a people who were *Hebrew*, and *Jesus* (*Yeshua* in Hebrew) was Hebrew, and the disciples (*talmidin* in Hebrew) were Hebrew — why weren't we looking at the Hebrew culture and texts for the depth of answers and language?

Another question was why a loving God (*Yehovah* in Hebrew) would take so much time and interest to provide specific teachings and rules for the welfare of His people, only to disregard or do away with some of them down the road? Why would people who had spent their lives following as closely as possible this *Torah* lifestyle turn away from it years and years later? I began to search for answers and eventually discovered information that began to shed light on these and other questions, too! The exciting journey began!

The aspect of *Torah* I was having the most confusion about is what is now called the *Hebrew* (or *Mosaic*) *Dietary Laws*. Yes, these were given to Moses at the time he was with God on *Mt. Sinai*, but was that the first anyone had known of these rules and others? The answer is 'no'.

I am blessed to have my grandfather's Bible, called *The* Sys*tem Bible Study or The Busy People's Bible* of 1922. This Bible is quite interesting and lists the various categories of *Torah*, or what is now called, in English, "Law." This includes additions from the *New Testament*. These are the categories and sub-categories listed in Section II, Part 1 of the "Laws of the Bible, Table of Contents." [4]

<u>Ten Commandments:</u>

- Duties toward God

- Duties toward Men
- Christ's New Commandment

The Organization of Civil Government:

- The King
- The Army
- Citizenship
- Privileges of Aliens
- The Judiciary
- Witnesses
- Authority and Its Limits
- Publication of the Law

Civil Laws:

- Parents and Children
- Rights of Women
- Marriage
- Divorce
- Marital Infidelity
- Master and Hired Servant
- Master and Slave
- Real Property
- Personal Property
- Love, Humanity to Animals

Criminal Laws:

- Individual Responsibility
- Crimes against Religion (The First Commandment)
- Crimes against Religion (The Second Commandment)
- Crimes against Religion (The Third Commandment)
- Crimes against Religion (The Fourth Commandment)
- Crimes against the Public Right
- Crimes against Public or Private Morals
- Crimes against the Person
- Crimes against Property Rights

Ceremonial Laws:

- Sacred Objects
- Sacred Persons
- Sacred Dues
- Sacred Offerings
- Sacred Times
- Ceremonial Cleanness and Uncleanness

The Ceremonial Cleanness and Uncleanness Encompasses Several Categories:

- Clean and Unclean Food
- Fat and blood are not to be eaten
- Fruit of young trees is not to be eaten
- Uncleanness from loathsome disease
- Uncleanness from Childbirth
- Uncleanness from contact with dead or unclean things
- Christ's teaching about cleanness and uncleanness
- Christian charity in matters of difference
- The fulfillment of the Law [4]

The overall *Torah* is involved in all areas of life. *Sha'ul* (Apostle Paul) describes the fulfillment of all the Law in *Romans* [13:8] "Don't owe anyone anything — except to love one another, for whoever loves his fellow human being has fulfilled *Torah.* [9] For the commandments '**Don't murder**,' '**Don't commit adultery**,' **Don't covet**,' and any others are summed up in this one rule: '**Love your neighbor as yourself**.' [10] Love does not do harm to a neighbor; therefore, love is fulfillment of *Torah.*" [2 (Page 1626)]

As we can see from all noted above, there is more involved in *Torah* scripture than just whether people can eat pork barbecue.

Let's start back at the beginning and look at the importance of each step of Creation. Our Creator was planning for our health and well-being from the very beginning. He put His plan, which we call Original Medicine, in place to bring people together and set apart for Him.

B'resheet (*Genesis*) [1:1] "In the beginning God created the heavens and the earth. [2] The earth was unformed and void, darkness was on the face of the deep, and the *Spirit of God* hovered over the surface of the water. [3] Then God said, 'Let there be light,' and there was light. [4] God saw that the light was good, and God divided the light from the darkness. [5] God called the light Day, and the darkness He called Night. So there was evening, and there was morning, one day." [2 (Page 2)]

On the first day, God created the earth, the heavens, and the water. All three of these components are necessary for the prospering of all other creations. The elements of the earth give everything life, and everything is made of the elements of earth, water, and air. All creation needs water to survive! The nutrients of the air are even more important to all life than we might know!

In *Dr. Jim Sharps* book, *Concepts of Original Medicine,* he writes, "The planet was designed to sustain life and, if used properly, provide good health and comfortable living for every creature. All God's natural laws were put in place so we could lead lives that are well-balanced. The air provides essential nutrients that are carried by the blood. We cannot live without air, but for as little as three minutes without serious damage to our health and life. Air provides oxygen for the combustion, or metabolism, of ingested nutrients. All cells need oxygen for all functions, including eliminating waste products." [5 (Page 34)]

From an original medicine standpoint, "any health treatment that does not encourage the use of good, clean, and fresh air will be significantly compromised in its effectiveness." [5 (Page 34)]

Dr. Sharps continues, "The rays of sun sterilize it (the air); and rainwater washes and cleanses it." There is a synergistic action between all of creation. "Impure air is one of the greatest causes of poor health." [5 (Page 35)]

"Air quality is best in the early morning and late evening. The best supply of clean, fresh air can be found in the mountains, in large, wooded areas, near large bodies of water, and in some remote places far from industry and automobiles. Clean, fresh air is negatively charged, but polluted air is positively charged." "Air contains electricity! Fresh air charges your nerves and muscles with electricity and increases your energy." [5 (Page 35)]

"Fresh air is an agent in producing a more positive mental attitude. It strengthens and nourishes the nervous system." "All bodily functions, including proper digestion, need clean air, and proper breathing aids in assimilation and metabolism." [5 (Page 36)]

In *The Book of Jubilees*, Chapter 2, page 481, it says that on day one, water was created. Over the next two days, the waters would be separated by sky into an area above the sky and below. And on day three, water was separated from dry land. The waters became great seas, lakes, rivers, and the dew of the earth. [1 (Page 481)]

B'resheet (*Genesis*) [1:6] "God said, 'Let there be a dome in the middle of the water; let it divide the water from the water.' [7] God made the dome and divided the water under the dome from the water above the dome, that is how it was, [8] and God called the dome Sky. So there was evening, and morning, a second day." [2 (Page 2)]

What a blessing water is to our lives and health. Water is the second nutrient in the healing process of Original Medicine.

We are created with 70%-75% of our bodies made of water, and the earth too is 70%-75% water. "Water is essential for the function of every cell of the body. Almost every cell and tissue of our body not only contains water and is continually bathed in fluid, but also requires water to perform its function!" An additional blessing of water for our health is that it regulates our body's temperature through the process of evaporation through the skin. [5 (Page 37)]

The water we drink, or get through our fruits and vegetables, is reabsorbed and recycled through the kidneys, and waste is carried out in the urine. Water must be constantly replenished as it is used throughout our bodies. Consider that our brain grey matter is 85% water, blood is 83% water, and our muscles are composed of 75% water. [5 (Page 37)]

Natural, pure water is the best. Clean water, distilled water, provides the best results. "Your body requires approximately 64-80 ounces of water (8 to 10 eight-ounce glasses) a day. A general rule is one ounce of water for every two pounds of body weight, modified to meet special circumstances such as activity level, outside temperature, and health status." [5 (Page 38)] More will be addressed about water when we look at foods and healing.

B'resheet (*Genesis*) [1:11] "God said, 'Let the earth put forth grass, seed-producing plants, and fruit trees, each yielding its own kind of seed-bearing fruit, on the earth'; and that is how it was. [12] The earth brought forth grass, plants each yielding its own kind of seed, and trees each producing its own kind of seed-bearing fruit; and God saw it was good. [13] So there was evening, and there was morning, a third day." [2 (Page 2)]

On the third day, all was put in place so that nourishment might be ready for all of Creation that would follow. God had provided rich soil in the earth, fresh, nutrient-filled air, and clean water infused with nutrients ready to welcome the brand-new crops into their home for prospering and growth. All God created had purpose, and the purpose of grasses, plants, and fruit would be to nourish the living creations to come! God provided the basics for all life, health, and healing days before they would be required by man or animals.

Dr. Sharps writes, "If we eat the foods God intended us to use in the way God intended us to use them, then we will have good, strong, healthy bodies. If we don't follow these dietary rules, then our bodies will suffer as a result and eventually become diseased." [5 (Page 42)] God provided whole, plant foods from seed and nourishing fruits from seed-bearing fruit trees for man to eat. His foods are full of nutrients, providing all the building blocks for repairing and creating healthy bodies. Foods "created by God and provided by nature... Nature, in the form of plant foods, supplies all the food and medicines we need for physical health." [5 (Page 42)]

"Fruits, vegetables, nuts, grains, seeds, and edible herbs, properly prepared and in adequate amounts, supply all the nutrients required for developing and maintaining optimum health." [5 (Page 41)] They are best eaten in as natural a state as possible.

We will touch on foods in the later sections. For now, it is enough to know that God's original plan for nourishing humankind and animals was through fresh, plant and fruit-based foods.

B'resheet (*Genesis*) [1:14] "God said, 'Let there be lights in the dome of the sky to divide the day from the night; let them be for signs, seasons, days, and years; [15] and let them be for lights in the dome of the sky to give light to the earth;' and that is how it was. [16] God made the two great lights — the larger to rule the day and the smaller light to rule the night — and the stars. [17] God put them in the dome of the sky to give light to the earth, [18] to rule over the day and over the night, and to divide the light from the darkness; and God saw that it was good. [19] So there was evening, and there was morning, a fourth day." [2 (Page 2)]

According to *The Book of Jubilees*, Chapter 2:10, the creation of this fourth day divided "the light from the darkness for prosperity that all things may prosper which sprout and grow on the earth. These three kinds He made on the fourth day." [1 (Page 482)]

"Sunlight is essential for radiant health."[5 (Page 39)] God knew this was a key to Creation for all life. "All life on earth depends on the energy of the sun; and all life on earth would cease to exist if there was no sunshine." [5 (Page 39)]

"Sunlight is composed of many different energy levels, transmitted in the form of electromagnetic waves. The rays of the sun expose the body to three types of light of different wavelengths:

1. Invisible light: The invisible light generated by the sun includes both ultraviolet and infrared light. Ultraviolet light (5 percent of solar radiation) provides the majority of the biological effects, both positive and negative, to the body. Infrared light (54 percent of solar emissions) provides warmth.
2. Visible light (40 percent of the solar radiation)
3. Other types of waves: shorter cosmic rays, gamma rays, and x-rays, longer radio waves, and electromagnetic waves." [5 (Page 40)]

"Sunshine helps maintain the ambient temperatures of the Earth. In this way, it supports both plant and animal existence and is a vital ingredient in our environment." [5 (Page 39)]

"Some of the obvious benefits of the sun are the production of vitamin D in the skin, improved vitamin and mineral absorption, particularly calcium, and overall improvement in metabolic function and efficiency." "As a secondary benefit, the abundant energy and life-giving properties that sunlight gives to the plant kingdom have similar positive effects on humans who eat those plants." [5 (Page 40)]

It is recommended that we get out in the sunshine for 20 minutes or more each day. "The full-spectrum light and energy provided by the sun supplies the subtle, vibratory energy underlying all plant and human function. Exposure to the sun results in a healthy-looking complexion, energized blood, and overall good health." [5 (Page 41)]

What a gift from God is the sun! There are so many important effects the sun has on our bodies. This is a brief summary:

Chemical: It participates in unlocking vitamins in foods. It is necessary for digestion and controls the chemistry of the blood.

Physical: The sun warms and energizes the body. It helps important functions of the body:

- Stores energy from the sun
- Our nerve endings absorb energy.
- It acts as a stimulant, tonic, and healer.
- It is a natural, effective healing agent, and much more!

Psychological: "Exposure to the sun offers the experience of peace, joy, happiness, and a feeling of relief and freedom. The mind immediately senses that the body is in its natural medium, and the thoughts begin to take on a more lofty aspect." [5 (Page 41)]

When lacking sunlight, complexions are pale; there is lowered physical vitality, and health is poor. One issue that affects many in winter is *Seasonal Affective Disorder*. Or S.A.D. The shorter days and less sunshine can bring on moodiness, lack of energy, and melancholy. We definitely need sunlight! *Dr. Sharps* says, "Sunshine is free, and its rays invigorates the body in many ways that promote radiant health." [5 (Page 42)]

B'resheet (*Genesis*) [1:20] "God said, 'Let the water swarm with swarms of living creatures, and let birds fly above the earth in the open dome of the sky.' [21] God created the great sea creatures— and every living thing that creeps, so that the water swarmed with all kinds of them, and there was every kind of winged bird; and God saw it was good. [22] Then God blessed them, saying, 'Be fruitful, multiply, and fill the water of the seas, let birds multiply on the earth.' [23] So there was evening, and there was morning, a fifth day. [24] God said, 'Let the earth bring forth each kind of living creature — each kind of livestock, crawling animals, and wild beast;' and that is how it was. [25] God made each kind of wild beast, each kind of livestock, and every kind of animal that crawls along the ground; and God saw that it was good." [2 (Page 2,3)]

Amazing creatures joined the new earth on day five! As with all God's creation to that point, each new plant or creature was brought forth with its own purpose, gifts, and abilities. Throughout the first week of the new earth, God created and wasted not a thing. His omniscient design had order and chemical and mathematical precision. And, at the end of each day, He saw that it was good.

Food to nourish and sustain all these incredible creatures of the seas, air, and land was already prepared and waiting. Grasses, seed-bearing plants, and fruits, ready for eating! In this new world, all glorified their Creator, and, along with all the angels, all nature lived in harmony.

B'resheet (*Genesis*) [1:26] "Then God said, 'Let us make humankind in our image, in the likeness of ourselves; and let them rule over the fish in the sea, the birds in the air, and the animals, and over all the earth, and over every crawling creature that crawls on the earth.' [27] So God created humankind in his own image; in the image of God, he created him: male and female he created them. [28] God blessed them: God said to them, 'Be fruitful, multiply, fill the earth, and subdue it. Rule over the fish of the sea, the birds of the air, and every living creature that crawls on the earth.' [29] Then God said, 'Here! Throughout the whole earth, I am giving you as food every seed-bearing plant and every tree with seed-bearing fruit. [30] And to every wild animal, bird in the air and creature that crawls on the earth, in which there is a living soul, I am giving as food every kind of green plant.' And that is how it was. [31] God saw everything that he had made, and indeed it was very good. So there was evening, and there was morning, a sixth day." [2 (Page 4)]

B'resheet (*Genesis*) [2:7] "Then *ADONAI*, God, formed a person (Heb. *Adam*) from the dust of the ground (Heb. *Adamah*) and breathed into his nostrils the breath of life, so that he became a living being. [8] *ADONAI*, God, planted a garden toward the east, and there he put the person whom he had formed. [9] Out of the ground *ADONAI*, God, caused to grow every tree pleasing in appearance and good for food, including the tree of life in the middle of the garden and the tree of knowledge of good and evil." [2 (Page 2)]

And God said all was "very good!" Humankind, a man named *Adam*, was formed, and a *help meet* to share life with him would soon join the picture. He was the image-bearer of the God Who created him. A set-apart creature to commune and be in fellowship with God Himself.

B'resheet (*Genesis*) [2:1] "Thus the heavens and the earth were finished, along with everything in them. [2] On the seventh day, God was finished with his work which he had made, so he rested on the seventh day from all his work which he had made. [3] God blessed the seventh day and separated it as holy; because on that day God rested from all his work which he had created, so that itself could produce." [2 (Page 5)]

Each day of Creation started in the evening and continued through morning to the late afternoon. Sundown to Sundown. The Hebrew calendar is set up this very way even today. I noticed that there was a time of rest each day, prior to the time of light and work. And after each six-day period of activity, was placed a day of rest. The day of rest started in the evening and continued through to the next evening on day seven; and then followed day one of the second week.

The *Seventh Day* was designed for rest, which brings us to another aspect of Original Medicine. *Shabbat*!

"*Shabbat* means 'rest,' which is the central theme of this important observance. From ancient to modern times, humans tend to become obsessed with work and 'getting ahead.' There is always more to do. Yet without proper rest and refreshment, human strength and creativity fail. In his infinite wisdom, God told the children of *Isra'el* to recharge themselves physically, emotionally, and spiritually. He demonstrated this principle when He created the universe. *Shabbat* is to be a perpetual reminder of God the Creator and our need to find rest in him. (*Exodus* 31:16-17)." [2 (page 5)]

"What does the *Torah* teach us when it says that 'God rested?" ..." It is to teach us that just as God stopped creating physical things on the seventh day, so is man to stop creating on this day." ..." By desisting from all such labors, we not only acknowledge the existence of a Creator, but also emulate the Divine example." [2 (Page 5)]

The Book of Jubilees says in Chapter 2, verse 21 "He created in it a sign in accordance with which they should keep the Sabbath with us (heavenly beings) on the seventh day, to eat and to drink, and to bless Him Who created all things as He has blessed and sanctified to Himself a particular exclusive people above all people, and that they should keep Sabbath together with us." [1 (Page 482)]

To Moses, God again stressed the importance of the Sabbath in *Exodus* [20:8] "Remember the day, *Shabbat*, to set it apart for God. [9] You have six days to labor and do all your work, [10] but the seventh day is *Shabbat* for *ADONAI* your God. On it, you are not to do any kind of work — not you, your son or daughter, not your male or female slave, not your livestock, and not the foreigner staying with you inside the gates to your property. [11]

For six days, *ADONAI* made the heaven and earth, the sea and everything in them; but on the seventh day he rested. This is why *ADONAI* blessed the day, *Shabbat*, and separated it for himself." [2 (Page 99)]

Although this Sabbath, *Shabbat*, rest has a very spiritual and relational aspect, it is also necessary physically too!

"Adequate rest is imperative for optimum health. Rest brings restoration, and it replenishes the resources we use. Without rest, the body's process of catabolism (breaking down) overrides that of anabolism (building up), resulting in disease and compromised health. Sleep is the most important medium for rest. Short naps, peaceful and relaxing environments, mental quietness, and the avoidance of stress also contribute to rest for your body." [5 (Page 47)]

"When God created the earth, He created night as a period of daily rest for both man and animals. The Lord our Creator knows that our bodies need a balanced daily rest — physically, mentally, emotionally, and socially. At the close of the creation week, God Himself 'rested' on the seventh day as an example to man of how to rest from his labors each week because He also knows that in order to function optimally, we also need a weekly rest. Not only did God 'rest' but He also blessed this day. 'Remember the Sabbath day, to keep it holy. Six days you shall labor and do all your work: but the seventh day is the Sabbath of the Lord your God: in it you shall do no work: you, nor your son, nor your daughter, nor your maidservant, nor your cattle, nor your stranger who is within your gates. (*Exodus* 20:8-10)" [5 (Page 50)]

"Rest at the appropriate time is beneficial and contains a blessing...The Sabbath was made for man and not man for the Sabbath! Regular sleep and weekly rest empower us to be receptive to the blessing of God so that He can fill our lives with His many blessings!" [5 (Page 50)]

As you can see, our Creator planned everything in an orderly fashion for our good and His glory.

So, where does *Torah* come into play, especially the laws regarding foods and even hygiene? In this harmonious place of creation, what could go wrong!?!

According to *The Book of Jubilees* Chapter 3, Adam, the 'man-person', named everything over the five days of the second week; and on day six of the second week, God created a 'woman-person' from the man's rib, a "companion suitable for helping the man-person." [1 (Page 485)]

After forty days in the place where God had created the man-person (in Hebrew *Ish*), he was brought to the *Garden of Eden*, which had been prepared for him. The woman-person, called Woman, or *Ishah*, was not taken to the *Garden of Eden* until the eightieth day. [1 (Page 485) and 2 (Page 6)]

The above bit of information cleared up a question I had regarding one of the scriptures in *Torah*.

Vayikra (*Leviticus*) [12:1] "*ADONAI* said to *Moshe*, [2]Tell the people of *Isra'el*: 'If a woman conceives and gives birth to a boy, she will be unclean for seven days with the same uncleanness as in *niddah*, when she is having her menstrual period. [3] On the eighth day, the baby's foreskin is to be circumcised. [4] She is to wait an additional thirty-three days to be purified from her blood; she is not to touch any holy thing or come into the sanctuary until the time of her purification is over. [5] But if she gives birth to a girl, she will be unclean for two weeks, as in her *niddah*; and she is to wait another sixty-six days to be purified from her blood." [2 (Page 143)]

The Book of Jubilees gives a bit more information on this. [3:10] "And for this reason the commandment is written on the heavenly tablets in regard to her that gives birth, 'If she bears a male, she shall remain unclean for seven days, and thirty-three days shall she remain in the blood of her purifying, and she shall not touch any holy thing, nor enter into the sanctuary, until she completes these days which are decreed in the case of a male child. [11] But in case of a female child, she shall remain unclean two weeks of days, according to the first two weeks, and sixty-six days in the blood of her purification, and they will be in all eighty days." [1 (Page 484)]

This time of purification was a time for the mother to recover and bond with the child. This also kept the child from anything unclean for this period of time. "She is to remain separated from marital relations and is forbidden to touch anything ritually pure...her infirmity refers to the discomfort felt following childbirth." [2 (Page 143)]

After living in the Garden for seven years, the serpent came to the woman and deceived her. That changed everything for all of Creation, and the first couple had to leave the Garden. According to *The Book of Jubilees*, the following took place:

- All flesh was sent out of the Garden, back to the land where they had been created.
- Everything was scattered according to its kinds and types.
- Humankind was the only creation that God had given "the ability to cover his shame."
- The mouths of all beasts, cattle, birds, etc., were closed and could no longer speak. [1 (Page 486)]
- Nothing would ever be the same.
- Adam gave Eve her name. (*Chava* in Hebrew)
- Adam and Eve begin to have children.

Keeping with the topic of childbirth, an additional command given to *Moshe* (Moses) in the *Torah*, *Leviticus* 12:3, regards circumcising the male child. Actually, this covenant was originally between God and Abraham (*Avraham*) in *Genesis* 17:10-14.

B'resheet (*Genesis*) [17:10] "Here is my covenant, which you are to keep, between me and you, along with your descendants after you: every male among you is to be circumcised. [11] You are to be circumcised in the flesh of your foreskin; this will be the sign of the covenant between me and you. [12] Generation after generation, every male among you who is eight days old is to be circumcised, including slaves born within your household and those bought from a foreigner not descended from you. [13] The slave born in your house and the person bought with your money must be circumcised; thus, my covenant will be in your flesh as an everlasting covenant." [2 (Page 22)]

Vayikra (*Leviticus*) [12:3] "On the eighth day, the baby's foreskin is to be circumcised." [2 (Page 143)]

Circumcision, or *cutting around*, perhaps has been important beyond creating a people set apart for God. The most important circumcision is the circumcision of our hearts as mentioned in *Deuteronomy* 30:6, Jeremiah 4:4, and *Galatians* 5:6, where the apostle Paul (*Sha'ul*) states, "When we are united with the Messiah *Yeshua*, neither being circumcised nor being uncircumcised matters; what matters is **trusting faithfulness expressing itself through love**." [2 (Page 1676)]

However, circumcision may have greater benefits to health as well. In *None of These Diseases*, by *S. I. McMillen*, we learn of a study done in 1954 that showed that Jewish women were relatively free of cervical cancer. At the time, cervical cancer was 25% of all cancers in women. Yet, Jewish women had less frequency of the cancer than non-Jewish women. The results of the study attributed the reason to the practice of circumcision in the Jewish men. God was setting aside a people. They were to teach other people groups and impact the world. "A number of recent studies have borne out the fact that freedom from cancer of the womb is not due to factors such as race or food or environment, but wholly to circumcision. Other convincing studies were made in India. Although the people there have similar racial backgrounds, eat the same types of food, and live in the same climate and environment, the population is divided into two religious groups. Those who worship *Mohammed*, also a descendant of Abraham, practice circumcision. Among that group there is a much lower incidence of cervical cancer than among other women of the same race who eat the same food and live in the same environment." A similar study was done of women in Fiji noting the same findings. Additionally, there is a lower incidence of cancer of the penis in circumcised men. So, it turns out that circumcision is a "perfect prophylaxis against this deadly cancer." [6 (Page 19-21)]

God gave instruction to Abraham regarding the day He chose for circumcision. It is the eighth day of life. Was that just a random choice of days? Was it for convenience? Or is it possible there were excellent reasons that only our Creator would know? God, *Elohim*, *Yehovah*, the Creator of all things, designed humankind with care and He chose the most perfect day for this procedure.

Again, in *None of These Diseases,* we learn that medical science spent many years trying to determine medically how to reduce cancers and found out the answer had been given over four thousand years earlier. So, why the eighth day for this effective procedure? "*L. Emmett Holt* and *Rustin McIntosh* report that a newborn infant has 'peculiar susceptibility to bleeding between the second and the fifth days of life... Hemorrhages at this time, though often inconsequential, are sometimes extensive; they may produce serious damage to internal organs, especially to the brain, and cause death from shock and exsanguination.' It is felt that the tendency to hemorrhage is due to the fact that the important blood-clotting element, vitamin K, is not formed in the normal amount until the *fifth* to the *seventh* day of life. If vitamin K is not manufactured in the baby's intestinal tract until the *fifth* to the *seventh* day, it is clear that the first safe day to perform circumcision would be the *eighth* day, the very day *Jehovah* commanded Abraham to circumcise Isaac." [6 (Page 21, 22)]

"A second element which is also necessary for the normal clotting of blood is prothrombin. A chart based on data discussed in *Holt Pediatrics* reveals that on the third day of a baby's life the available prothrombin is only thirty percent of normal. Any surgical operation performed on a baby during that time would predispose to serious hemorrhage...the prothrombin skyrockets on the eighth day to a level even better than normal – 110 percent. It then levels off to 100 percent. It appears that an eight-day old baby has more available prothrombin than on any other day in its entire life." [6 (Page 22)]

God, the Maker of All, created vitamin K and prothrombin, and knew just which day was the safest for His little image-bearers. All God's Word is written by a Father who cares for all His creation and especially His image-bearers!

Today, I understand in most hospitals, newborn male babies are given injections of vitamin K in order to do the circumcision procedure almost immediately after birth.[9] We would be wiser to follow God's leading and wait for the eighth day.

Often, we think that the *Torah* was given to Moses for the Hebrews only. As we can see in just these few examples regarding hygiene, God, "Who is the same yesterday, today and forever" had every little detail taken care of before He rested. (*Malachi* 3:6, *Hebrews* 13:8, *Revelation* 1:8)

Torah deals with all issues of life. Especially of interest in this paper are the areas that deal with health, hygiene, and healing. We have looked at a couple of the areas of hygiene. Now we turn our attention to areas of the *Torah* that teach about health looking at what is called "Clean" and "Unclean."

Many times, we think that all the information God provided to Moses was new at that time. But there are hints from preflood times that the children of God had previously been given these details many generations before the flood of Noah's time.

As God called Noah, we see he was to take with him seven pair of 'clean' animals and birds, but only one pair of what God called 'unclean.'

B'resheet (*Genesis*) 7:1 "*ADONAI* said to *Noach*. 'Come into the ark, you and all your household; for I have seen that you alone in this generation are righteous before me. 2 Of every clean animal you are to take seven couples, and of the animals that are not clean, one couple; 3 also of the birds in the air take seven couples — in order to preserve their species throughout the earth.'" [2 (Page 11)]

Prior to the flood, men who followed God through the generations had possibly still eaten a plant-based diet, as God had commanded in the beginning. There is no mention of any change in the scriptures. There was knowledge of what was considered 'clean' and those considered 'unclean.' 'Clean' beasts and cattle were given in sacrifice to God. Only those considered clean would be acceptable as good and pleasing fragrance in sacrifice.

'Clean' at that time had to do with the purpose of the animal and issues of sacrificial appropriateness. The terms 'clean' and 'unclean' are used with spiritual cleanliness matters, as well as hygienic cleanliness. It wasn't until after the flood that it would be an issue of food as well.

"The terms used in Hebrew to designate the clean and unclean animals are *tahor* (clean) and *tamai* (unclean). These terms are never used to describe physical cleanliness or uncleanliness, but rather a spiritual or moral state of being." [2 (Page 142)]

"The term *tamai* (unclean) is used only in relation to moral and religious deficiencies that contaminate the soul and character of man, particularly incest and idol worship, and to characterize the absence of ritual purity. It is often translated as defilement.
The creatures designated as *tamai* were not only forbidden as food, but also for sacrificial purposes. The English words *clean* and *unclean* are therefore to be understood as purity and defilement in a spiritual-ritual sense." [2 (Page 142)]

After the flood, a new rule was instituted by God regarding the proper way to eat the clean animals that would now become part of their food source. Aside from providing milk, the clean animals would now be used for food. As all was destroyed in the flood, it would be a while before the grasses, plants and fruit trees would be ready again to provide food.

Vayikra (*Leviticus*) [19:23] "'When you enter the land and plant various kinds of fruit trees, you are to regard its fruit as forbidden — for three years it will be forbidden to you and not eaten. [24] In the fourth year all its fruit will be holy, for praising *ADONAI*. [25] But in the fifth year you may eat its fruit, so that it will produce even more for you; I am *ADONAI* your God.'" [2 (Page 155)]

This rule for growing and consuming fruit from the trees is noted in *Jubilees* chapter 7 regarding Noah planting his vineyards and trees.

Jubliees [7:1] "In the seventh week in the first year of it, in this jubilee, Noah planted vines on the mountain on which the ark had rested, named Lubar, one of the Ararat Mountains, and they produced fruit in the fourth year, and he guarded their fruit, and gathered it in that year in the seventh month. [2] He made wine from it and put it into a vessel, and kept it until the fifth year, until the first day, on the new moon of the first month." [1 (page 494-495)]

This is a rule even today! My husband and I purchased a grapefruit tree years ago in Florida. We were told not to take any fruit from the tree until at least the fourth year. At that time, the tree was loaded with beautiful, tasty fruit!

From this, we can see that for at least a period of time, they would have no fruits or plants to nourish them. As a result of this, men would be allowed to eat meat as well as sacrifice the animals.

B'resheet (*Genesis*) 9:1 "God blessed *Noach* (Noah) and his sons and said to them, 'Be fruitful, multiply and fill the earth. 2 The fear and dread of you will be upon every wild animal, every bird in the air, every creature populating the ground, and all the fish in the sea; they have been handed over to you. 3 Every moving thing that lives will be food for you; just as I gave you green plants before, so now I give you everything — 4 only flesh with its life, which is its blood, you are not to eat." [2 (Page 13)]

A rule regarding eating the blood of the animals was instituted. In *Leviticus*, God reiterates this to Moses.

Vayikra (*Leviticus*) 17:11 "'For the **life of a creature is in the blood**, and I have given it to you on the altar to make atonement for yourselves; **for it is the blood that makes atonement because of the life**.' 12 This is why I told the people of *Isra'el*, 'None of you is to eat blood, nor is any foreigner living with you to eat blood.' 13 When someone from the community of *Isra'el* or one of the foreigners living with you hunts and catches game, whether animal or bird *that may be eaten*, he is to pour out its blood and cover it with earth. 14 For the life of every creature — its blood is its life. Therefore, I said to the people of *Isra'el*, 'You are not to eat the blood of any creature, because the life of every creature is its blood. Whoever eats it will be cut off.'" [2 (Page 153)]

Note that He makes a differentiation by stating "*that may be eaten.*" Here we see that there was knowledge of the purpose of all the creatures and not all of them were for food. Throughout the generations from creation to the time of Noah, knowledge was passed down from generation to generation, from father to son until the time of the flood. It is something to consider that Adam was still alive at the time Noah's father was born. Noah followed his lineage back to Adam through Seth. Noah's great-grandfather was *Enoch*, his grandfather was *Methuselah*, and his father was *Lamech.*

It is believed that Noah was born in the year 1056 after creation. *Enoch*, *Methuselah* and *Lamech* would all have known Adam and *Seth*, Adam's son; and spent many years with them before they died. [1 (Page 488)]

How glorious it is to realize the continuation of life from Adam on. This would lead us to believe that all God taught Adam would have been passed down to all generations until Noah. *Enoch*, Noah's great-grandfather, was "the first to write a testimony and he testified to the sons of men...and recounted the weeks of the jubilees and made known to them the days of the years and set in order the months and recounted the Sabbaths of the years as we made them known to him." [1 (Page 487)]

This is the same *Enoch* that was written about in *Genesis* 5:21 "*Hanokh* (Enoch) lived sixty-five years and fathered *Methushelach* (Methuselah). 22 After *Methushelach* was born, *Hanokh* walked with God for 300 years and had sons and daughters. 23 In all, *Hanokh* lived 365 years. 24 *Hanokh* walked with God, and then he wasn't there, because God took him." [2 (Page 10] *The Book of Jubilees* Chapter 4 verse 23 says "And he was taken from among the children of men, and we conducted him into the *Garden of Eden* in majesty and honor, and there he wrote down the condemnation and judgement of the world, and all the wickedness of the children of men." [1 (Page 488)]

The Book of Jubilees says in chapter [7:20] "In the twenty-eighth jubilee Noah began to direct his sons in the ordinances and commandments, and all the judgements that he knew, and he exhorted his sons to observe righteousness, and to cover the shame of their flesh, and to bless their Creator, and honor father and mother, and love their neighbor, and guard their souls from fornication and uncleanness and all iniquity." [1 (Page 496)]

Again, in *The Book of Jubilees*, Chapter [10:12] "We (the angels) explained to Noah all the medicines of their diseases, together with their seductions, how he might heal them with herbs of the earth. [13] Noah wrote down all things in a book as we instructed him concerning every kind of medicine. Thus, the evil spirits were precluded from hurting the sons of Noah. [14] He gave all that he had written to *Shem*, his eldest son, for he loved him greatly above all his sons." [1 (Page 502)]

Knowledge was passed down and continued to be shared. *The Book of Jasher* tells the history of the life of Abram. It says that Abram, at age ten, with his mother and *Sarai*, who was just born, went to live with Noah and Shem. Noah and Shem shared with them about the God of Creation. [8 (Page 26)] Then, Abram shared with *Isaac*, *Ishmael*, and *Ya'akov* (Jacob). And *Ya'akov* shared with his sons and so it went until God called Moses. [8]

During the time the Hebrew children were in Egypt, they began to take on the lifestyle of the Egyptians. By the time Moses came to call them out, much of God's Word probably had been forgotten or put aside. Abraham, Isaac, and Jacob's descendants were not following after the One God.

Through Moses, God of Creation would bring His Word and Wisdom in the form of tablets that became the *Torah* and thus continued the history of the nation of Hebrew people. (The word Hebrew (*Ivrim, Ibrim*) may have come from *Eber*, a biblical ancestor or Abraham; or from the Hebrew word for '*he crossed over*, *Or traversed*'.) As this book focuses primarily on the scriptures of *Torah* that were guidelines for healthy eating as a key to Original Medicine, let's take a look at what the scripture says.

Vayikra (*Leviticus*) [11: 1] "*ADONAI* said to *Moshe* and *Aharon*, [2] "Tell the people of *Isra'el*,
'These are the living creatures which you may eat among all the land animals: [3] any that
has a separate hoof which is completely divided and chews the cud — these animals you
may eat. [4-6] But you are not to eat those that only chew the cud or only have a separate
hoof. For example, the camel, the coney and the hare are unclean for you, because they
chew the cud but don't have a separate hoof; [7] while the pig is unclean for you, because
although it has a separate and completely divided hoof, it doesn't chew the cud.

[8] "'You are not to eat meat from these or touch their carcasses; they are unclean for you.

[9] "'Of all the things that live in the water, you may eat these: anything in the water that
has fins and scales, whether in seas or rivers – these you may eat. [10] But everything in the
seas and rivers without both fins and scales, of all the small water-creatures and of all the
living creatures in the water, is a detestable thing for you. [11] Yes, these will be detestable
for you – you are not to eat their meat, and you are to detest their carcasses. [12] Whatever
lacks fins and scales in the water is a detestable thing for you.

13 "'The following creatures of the air are to be detestable for you – they are not to be
eaten, they are a detestable thing: the eagle, the vulture, the osprey, 14 the kite, the various
kinds of buzzards, 15 the various kinds of ravens, 16 the ostrich, the screech-owl, the
seagull, the various kinds of hawks, 17 the little owl, the cormorant, the great owl, 18 the
horned owl, the pelican, the barn owl, 19 the stork, the various kinds of herons, the hoopoe
and the bat.

20 "'All winged, swarming creatures that go on all fours are a detestable thing for you; 21
except that of all winged swarming creatures that go on all fours, you may eat those that
have jointed legs above their feet, enabling them to jump off the ground. 22 Specifically,
of these you may eat the various kinds of locusts, grasshoppers, katydids and crickets. 23
But other than that, all winged swarming creatures having four feet are a detestable thing
to you.

24 "'The following will make you unclean; whoever touches the carcass of them will be
unclean until evening, 25 and whoever picks up any part of their carcass is to wash his
clothes and be unclean until evening: 26 every animal that has a separate but incompletely
divided hoof or that doesn't chew the cud is unclean for you; anyone who touches them
will be unclean. 27 Whatever goes on its paws, among all animals that go on all fours, is
unclean for you; whoever touches its carcass will be unclean until evening; and whoever
picks up its carcass is to wash his clothes and be unclean until evening — these are
unclean for you.'"

29 "'The following are unclean for you among the small creatures that swarm on the
ground: the weasel, the mouse, the various kinds of lizards, 30 the gecko, the land
crocodile, the skink, the sand-lizard, and the chameleon. 31 They are unclean crawling
creatures; whoever touches them when they are dead will be unclean until evening. 32
Anything on which one of them falls when dead will become unclean – wooden utensils,
articles of clothing, leather, sacking – any utensil used for work; it must be put in water,
and it will be unclean until evening; then it will be clean. *(vii)* 33 If one of them falls into
a clay pot, whatever is in it will become unclean, and you are to break the pot. 34 Any
food permitted to be eaten that water from such a vessel gets on will become unclean, and
any permitted liquid in such a vessel will become unclean. 35 Everything on which any
carcass-part of theirs falls will become unclean, whether oven or stove; it is to be broken
in pieces – they are unclean and will be unclean for you; 36 although a spring or cistern
for collecting water remains clean. But anyone who touches one of their carcasses will
become unclean. 37 If any carcass-part of theirs falls on any kind of seed to be sown, it is
clean; 38 but if water is put on the seed and a carcass-part of theirs falls on it, it is unclean
for you.'"

39 "'If an animal of a kind that you are permitted to eat dies, whoever touches its carcass
will be unclean until evening. 40 A person who eats meat from its carcass or carries its
carcass is to wash his clothes; he will be unclean until evening.'"

41 "'Any creature that swarms on the ground is a detestable thing; it is not to be eaten – 42
whatever moves on its stomach, goes on all fours, or has many legs – all creatures that
swarm on the ground; you are not to eat them, because they are a detestable thing. 43 You
are not to make yourselves detestable with any of these swarming, crawling creatures; do
not make yourselves unclean with them, do not defile yourselves with them. 44 For I am

Adonai your God; therefore, consecrate yourselves and be holy, for I am holy; and do not defile yourselves with any kind of swarming creature that moves along the ground. [45] For I am *Adonai*, who brought you up out of the land of Egypt to be your God. Therefore, you are to be holy because I am holy.'"

[46] "'Such, then, is the law concerning animals, flying creatures, all living creatures that move about in the water, and all creatures that swarm on the ground. [47] Its purpose is to distinguish between the unclean and the clean, and between the creatures that may be eaten and those that may not be eaten.'" [2 (Page 141-143)]

Chapter 12 of *Vayikra* (*Leviticus*) moves into guidelines for hygiene in childbirth, circumcision, and menstruation.

Chapter 13 of *Vayikra* (*Leviticus*) begins a look at how to deal with a variety of skin conditions. The word *tzara'at*, is noted for issues of leprosy. Interestingly, it seems it was the priest, the *cohen*, that made recommendations and rulings on all skin diseases, and other ailments. The person would show themselves to the priest every seven days until the condition cleared up, or they would need to be separated from others indefinitely. Some conditions required temporary separation from other people, others did not. In issues of molds and fungus, there were inspections every seven days on the walls and other items in the home. In extreme cases, the homes would need to be completely destroyed and burned to eliminate the problem. A variety of remedies and sacrifices were recommended to heal the person and cleanse, purify and restore the person to community and to God.

As you can see, none of the guidelines God, *Adonai*, provides in *Torah* are unusual or hard. Noting the entirety of *Torah*, it is a handbook for healthy living and living in community with others. So back to our question of whether or not these very specific rules would be rescinded or removed is questionable at best. In the remainder of this book, we will look at the possibilities of Jesus, Peter, Paul, and James eliminating these practices from their lives and recommending we take no care for following them.

Nowhere that I can see is keeping *Torah* a qualification for salvation for the Hebrews, nor for the followers of Jesus. What could be the reason for the confusion? In Section Two, we take a look at a variety of scriptures from Jesus and see what we can learn there.

CHAPTER TWO

DID JESUS (*YESHUA*) REALLY DO AWAY WITH *TORAH*, INCLUDING THE DIETARY LAWS

As we begin the study of Jesus' words, we need to start at the beginning and seek to know who he is, why he came and what his message was to his followers then and now.

According to *Michael Rood*, in *The Chronological Gospels*, "The modern Christian world has grown up with a Greek perception of the personality commonly known as 'Jesus Christ'". [1 (page 1)] However, "the life and ministry of *Yeshua* of *Nazareth*" is that of "an *Israelite* from the tribe of *Judah* and of the lineage of *King David*." [1 (page 1)]

Could it be that *Yeshua* was not only the *One* we call Savior, but also the "***The Prophet*** Whom *we must hear and obey*" as spoken of in *Deuteronomy* 18:15? [1 (page 1)]

D'varim (*Deuteronomy*) [18:15] "*ADONAI* will raise up for you a prophet like me (*Moses*) from among yourselves, from your own kinsmen. You are to pay attention to him," [2 (page 251)]

"It is impossible to understand the *Gospel of the Kingdom* that *Yeshua* and his disciples taught throughout the *Galilee* or to comprehend the significance of the conflict between *Yeshua* and the religious leaders of *Israel* without a fundamental understanding to both the instructions in the *Torah* (the commandments given directly by the Almighty to Moses) and the man-made laws of first century *Judaism* as they were being developed by the *Pharisee*-ruled *Sanhedrin*." [1 (page 1)] "It is likewise impossible to establish the order of events in *Yeshua's* ministry without an accurate understanding of both the *Feasts of the LORD* and the Creator's celestial calendar. [1 (page 1)]

"Each one of the Creator's Feasts is embedded with detailed prophetic shadow pictures that the Messiah *must* fulfill. *The Gospels* of *Matthew*, *Mark*, *Luke*, and *John* detail how the Messiah fulfilled the *Spring Feasts of the LORD* as the *Suffering Servant* – the picture of the substitutionary Lamb of God – the acceptable sin offering." [1 (page 2)]

"Without a knowledge of the *Spring Feasts of the LORD*, the first four *Gospels* remain shallow and confusing; and without knowledge of the *Fall Feasts of the LORD*, the fifth Gospel, the book of *Revelation*, will remain to the Western mind an indecipherable time-warp continuum… the basic recognition that the book of *Revelation* details how the

Messiah will fulfill the *Fall Feasts of the LORD* as the Almighty Judge, who rules the earth with absolute justice." [1 (page 2)]

There is so much to know about *Yeshua*. As *John* (*Yochanan*), his *talmid* (disciple) states in *Yochanan* (*John*) [21:24] "This one is the *talmid* who is testifying about these things and who has recorded them. And we know that his testimony is true. [25] But there are also many other things *Yeshua* did; and if they were all to be recorded, I don't think the whole world could contain the books that would have to be written!" [2 (page 1556)]

For this book, we will be looking at who *Yeshua* Jesus is in relation to the *Torah*, what his message is, and any possibility that He might have done away with Dietary Laws in *Torah,* or *Torah* itself.

Throughout the Scriptures, Jesus is referred to as The *Word of God* or *The Word*. Why do we refer to Jesus this way? The books of John, 1 John, and Revelation all refer to Him as *The Word*. 'The Word that Became Flesh and Tabernacled among us'. The use of the term *The Word* or something similar appears seven times throughout the Bible. The Apostle John (*Yochanan*) brings to our attention the deity of *Yeshua* Jesus and the overarching idea that *Yeshua* was the *Word* shared with humankind from the very beginning of the Creation. [3]

Yochanan (*John*) [1:1] "In the beginning was the *Word*, and the *Word* was with God, and the *Word* was God. [2] He was with God in the beginning. [3] All things came to be through him, and without him nothing made had being. [4] In him was life, and the life was the light of mankind. [5] The light shines in the darkness, and the darkness has not suppressed it." … [9] "This was the true light, which gives light to everyone entering the world. [10] He was in the world – the world came to be through him – yet the world did not know him." [2 (page 1518, 1519)]

Yochanan (*John*) [1:14] "The *Word* became a human being and lived with us, and we saw his *Sh'khinah*, the *Sh'khinah* of the Father's only Son, full of grace and truth." [2 (page 1519)]

1 Yochanan (*John*) [1:1] "The *Word*, which gives life!... He existed from the beginning. We have heard him, we have seen him with our eyes, we have contemplated him, we have touched him with our hands!" [2 (page 1770)]

Revelation of Yeshua the Messiah to Yochanan (*John*) [19:13] "He was wearing a robe that had been soaked in blood, and the name by which he is called is, '*THE WORD OF GOD'*." [2 (page 1805)]

What do we think of when we speak of the term 'word'? Many times, we mean the actual words given on stone tablets to Moses. It also encompasses the words given to the various prophets throughout the Old Testament (Heb. *Tanakh*). It includes all the words of the letters, called epistles, in the New Testament written and spoken by the students, or disciples of *Yeshua*.

Looking at the Greek meaning, we see the actual translation for 'word' is *logos*. *Logos* can be used in contexts such as spoken word, talk, to preach, to reason, utterance, and more. The logo can be a symbol or identifying design. It represents the person who is speaking or writing. It is the entire message.

Yeshua Jesus reveals to us the message from the Father through His words, actions, and lifestyle. He encompasses all that is The Word of *Yehovah* God. Jesus himself told us, "My teaching is not my own, it comes from the One who sent me. (*Yochanan*, John 7:16) Yeshua is the part of the God-Head that is the Speaker, the Spokesperson. He brings us the Word of the Father. He is the Way, the Truth, and the Life! (*Yochanan John* 14:6)

The Word of God is also a title of the *Holy Scriptures*. *Hebrews* 4:12, for example: "See, the Word of God is alive! It is at work and is sharper than any double-edged sword to judge the inner reflections and attitudes of the heart." [2 (page 1734)] The communication from God in Scripture is the written word that helps us know *Yeshua*, who is called the Living Word of God.

Let's take a look at some of the *Word* written and spoken in the *Holy Scriptures*. The *Torah* is our primary focus in this book, and from what we just learned, the *Torah* was written and spoken by the pre-incarnate *Word of God*, *Yeshua*!

"*Moses* told us clearly and repeatedly that no one is ever allowed to add to, or to subtract one single commandment from the *Torah* (*Deuteronomy* 4:2)." [1 (page 7)]

D'varim (*Deuteronomy*) 4:2 "In order to obey the *mitzvot* of *ADONAI* your God which I am giving you, do not add to what I am saying, and do not subtract from it." [2 (page 230)]

In the *New Testament*, *Revelation* 22:12-13, 16-19 gives definitive instructions directly from Jesus, *Yeshua*, to share with the Messianic communities. These are almost the very last words of Jesus.

Revelation 22:12 "'Pay attention!' [*says Yeshua*,] 'I am coming soon, and my rewards are
with me to give to each person according to what he has done. 13 I am the *Alef* and the
Tav, the First and the Last, the Beginning and the End.' … 16 'I, *Yeshua*, have sent my
angel to give you this testimony for the Messianic communities, I am the Root and the
Offspring of David, the bright and Morning Star. 17 The Spirit and the Bride say, 'Come!'
Let anyone who hears say, 'Come!' And let anyone who is thirsty come – let anyone who
wishes, take the water of life free of charge. 18 I warn everyone hearing the words of the
prophecy in this book that if anyone adds to them, God will add to him the plagues
written in this book. 19 And if anyone takes anything away from the words in the book of
this prophecy, God will take away his share in the *Tree of Life* and the holy city, as
described in this book.'" [2 (page 1811)]

As we can see from these verses, we are told in no uncertain words not to make any changes to God's word! Therefore, it is hard to believe that Jesus would have changed, subtracted, or added to the *Torah* given by the *Father* through the *Word* to *Moses*.

Another topic we need to address is what is meant by "traditions of men". Just as many traditions not directed by God have entered into Christianity today, traditions and other festivals had been added to what God had instructed *Israel*. Jesus addresses this issue in the *Book of Mark* in chapter 7.

Mark 7:1 "The *P'rushim* and some of the *Torah*-teachers who had come from
Yerushalayim gathered together with *Yeshua* 2 and saw that some of his *talmidim* ate with
ritually unclean hands, that is, without doing *n'tilat-yadayim*. 3(For the *P'rushim*, and

indeed all the *Judeans*, holding fast to the *Tradition of the Elders*, do not eat unless they have given their hands a ceremonial washing. [4] Also, when they come from the marketplace, they do not eat unless they have rinsed their hands up to the wrist; and they adhere to many other traditions, such as washing cups, pots, and bronze vessels.)

7:5 "The *P'rushim* and the *Torah*-teachers asked him, 'Why don't your *talmidim* live in accordance with the *Tradition of the Elders*, but instead eat with ritually unclean hands?'
6 *Yeshua* answered them, '*Yesha'yahu* (*Isaiah*) was right when he prophesied about you hypocrites – as it is written,

'**These people honor me with their lips, but their hearts are far away from me.** 7
Their worship of me is useless, because they teach man-made rules as if they were doctrines. '(a *Isaiah* 29:13)

7:8 "'You depart from God's command and hold onto human tradition.' 9 'Indeed,' he said to them, 'you have made a fine art of departing from God's command in order to keep your tradition! 10 For *Moshe* said, '**Honor your father and your mother**, [b] and '**Anyone who curses his father or mother must be put to death.**' [c] 11 But you say, 'If someone says to his father or mother, 'I have promised as a *korban*' (that is, as a gift to God) 'what I might have used to help you,' 12 then you no longer let him do anything for his father or mother. 13 Thus, with your tradition which you had handed down to you, you nullify the *Word of God*! And you do other things like this.'" (b Exodus 20:12; Deuteronomy 5:16) (c Exodus 21:17; Leviticus 20:9) 2 (page 1450)

This passage has been difficult to understand until read from the Hebrew and with an understanding of *Torah* and *Hebrew* culture. *Nehemia Gordon*, in his book *The Hebrew Yeshua vs The Greek Jesus,* addresses this issue and other places where, over the years, translations and translators have misunderstood the situation. I highly recommend this book for a deeper understanding of scripture.

What is happening in Mark 7? The issue is about a perception of violating something, but is it *Torah*? No, actually, the *talmidim* were not violating *Torah*, but they were violating the 'traditions of men" created by the rabbis and Pharisees. This "tradition of men" is a doctrine highly regarded by the Pharisees. It is said this is a second law given on Mt. Sinai during a second revelation to Moses, and it was received orally rather than written. The belief is it was oral to keep it from getting into the hands of peoples of other nations. [4]

The issue of washing the hands in *Mark* 7 is a "*tradition of the elders*". We always hear about how the *Hebrews* had been given so very many "laws" by God. But was God the one who gave all the laws to them, or did the "*traditions of the elders*" become "laws" as they were added by the rabbis? Did you know that there is another rule book separate from the *Torah* of Moses?

There is another book! It is a book called the *Talmud.* It comprises what the rabbis called the *Oral Torah* and other writings by rabbis over the years. The *Oral Torah* is the most fundamental doctrine of the Pharisees. "One of the most profound changes in *Phariseeism* since the 1st Century CE is that the *Oral Torah* has been written down." "About 200 CE, *Rabbi Judah the Prince* wrote down the *Mishnah*, a compilation of

Pharisaical doctrines and practices discussed in the rabbinical academies. During the following centuries, the Rabbis debated the meaning of various *Mishnaic* passages, and these debates and explanations were written down as the *Talmud*." [4 (page 13)] These writings are called the *Jerusalem Talmud* and the *Babylonian Talmud*. Both were written down after the life of Jesus, but the Rabbi's rules and traditions had been added orally for years prior to Jesus' birth.

"The problem is that the Rabbis interpret Scripture using what is known today as *midrashic* interpretation. *Midrashic* interpretation consists of taking words out of context and reading meaning into them." [4 (page 18)]

"The Rabbis believe that if something is done by an entire Jewish community for an extended period of time, then this custom, called *minhag*, becomes binding upon the community." "This principle is enshrined in the Rabbinical maxim 'A custom of Israel is a law' ...literally says, 'A custom of Israel is ***Torah***'!" An example of this is the wearing of the *kippah*, or skullcap. [4 (page 19)]

"Sanctified customs such as these are in direct violation of the *Torah,* which commands us: 'You shall not add unto a matter which I command you today nor shall you diminish aught from it, to keep the commandments of *YHWH* your God which I am commanding you. (*Deuteronomy* 4:2)" Other places this rule of *Torah* is mentioned is in *Deuteronomy* 12:32, and *Proverbs* 30:6." [4 (page 20)]

"These invented Rabbinic laws are called *takanot* ('enactments, reforms') or *mitzvot derbanan* ('commandments of the Rabbis')." [4 (page 20)]

This is where the rule for the washing of the hands comes in. "Because the Rabbis enacted this law, and because God supposedly commanded us to obey the Rabbis (at least according to the *Oral Law*), the blessing can be made: 'Blessed art thou Lord, King of the universe, who has sanctified us with his commandments **and commanded** **us** to wash the hands.'" [4 (page 20-21)]

As Christians, our lack of understanding of the *takanot* in the *Talmud* confuses us when we picture that Jesus is removing rules from what is perceived to be God's laws in *Torah.* However, now seeing that the *Talmud* is an extraneous rule book, not written by our *Word*, we can delve a bit deeper into what *Yeshua* the Messiah was accomplishing by "breaking" the *takanot*.

What is this *washing of the hands* rule? According to *Nehemia Gordon*, "When the Rabbis talk about 'washing the hands' they do not mean to take a bar of soap and cleanse oneself: that's just common-sense hygiene. What the Rabbis mean is a very specific ritual-washing of the hands. The Rabbinical ritual begins with a special jug that fulfills certain requirements and specifications. This jug is filled with water and then placed in the left hand and used to pour water over the right hand. Then the jug is passed to the right hand, and water is poured over the left hand. The process is repeated a second time, and according to some traditions, a third time. At the end, a blessing must be recited: 'Blessed art thou, Lord, king of the universe, who has sanctified us with His commandments **and commanded us to wash the hands**." [4 (page 8-9)]

Now we begin to make a bit more sense of *Matthew* 15:2-3 (and *Mark* 7), which says, "Why is it that your *talmidim* break the *Tradition of the Elders*? They don't do *n'tilat-yadayim* before they eat!' [3] He answered, 'For God said, '**Honor your father and mother**,' and '**Anyone who curses his father or mother must be put to death**.' [5] 'But you say, 'If anyone says to his father or mother, 'I have promised to give to God what I might have used to help you,' [6] 'then he is rid of his duty to honor his father or mother.' 'Thus, by your tradition, you make null and void the word of God! [7] You hypocrites! *Yesha'yahu* (*Isaiah*) was right when he prophesied about you, [8] '**These people honor me with** their **lips, but their hearts are far away from me.** [9] **Their worship of me is useless, because they teach man-made rules as if they were doctrines.'"** [2 (page 1412)]

What is interesting to me in this passage is the confusion that comes from the next part of this scripture in *Matthew* 15:10 (and *Mark* 7:14-23). As you can see, Jesus, *Yeshua*, was not addressing the issue of foods, clean or unclean. It was a discussion about man-made rules that had become *traditions of men* and distractions from *Torah.*

In *Matthew* [15:10,] *Yeshua* continued to speak to the crowd and said: "Listen and understand this! [11] What makes a person unclean is not what goes into his mouth; rather, what comes out of his mouth, that makes him unclean!" [2 (page 1413)]

As the scripture was dealing with ritual purity of hands, it would be the lack of the ritual process that would make the person *ritually unclean.* It was not even about dirt on the hands, and no one in that community would have thought of eating anything not specified in *Torah*; this was not about removing something from *Torah* but separating *Torah* from the man-made traditions. Specific foods were not discussed.

"He is not saying that it is now permissible to violate *Torah* and eat cats, rats, lizards, pigs, or tarantulas (which are all delicacies in various cultures). *Yeshua* is upholding the sanctity of the *Torah* and defending it against the man-made rules of a system that was manipulating and controlling the masses with a hybrid religion." [1 (page 143)]

Michael Rood, in *The Chronological Gospels* writes this note for *Mark* 7:16.1. "The *takanot* of the Pharisees (or any other religion) is a violation of the *Torah* – and sin is the violation of the *Torah* (*1 John* 3:4). *Yeshua* clearly and pointedly commanded his disciples 'Do not follow the *takanot* of the Pharisees' and gave added clarification in his last message to *Israel* (recorded in *Matthew* 23.)" [1 (page 143)]

"*Yeshua* vociferously violated the man-made rules of the Pharisees at every turn – that is why they started making plans to kill him at *Shavuot* (*John* 5:1-47) when he healed a man and then immediately commanded him to break the law of the *eruv* by picking up his mat on the *Sabbath* and carrying it away. If we miss this one principle – we have missed the entire teaching ministry of the Messiah who came to declare the truth that sets men free from bondage of religion." [1 (page 142)]

One of the next areas of confusion is *Matthew* 23: 1-7. Let's take a look.

Mattityahu (*Matthew*) [23:1] "Then *Yeshua* addressed the crowds and his *talmidim*: [2] 'The *Torah*-teachers and the *P'rushim*,' he said, 'sit in the seat of *Moshe* (*Moses*). [3] So whatever they tell you, take care to do it. But don't do what they do because they talk but don't act! [4] They tie heavy loads onto people's shoulders but won't lift a finger to help carry them. [5] Everything they do is done to be seen by others; for they make their *t'fillin* broad and their *tzitziyot* long, [6] they love the place of honor at banquets and the best seats in the synagogues, [7] and they love being greeted deferentially in the marketplaces and being called 'Rabbi.'" [2 (page 1424)]

This is a lot to understand from a Greek and English perspective. What is this *seat of Moses*? And is there a contradiction? According to *Nehemia Gordon*, the Greek and the English translations are the same. But now that *Hebrew* scrolls of *Hebrew Matthew* have been revealed, how do these scrolls read?

As Nehemia states, "I knew all about Hebraisms from my study of the *Septuagint*, the ancient Greek translation of the *Tanach*. World-renowned experts in classical Greek find the *Septuagint* incomprehensible, while an Israeli student can read it after only a couple of years of learning Greek. The reason is that the *Septuagint* was translated by very bad translators. Rather than translate the *Tanach* into proper Greek, they mechanically translated the words, leaving behind numerous *Hebrew* thought patterns. To someone who is familiar with the *Tanach* in Hebrew, this Greek is relatively easy to read. But to a Classical Greek specialist who expects to find elegant Greek syntax, it sounds like gibberish. And in ancient times, it was no better. As one of my (*Nehemia Gordon's*) professors says, 'On the streets of Athens they did not understand the *Septuagint*.'" "To complicate matters, numerous Greek copyists who did not know any Hebrew tried to 'improve' what was clearly poor Greek. The result was a translation which at times mimics the Hebrew word-for-word and at other times wildly differs from it." [4 (page 33-35)]

Nehemia, a *Karaite Jew*, continued to research the scriptures for these areas of confusion to help a Christian friend, *Michael Rood*. He learned through colleagues that a copy of the *Book of Matthew* exists in Hebrew and is called *Shem-Tov's Hebrew Matthew*. That was the first copy of *Hebrew Matthew* he found. At the time of this writing, there are more than 28 copies Nehemia has researched from around the world. How exciting that the *Word of God* in *Hebrew* is coming to the forefront!

Shem-Tov's Hebrew Matthew manuscript was known about for centuries, but it was always assumed that *Shem-Tov* simply translated his version of *Matthew* from Greek or Latin into Hebrew. Then, in the 1980s, *George Howard* of *Mercer University* in Georgia carried out a detailed linguistic study in which he showed that there were parts of *Shem-Tov's Hebrew Matthew* which could not be easily explained as translations from Greek.

We looked at Hebrew *word puns* in our first section, looking at *Torah*. Guess what? Hebrew *word puns* show up in *Shem-Tov's Hebrew Matthew,* too! They give even more credence to the Hebrew scripture of *Matthew* being translated into Greek and not the other way around.

Here are a few examples. "In *Hebrew Matthew* 18:9 *Yeshua* says, 'If your eye causes you to stumble (*tacbshilcha*) … cast it from you (*tashlicheha*).'" [4 (page 40)] Two words that sound much alike but have very different meanings. That is a *word pun*!

"A more complex example can be found in *Matthew* 12:13, 15:

(13) "Then he said to the man, 'stretch out your hand,' and he stretched out (*vayet*) his hand … (15) And it was after this that *Yeshua* knew, and he turned from there (*vayet*) and many sick people went after him… [4 (page 41)]

Here, the word *vayet* is used twice with two different meanings ('and he stretched out'; 'and he turned') in close proximity. A similar example can be found in *Matthew* 14: 35-36:

(35) … and they brought him everyone who was sick (*hacholim*) with all types of illnesses. (36) And they entreated (*ve-vhilu*) him…

In this example, the root *chlh* is used with two distinct meanings ('sick', 'entreated'). A typical Hebrew *word pun*." [4 (page 41)]

"One of the main proofs cited by those who believe that *Matthew* was written in Greek is actually a *word pun* in the Greek itself. In *Matthew* 16:18, *Yeshua* says to *Simeon*, '…You are Peter (*Petros*), and upon this rock (*petrai*) I will build my church…' (*Matthew* 16:18). This *word pun* is based on the Greek word *petra,* meaning 'rock' from which Peter's name (*Petros*) is derived. This is usually brought as a decisive proof for a Greek *Matthew* original since it is clear that the Greek *word pun* is interwoven with the content of the passage. But in the Hebrew, there is a different *word pun* not found in the Greek! In Hebrew, *Matthew* 16:18, *Yeshua* says, '…You are a stone (*even*), and I will build (*evneh*) my house of prayer upon you.' In Hebrew, the *word pun* is between *'even'* 'stone' and the verb *'evneh'* 'I will build.' This *word pun* is significant because it is based on a similar *word pun* in *Psalms* 118:22, 'The stone (*even*) that the builders (*bonim*) refused, has become the chief cornerstone' which is later quoted in *Matthew* 21:42, 44.

"Why are all these *word puns* important? If *Shem-Tov's Hebrew Matthew* was a translation from Greek, then where did these *word puns* come from? The purpose of a *word pun* is to beautify the text. … There is other evidence besides *word puns* which seem to support a Hebrew original. In some instances, it seems as if the Greek *Matthew* does not make sense or presents a difficult reading, while *Shem-Tov's Hebrew Matthew* makes perfect sense. For example, in Greek it says, 'For all the prophets and the law prophesied **until** *John*.' (*Matthew* 11:13 [KJV]). If I (Nehemia) were *Shem-Tov* writing a polemic against Catholic Christianity' [and that was what *Shem Tov* was writing], 'I would have brought this verse as my first argument. Here in black and white, the Greek *Matthew* says that the *Tanach* was not talking about *Yeshua*; the *Tanach* only prophesied up until *John the Baptist,* while *Yeshua's* ministry was not foretold by the *Tanach*. That's what it says in the Greek *Matthew*! The Hebrew *Matthew*, though, has a slight but highly significant change. The Hebrew says, 'For all the prophets and the *Torah* spoke concerning *John*' (*Hebrew Matthew* 11:13). This Hebrew text makes more sense. The Hebrew is saying that throughout the *Tanach,* there are references to a prophet such as *John the Baptist* (perhaps one can point to *Malachi's* final prophecy as an example). In Greek, the words for 'until' and 'concerning' are substantially different (*heos* vs. *peri*), but in Hebrew the difference is only one single letter (*'ad* vs *'al*). So, if then *Shem-Tov's Hebrew Matthew* were just a translation from Greek, then the Greek text on which it was based had substantially different reading from the Greek *Matthew* known today. But if the Greek *Matthew* is a translation from Hebrew, then the Hebrew original it was based on was very similar to *Shem-Tov's Hebrew Matthew*." [4 (page 43-44)]

A possible conclusion is that even if "*Shem-Tov's Hebrew Matthew* is not the original Hebrew *Matthew*, it may have original elements left behind from the original *Matthew*…These mistakes of differences were actually in the Greek, while the Hebrew had the original pure text written by *Matthew* himself. But these people versed in the Greek *Matthew* failed to realize this, so inadvertently 'corrected' the Hebrew based on the Greek. So, when *Shem-Tov's Hebrew Matthew* is identical to our modern Greek text, we can learn nothing new; it could just be a 'correction' from the Greek. But when *Shem-Tov's Hebrew Matthew* differs from the Greek text, it may contain 'original readings' which were lost in the Greek." [4 (page 45)]

Although *Shem-Tov's Hebrew Matthew* was the original document studied, many additional Hebrew *Matthew* manuscripts have been brought to light in recent years.

Now, let's revisit a question asked regarding *Matthew* 23:2-3. What is *Moses' seat*? The *King James* version reads, "'(2) The scribes and the Pharisees sit in *Moses' seat*: (3) All therefore whatsoever they bid you observe, that observe and do; but do not ye after their works: for they say, and do not.' But when *Nehemia* went to look in the Hebrew text of *Matthew,* he found something quite different.' … The Hebrew translates '(2) The Pharisees and sages sit upon the *seat of Moses*. (3) Therefore, all that **he** says to you, diligently do, but according to **their** reforms (*takanot*) and **their** precedents (*ma'asim*) do not do, because they talk but they do not do.'

"In the Hebrew *Matthew*, *Yeshua* is telling his disciples *not* to obey the *Pharisees*. If their claim to authority is that they sit in the *Moses' Seat*, **then diligently do as Moses says!**' [4 (page 47-48)]

What is this '*Moses' Seat'*? *Michael Rood* "explained that there were two main opinions on the meaning of the phrase '*Moses' seat*.' Some said that in every synagogue there was an actual chair called a '*Moses' seat'* in which the leaders of the congregation would sit and teach with authority. The other opinion was that '*Moses' seat'* was a figure of speech indicating someone who teaches with authority of *Moses*. Either way, the statement that the *Pharisees* sit in '*Moses' seat*' meant that they have some kind of *Mosaic* authority." [4 (Page 2)]

From the Hebrew translation, it would seem that if the *Pharisees* and *Torah*-teachers were in fact teaching from the *Torah*, people were to listen to them. However, when the *Pharisees* and others were teaching and doing things not included in *Torah*, they were not to be followed. "*Yeshua* is warning his disciples not to look to the *ma'asim*, the precedents of the Rabbis, as the standard for proper behavior. Nor are they to follow the *takanot*, the invented laws of the Rabbis. Instead, they are to listen to what Moses says, because after all, the Rabbinic claim to authority is that they sit in *Moses' seat*." [4 (page 53-53)]

"If *Shem-Tov's* text of *Matthew* is correct, then *Yeshua* was warning his disciples not to follow the *takanot* or man-made laws of the Rabbis. Of course, this is consistent with what *Yeshua* taught his disciples in *Matthew* 15:3ff., 'Why do ye also transgress the commandment of God by your tradition? … Ye made the commandment of God of none effect by your tradition.' [KJV]. Like the *Karaite* sages of the Middle Ages, *Yeshua* accused the Pharisees of putting their own invented laws above the law of the *Torah*. Interestingly, in the Hebrew of *Matthew* 15:3, the word translated as 'tradition' is also *takanot*, 'reforms that change biblical law'! So, in Hebrew *Matthew*, there is a consistent thread throughout the book. *Yeshua* is preaching against the *takanot*, the *Pharisaic* reforms that change biblical law." [4 (page 50)]

"In the Greek *Matthew* 15:8-9, *Yeshua* then accuses the *Pharisees* of 'teaching for doctrine the commandments of men,' supposedly a quote from *Isaiah* 29:13. However, this is not exactly what *Isaiah* says. *Isaiah* actually talks about 'learned commandments of men.' Incredibly, the Hebrew *Matthew* has the precise quote from *Isaiah*, word for word.

Greek *Matthew* 15:9 : 'teaching for doctrines the commandments of men'

Hebrew *Matthew* 15:9 : 'learned commandments of men'

Hebrew *Isaiah* 29:13: 'learned commandments of men'" [4 (page 50)]

An additional witness to *Matthew* being written in Hebrew is a notation from a church father named *Papias*. "*Papias* had been the bishop of *Hierapolis*, a town in *Asia Minor*, and lived about 60-130 CE. Much of what *Papias* knew about *Yeshua* and his disciples came directly from the testimony of people who had studied under the original disciples. Among the people *Papias* spoke to directly was '*John the presbyter*,' the author of the *Gospel of John*. Based on his inside information, *Papias* reports matter-of-factly: '*Matthew* collected the oracles [literally: 'words'] in the Hebrew language, and each interpreted them as best he could.' …'So, there it was in black and white. *Papias* was saying *Matthew* wrote his gospel in Hebrew, and speakers of different languages did their best to interpret or translate it into their own languages. Apparently, *Papias* realized that some of the ancient translations of *Matthew's Hebrew Gospel* were none to accurate, and this is why he says that 'each translated them as best he could.' So not only was it known in ancient times that *Matthew* was originally written in Hebrew, but it was also widely recognized that the Greeks and other non-Hebrews had a difficult time translating *Hebrew Matthew* into Greek and other languages." [4 (page 76-77)]

As we can see, without proper understanding of a culture, the writings of those not familiar with the culture will tend to miss some of the very important aspects of what is really happening and being said. To see this more clearly, let's take a look at two miracles performed by Ye*shua* and see if there is a message in the miracles themselves.

The first miracle we learn about is during the wedding at *Cana* in the 2nd chapter of the *Book of John.*

Yochanan (*John*) 2:1 "On Tuesday * there was a wedding at *Kanah* in the *Galil*; and the mother of *Yeshua* was there. 2 *Yeshua* too was invited to the wedding, along with his *talmidim*. 3 The wine ran out, and *Yeshua's* mother said to him, 'They have no more wine.' 4 *Yeshua* replied, 'Mother (My lady), why should that concern me?' – or you?' My time hasn't come yet.' 5 His mother said to the servants, 'Do whatever he tells you.'
6 Now six stone water jars were standing there for the Jewish ceremonial washings, each with a capacity of twenty or thirty gallons. 7 *Yeshua* told them, 'Fill the jars with water.'

And they filled them to the brim. [8] He said, 'Now draw some out, and take it to the man in charge of the banquet'; and they took it. [9] The man in charge tasted the water; it had now turned into wine! He did not know where it had come from, but the servants who had drawn the water knew. So, he called the bridegroom [10] and said to him, 'Everyone else serves the good wine first and the poorer wine after people have drunk freely. But you have kept the good wine until now!' [11] This, the first of *Yeshua's* miraculous signs, he did at *Kanah* in the *Galil*; he manifested his glory, and his *talmidim* came to trust in him. [12] Afterwards, he, his mother and brothers, and his *talmidim* went down to *K'far-Nachum* (*Capernaum*) and stayed there a few days." [2 (page 1523)]

In *The Chronological Gospels*, *Michael Rood* has several explanatory notes. Regarding *John* 2:4.1, "*Yeshua's* mother is in a position of responsibility at this wedding, and the servants are at her command. When she informs *Yeshua* that they have run out of wine, he responds to her in respect of her official capacity (my lady – not 'woman') and then states, according to wedding custom, that he is ranked lower on the guest list and is, therefore, not among those who are expected to provide wine for the wedding party. The KJV sounds a bit disrespectful: 'Woman, what have I to do with you? Mine hour is not yet come!'" [1 (page 77)]

The note for *John* 2:6.1 tells the following. "We are informed that this is an orthodox *Pharisee* wedding reception by the notation that the six stone waterpots are for 'the purifying of the Jews', (KJV), which speaks of a water purification ritual invented by the *Pharisees*. These stone water-purification pots are never mentioned in the *Torah*, but they are meticulously detailed in the ancient *Talmudic* writings of the *Pharisee* sages. These hand-hewn stone waterpots held approximately 2 liters of liquid. Many of these ancient relics are preserved in the museums of *Israel* today, and their prescribed use by the *Pharisees* is well documented. (Modern interpretations of a '*firkin*' (KJV) incorrectly interpret the capacity of each stone vessel to be between 20 and 30 gallons. Even empty, the size and enormous weight of stone waterpots of this capacity would make them utterly impossible to utilize for their designed purpose.) *John* records that the wedding reception was filled with religious partygoers who apparently expected everyone else to provide the wine for their good time. After an undocumented discussion with her son, *Miriam* (*Mary*) turns to the servants and tells them to do whatever he instructs them to do. *Yeshua* then directed them to violate the 'holy' function of these stone waterpots – and it was kept a secret from the head rabbi, who was typically the master of ceremonies at *Pharisee* weddings. If the rabbi had known where the 'best wine' had come from, he would have indignantly ended the party right then and there!" An additional note for *John* 2:7.1 regards the description of the actions of the servants. "The servants are literally following the instructions documented in the *Talmud* (*Chillin* 26b) as they fill the stone vessels *to the brim*." [1 (page 77-78)]

So once again, we see a much deeper message in this first miracle. If we continue to uncover additional healings and situations, we will continue to see that throughout his ministry, *Yeshua* is separating *Torah* from *Talmud* to release his people from the burdens of these extraneous rules.

Even when he heals, there is a greater message that explains even further why the *Pharisees* were insistent in bringing down our Savior!

In *Mark* 8:22-26, *Yeshua* heals a blind man at *Beit Saida*. The scripture reads, "When he came to *Beit Saida*, they brought a blind man to *Yeshua* and begged him to touch him. [23] He took the blind man by the hand and led him out of town. He put spit on his eyes, and putting his hands on him, he asked the man if he saw anything. [24] He looked up and said, 'I see men like trees, walking.' [25] Again, he put his hands on his eyes and made him look up, and he was restored and saw every man clearly. [26] *Yeshua* sent him away to his house, saying, 'Do not go into town, nor tell it to any from the town." [1 (page 147)]

I have always wondered at this strange process of healing the blind. However, I just thought that Jesus certainly knew better than I on these matters, so we were to be thankful for the man's healing! However, as we shall see, *Michael Rood* sheds light on this healing process as well!

His note for *Mark* 8:23.1 is as follows: "Rabbinic *takanot* absolutely forbids putting saliva on the eyes on *Sabbath* (*Talmud*, tractate *Shabbat* 108b)." Yet *Yeshua* did just that! [1 (page 147)]

Again, we see the connection between the miracles and *Yeshua's* focus on separating *Torah* from the *Talmud.*

"According to noted Messianic Jewish scholar *Arnold Fruchtenbaum*:" *Yeshua's* first *Sermon on the Mount* address, "in its context – in the Jewish frame of reference in which it was spoken – the *Sermon on the Mount* is the Messiah's interpretation of the standard of righteousness which the *Torah* demanded, put in contrast with some of the *Pharisaic* interpretations. A better title for this 'sermon' would be '*The Messiah's Interpretation of the Righteousness of the Torah.*' Simplistically stated, the difference is between mere external conformity in contrast to internal conformity that naturally lends itself to external conformity to *Torah*." [2 (page 1389)]

As part of the "*Sermon on the Mount*," *Yeshua* clearly addresses his view on *Torah.*

Mattityahu (*Matthew*) [5:17] "Don't think that I have come to abolish the *Torah* or the *Prophets*. I have not come to abolish but to *complete*. [18] Yes indeed! I tell you that until heaven and earth pass away, not so much as a *yud* or a stroke will pass from the *Torah* – not until everything that must happen has happened. [19] So whoever disobeys the least of these *mitzvot* and teaches others to do so will be called the least in the *Kingdom of Heaven*. But whoever obeys them and so teaches, will be called great in the *Kingdom of Heaven*. [20] For I tell you that unless your righteousness is far greater than that of the *Torah*-teachers and *P'rushim*, you will certainly not enter the *Kingdom of Heaven*!'" [2 (page 1390)]

"These verses provide crucial insight into *Yeshua's* understanding of *Torah* and its meaning. Here, he is not canceling the *Torah*, instead he is stating that he came to *interpret it correctly*. *Romans* 10:4 is misinterpreted by many, making *Yeshua's* words in *Matthew* 5 difficult to understand. Some teach that his use of the word *telos*, often translated 'fulfill', means that his life, or perhaps his death, meant the termination or end of the law. Yet as *David Stern* notes, 'An error made by all major English versions and by most commentators – and one with profound anti-Semitic implications even when none are intended – is the rendering of the Greek word *telos* as 'end' in the sense of termination.' (*Jewish New Testament Commentary 395*). Yet *telos* is used forty-two times in the *New Testament*, but only five times (*Mark* 3:26; *Luke* 1:33; *2 Cor.* 3:3; *Heb*. 7:3; *1 Pet.* 4:7) is it translated 'finish,' 'cessation,' or 'termination.' In all other cases (including *Rom.* 10:4), *telos* is understood as 'outcome,' 'result,' or 'consummation.' Moreover, the statement that *Yeshua* did not come to abolish the *Torah* is a first-century rabbinic idiom. To 'abolish' the *Torah* meant to misinterpret it, not cancel it. Second, *Yeshua's* expression, to 'complete' *Torah*, meant that he came to teach it correctly. *David Friedman* reinforces this: '*Yeshua* is here stating that it is not his intention to teach the *Torah* incorrectly, but quite the opposite, to affirm its fullness and truth by teaching all of it in a way that is true to its intended meaning' (*Friedman, 'Jewish Idioms in the New Testament'*)." [2 (page 1391)]

At the beginning of his ministry, *Yeshua* went to the wilderness to be tempted by the *Adversary*. After his time overcoming the *Adversary*, "*Yeshua* began proclaiming, "Turn from your sins to God, for the *Kingdom of Heaven* is near!" *Mattityahu* (*Matthew* 4: 17) [2 (page 1388)]

The *Kingdom of Heaven* was at hand. *Yeshua* would be the *One who* would fulfill *Isaiah* [61:1] "The Spirit of *ADONAI ELOHIM* is upon me, because *ADONAI* has anointed me to announce good news to the poor. He has sent me to heal the brokenhearted; to proclaim freedom to the captives, to let out into light those bound in the dark; [2] to proclaim the year of the favor of *ADONAI*." [2 (page 594)]

In *Luke* 4:18-19, *Yeshua* reads these words from *Isaiah*. [18] "The Spirit of *ADONAI* is upon me; because he has anointed me to announce Good News to the poor; he has sent me to proclaim freedom for the imprisoned and renewed sight for the blind, [19] to proclaim a year of the favor of *ADONAI*." [2 (page 1479)]

Throughout his ministry, *Yeshua* shared the good news of this *Kingdom* through his actions and his teachings. This Kingdom brought healing to people and set them free of various diseases, demonic oppression, and more. *Yeshua* is the fulfillment of many prophecies, especially *Isaiah* 53.

Isaiah [53:4] "In fact, it was our diseases he bore, our pains from which he suffered; yet we regarded him as punished, stricken, and afflicted by God. [5] But he was wounded because of our crimes, crushed because of our sins; the discipling that makes us whole fell on him, and by his bruises we are healed." [2 (page 579)]

He purchased everything for us, and now we *are* (always present tense) healed!

Let's look at another of *Yeshua's* healing miracles and see the gift he provided for us by fulfilling the Spring Feasts of the LORD.

This testimony is shared in three of the Gospels and is the story of healing both a twelve-year-old girl and a woman who had been suffering for twelve years. Both these healings took place on the same day! We will take a look at this story in the gospel of *Matthew*, but it is also in *Mark* 5:22-34 and *Luke* 8:41-48 as well.

Matthew [9:18] "While *Yeshua* spoke to *Yochanan's disciples*, there came to *him* a certain ruler. He worshiped him and said, 'My daughter is dying right now. Please, come and lay your hand on her, and she shall live.' [19] *Yeshua* arose and followed him, and so did his disciples. [20] [As *Yeshua* approached *Yairus'* house], a woman who was diseased with an issue of blood for twelve years came behind him and took hold of the hem of his garment. [21] She spoke within herself, 'If I may but touch his garment, I shall be whole.' [22] But *Yeshua* turned around, and when he saw her, he said, 'Daughter, be of good comfort! Your faith has made you whole!' The woman was made whole from that hour. [23] When *Yeshua* came into the rabbi's house and saw musicians and others making a commotion, [24] he said to them, 'Step aside. The maid is not dead. She is just sleeping.' They laughed him to scorn, [25] but after they were thrown out, he went back in and took her by the hand and the maid arose. [26] The notoriety of this incident was spread throughout the land." [1 (page 126-128)]

Thankfully, the young girl was healed, and her story is told even today. The story of the woman with the issue of blood is also told, but there is much to that story that can get lost in the translation without additional information.

"The garment *Yeshua* is wearing is a *tallit* – a four-cornered, seamless garment worn by the Israelites over their white linen *haluq*. We were instructed at *Sinai* (in the *Torah*) to put a braided ribbon (*tzit-tzit*) of blue on each corner of our outer garment as a constant reminder to keep the commandments (*Numbers* 15:38). *Malachi* prophesied that the *Messiah* would have healing in his wings – *kanaph* – the heaven-blue ribbons on the corners of the *tallit* (*Malachi* 4:2). This is one of the most profound Messianic prophecies that was fulfilled and reported time and again in the Gospel records." [1 (page 127)]

"In *Numbers* 15:38, the word translated 'border' or 'corner' is the Hebrew word *kanaph*, which can also be translated 'wings,' as it is seventy-six times in the biblical text. The same word is used in *Malachi* 4:2 and translated as 'wings.' For this reason, the corners of the prayer shawl are often called 'wings.' Hanging from the end of each corner was a *tzitzit* (fringe) in obedience to the biblical command." [2 (page 1400)]

"During the first century, there were several traditions associated with the *tzitzit* concerning the Messiah. One was that these knotted fringes possessed healing powers. Another suggested that the *tzitzit* served as a sort of talisman or amulet. Both of these traditions may have had their roots in the prophecy of *Malachi* 3:20(4:2), where the Messiah is said to be coming 'with healing in [his] wings.' Certainly, the woman with the hemorrhage knew of these traditions, which might explain why she sought to touch the corner (the 'wings') of *Yeshua's* prayer garment. When one realizes the significance of the concept to the first-century *Hebraic* mind, it becomes clear why this woman was instantly healed. She was expressing her faith in *Yeshua* as the sun of righteousness with healing in his wings and declaring her faith in God's prophetic Word." [2 (page 1400)]

Another note brings to light the desperation of her situation. *Luke* [8:43] states, "A woman, having an issue of blood for twelve years, spent all her living on physicians but could not be healed by any. [44] She came from behind and grabbed the *tzit-tzit* on his tallit, and immediately her issue of blood stanched." [1 (page 127)]

"The woman was deliberately breaking the *Torah's* quarantine restrictions, but she knew that if *Yeshua* was the true Messiah, she would be healed. Messianic prophecy fulfilled – *Malachi* 4:2" [1 (page 127) [see End Note Vayikra (Leviticus) 15:19-31]]

Another note of importance to all of us is *Matthew* 9:22, in which *Yeshua* says, "Your faith has made you whole!" [1 (Page 127)]

How encouraging to all of us to come to our Messiah with faith and trust for our own wholeness!

No discussion of *Yeshua* and his healing would be complete without a look at the great exchange he made for us with his scourging and crucifixion. He exchanged his righteousness and wholeness for our sin nature, our diseases, struggles, and iniquities. We now have his righteousness and healing! He purchased us with his blood, body, and life! I will write more on this when looking at a scripture from Paul.

As we have learned in Section Two, *Yeshua*, Jesus, **did not** come to do away with the *Torah* and **did not** teach his disciples to disregard it either. With that, He came to teach *Torah* correctly and separate it from man's added rules and traditions. I contend that the *Dietary Laws* in *Torah* still stand, along with all the *Torah*. *Torah* stands, not to determine whether or not someone has salvation, but to give us guidelines for a set apart, holy life; and save us from a life of struggle and disease.

In Section Three, I will tackle a few additional scriptures that seem to cause confusion. We will look at three of *Yeshua's talmidim* – Peter (*Kefa*), Paul (*Sha'ul*), and James (*Ya'akov*). Did they do away with *Torah*? We shall see!

CHAPTER THREE

YESHUA'S TALMIDIM – *KEFA* (*PETER*), *YA'AKOV* (*JAMES*), AND *SHA'UL* (*PAUL*) – DID THEY CONTINUE TO FOLLOW *TORAH*? AND DID THEY FOLLOW DIETARY TEACHINGS?

These questions need answering, and in order to get to the answers, we will look first at what the disciples learned from *Yeshua* and then how they carried out *Yeshua's* instructions after His crucifixion. Various statements made by each of these men have been touted in making the case that the *Torah* had been negated. But is that true?

The writings of the apostles were letters to various individuals and Messianic communities, clarifying issues and answering questions. The *talmidim* would have a big job on their hands once the Holy Spirit, *Ruach Hakodesh*, empowered them to carry out the *Words of the Lord*. Their assignment would be clear.

The various testimonies were not always documented in chronological order. According to *The Chronological Gospels*, the story in *Matthew* chapter ten took place in weeks twenty-eight to thirty of *Yeshua's* ministry. *Michael Rood* believes *Yeshua's* ministry lasted seventy weeks and was extended to three and one-half years due to a scriptural addition and a misunderstanding of the Jewish Feasts by the Greek transcriptionist. The scripture in question is *John* 6:4. It was probably added by a *Greek* scribe who didn't know the order of the Hebrew feasts and picked Passover incorrectly. "All of the words found in *John* 6:4 were added in the third century (after *Yeshua's* resurrection) and are absent from the ancient *Greek* manuscripts *MSS 472* and *850*." [2 (page 135)]

In chapter ten of *Matthew's* account, "*Yeshua* sent out the twelve, in pairs of two, after the *Rosh Kodesh* (New Moon)". *Yeshua* instructed the *talmidim* in what they were to do on their journey. [2 (page 130)]

Mattityahu (*Matthew*) [10:1] "*Yeshua* called his twelve *talmadim* and **gave them authority**
to drive out unclean spirits and to heal every kind of disease and weakness. [2] These
are the names of the twelve emissaries: First, *Shim'on*, called *Kefa*, and *Andrew* his
brother, *Ya'akov Ben-Zavdai* and *Yochanan* his brother, [3] *Philip* and *Bar-Talmai*, *T'oma*
and *Mattityahu* the tax collector, *Ya'akov Bar-Halfai* and *Taddai*, [4] *Shim'on* the Zealot,
and *Y'hudah* from *K'riot*, who trusted him. [5] These twelve *Yeshua* sent out with the
following instruction: 'Don't go into the territory of the Gentiles, and don't enter any
town in *Shomron*, [6] but **go rather to the lost sheep of the house of *Isra'el*.** [7] As you go,

proclaim, 'The Kingdom of Heaven is near,' [8] **heal the sick, raise the dead, cleanse those afflicted with *tzara'at*, expel demons**. You have received without paying, so give without asking payment. [9] Don't take money in your belts, no gold, no silver, no copper; [10] and for the trip don't take a pack, an extra shirt, shoes, or a walking stick – a worker should be given what he needs.'" [3 (page 1401)]

There was another time during His earthly ministry that *Yeshua* sent His disciples on a mission to the surrounding towns. He appointed seventy disciples, or talmadim, for this mission. *Kefa* was one of these students. We can read about this in *Luke 10.* In *Luke* 10:8, they were told that when they "enter a town where they are welcomed, they may eat as it is put in front of them."

"Among the *Israelites* to whom *Yeshua* is sending the seventy disciples, you would never find **abominable flesh** set before anyone. *Yeshua* is speaking of eating whatever *oklah* – food – that is set before you, not *pharmakia* (inorganic substances created in a laboratory) nor animals that are classified as an *abomination* by the Creator. It is sin to eat anything that is expressly forbidden by our Creator, regardless of the intention of the provider." [2 (page 162)]

Yeshua was continuously teaching his students even up to the last meal they would share together. This took place on the night **before** the *Passover Feast* and *Feast of Unleavened Bread.*

John [13:1] "Now, **<u>before the Feast of the Passover</u>**, *Yeshua* knew that the hour was come that he should depart out of this world to the Father. He, having loved his own which were in the world, loved them to the *very* end. [2] **And after [the last] supper had ended**..." [2 (page 222)]

The details of the evening are noted in *Matthew* 26, *Mark* 14, and *Luke* 22. Valuable information is in each Gospel. As we look at their last meeting before the crucifixion, we will glean bits and pieces from the various writers.

Matthew [26:20] "Now when the even was come, he reclined with the twelve [*in the upper room where they had been making Passover preparations*]." [2 (page 222)]

Luke [22:14] "When the evening dinner hour was come, he reclined with his twelve apostles. [15] He said to them, 'With great desire I have desired to eat this *Passover* with you before I suffer, [16] but I now tell you that I will not again eat of the *Passover* until it is fulfilled in the *Kingdom of YHWH.*'" [2 (page 222)]

A note on *Luke* 22:16 reads, "*Yeshua* will literally fulfill all of the prophetic shadow pictures embedded in the *Passover* in less than twenty-four hours. The rehearsal in the Temple was just a shadow of the fulfillment that was about to occur in the *Kingdom of YHWH* as the *Lamb of YHWH* was about to be the substitution for the sins of the nation of *Israel* and the transgressions of the entire world." [2 (page 222)]

Matthew [26:26] "As they were eating, *Yeshua* took bread, blessed the *Most High*, and **broke the bread**, and gave it to the disciples, and said, '**Take, eat; this is my body**.' [27] He took the cup and gave thanks again and gave it to them, saying, 'Drink all of it [28] for **this is the renewed covenant in my blood, which is shed for many for the remission of sins**. [29]

But I say to you, from this day forward, I will not drink of the fruit of the vine, until the new day when I drink with you in my Father's kingdom.'" [2 (page 223)]

"*Yeshua* spoke the blessing with which the *Melek Tzadek* blessed the *Most High* when he brought forth bread and wine to *Avraham* when he returned from the slaughter of the kings. This is the same blessing that *Avraham* taught *Yitzhak*, who taught *Ya'akov*, who taught his twelve sons, who still speak this blessing every *Shabbat* over the bread." … "'*Blessed are you YHWH, King of the universe, who brings forth bread from the earth.*' *Yeshua* then explained that this had always – even from the time of *Melek Tzadek* – represented his body, which would be the provision for our ultimate healing. *Avraham* had indeed seen *Yeshua's* day in the representation of the shed blood and the broken body that the *Melek Tzadek* shared with him. *Avraham* rejoiced and laid a tenth of his vast wealth at the feet of the *Priest of the Most High Elohim*." [2 (page 223)]

"After the bread, *Yeshua* took the cup and blessed the *Most High* with the blessings that *Melek Tzadek* blessed *Elohim* of *Avraham*: '*Blessed are you YHWH, King of the universe, creator of the fruit of the vine*.' This represents the payment for the broken blood covenant that we entered into at *Mount Sinai*. We broke the covenant, ratified with the blood of bulls, and for that transgression, the guilty party must die. *Yeshua*, who never once violated that covenant, offered himself and died in our place. Through the substitutionary payment of the death penalty, which is the curse for breaking the blood covenant, he can renew that covenant with us, write the *Torah* on our hearts, and actually live in us through the gift of the Holy Spirit (*Jeremiah* 31:31-34)." [2 (page 223)]

One additional note for *Luke* 22:18 provides "an important detail. *Yeshua* did not drink the wine that evening, and prophetically proclaimed his abstinence until the marriage supper of the *Lamb* – an important part of this remembrance." [2 (page 223)]

Graciously, *Yeshua* also taught them servant leadership skills. *John* [13:1] "Before the *Feast of the Passover*, *Yeshua* knew that his hour was come that he should depart out of this world to the Father, yet he loved his own which were in the world to the very end. [2] After [*the last*] supper had ended, *Hasatan* had already put *enmity* into the heart of *Yehudas ben Shimon of Ascareyotah* to betray him. [3] But *Yeshua* knew that the Father had given all things into his hands, and *did not doubt* that he came from *YHWH*, and would go to *YHWH*. [4] So, he arose from supper, laid aside his garments, and took a towel to clothe himself. [5] Then he poured water into a basin and began to wash the disciples' feet and to wipe them with the towel with which he was clothed. [6] When he came to *Shimon, Kefa* said to him, 'Master, are you going to wash my feet?' [7] *Yeshua* answered, 'You do not understand what I am doing now, but you will understand later.' [8] *Kefa* said to him, 'You shall never wash my feet!' *Yeshua* answered him, 'If I do not wash you, you will have no future with me.' [9] *Shimon Kefa* said to him, 'Master, wash not my feet only, but also *my* hands and *my* head.' [10] *Yeshua* said to him, 'He that is washed needs only to wash his feet and is completely clean. And you are clean, but not all of you.' [11](for he knew who should betray him – that is why he said, 'You are not all clean.') [12] After he had washed their feet and donned his garment, he reclined again and said to them, 'Do you understand what I have done to you? [13] You call me Rabbi and master, and you say well; for so I am. [14] If I then, *your* Rabbi and master, have washed your feet; you also ought to wash one another's feet. [15] **I have just given you an example, that you should do as I**

have done to you. [16] **TRUTH**, I say to you, the servant is not greater than his master; neither is he that is sent greater than he that sent him. [17] If you know these things, happy are you if you do them. [18] I speak not of you all. I know whom I have chosen, but that the Scripture may be fulfilled. 'He that eats bread with me has lifted his heel against me.' [a] [19] Now I tell you before it comes to pass, so that when it does come to pass, you will believe that I am *the One*. [20] **TRUTH** I say to you, he who receives whoever I send, receives *the One* who sent me.' [21] When *Yeshua* had said this, he was troubled in spirit, and he again testified, '**TRUTH** I say to you, one of you will betray me. [23] Then the disciples looked one on another, again wondering of whom he spoke." [2 (a Psalm 41:10 (9), page 225)]

We know who he was referring to, but they did not. The disciples thought perhaps *Yehudas* (*Judas*) was going to purchase provisions for Passover, or to give something to the poor. "The day of the preparation of the *Passover* sacrifice had now begun." [2 (page 226)]

John [13:31] "When *Yehudas* had left *the house*, *Yeshua* said, 'Now the *Son of Man* will be glorified, and *YHWH* will be glorified in him. [32] If *YHWH* is glorified in him, *YHWH* shall also glorify the *Son of Man* in himself and will soon glorify him. [33] My dear children, I will only be with you yet for a little while. You will seek me, but just as I said to the sages and *Prushim*, 'Where I go, you cannot come.' Now I say the same thing to you. [34] **I am also giving you a new commandment: love one another. Just as I have loved you, love one another**. [35] By this shall all men know that you are my disciples – if you have love one for another.'" [2 (page 226)]

Luke [22:31] "The master said, '*Shimon*! Look, *hasatan* has desired to have you, that he may sift you like wheat. [32] But I have prayed for you, that your faith does not fail. When you return from your sifting, strengthen your brothers.' [33] *Kefa* said to him, 'Master, I am ready to go with you both into prison and to death.' [34] *Yeshua* warned, 'I tell you, *Kefa*, the cock will not crow this day, before you will deny three times that you know me.' [35] *Yeshua* asked them, 'When I sent you without a money purse, a bag of provisions, or extra sandals, did you lack anything?' They replied. 'Not a thing!' [36] Then he said, 'Now, whoever does not have a sword, let him take his purse or his bag of provisions, or even sell a garment and buy one, [37] because I am telling you that which is written, '*He was reckoned among the transgressors*', [a] and this must still be accomplished by me. There is a reason for everything that is written concerning me.' [38] They said, 'Master, look; we have two swords,' He said, 'It is enough.'" [2 (a Isaiah 53:12; page 227)]

To this point, there has been no mention of changing any teaching of the *Torah*, nor suggestion on how to eat differently. They have been taught to go only to the house of *Isra'el*, to declare the *Kingdom of Heaven* is near, to love one another, and are to heal every disease and infirmity, raise the dead, and cast out demons! To do as they had seen him do. All of this is to be done willingly without asking for payment. These teachings took place before *Yeshua* was crucified.

An additional instruction, called The *Great Commission*, took place after *Yeshua's* resurrection, and happened right before his ascension to the Father. Although the *Book of Matthew* may have been written thirty to forty years after the Crucifixion (between years 58c.e. and 68c.e.), the disciples were evidently careful to write down their experiences within the first few years and possibly during their tutelage with *Yeshua*. The formal *Gospels* and letters were all completed many years later.

Mattityahu (*Matthew*) [28:16] "So the eleven *talmidim* went to the hill in the *Galil* where *Yeshua* had told them to go. [17] When they saw him, they prostrated themselves before him, but some hesitated. [18] *Yeshua* came and talked to them. He said, 'All authority in heaven and on earth has been given to me. [19] Therefore, **go and make people from all nations into *talmidim*, immersing them** into the reality of the *Father*, the *Son* and the *Ruach HaKodesh*, [20] and **teaching them to obey everything that I have commanded you**. And remember! I will be with you always, yes, even until the end of the age.'" [3 (page 1438)]

The Chronological Gospels reads as follows: *Matthew* [28:18] "Then *Yeshua* came and spoke to his disciples, 'All power and authority has been given to me in Heaven and in Earth. [19] Go! [20] Teach all nations to carry out all the things that I have commanded you – forever.' According to *Mattityahu* [[Amen]]" [2 (page 273)]

The note for this scripture states: "{*Mt.* 28:19.1} The *KJV* and late Greek manuscripts add the phrase 'baptizing them in the name of the Father, and of the Son, and of the Holy Spirit.' *Eusebius*, in his ***Oration in Praise of the Emperor Constantine*** chapter XVI, quoted this passage from *Matthew* (and did so another 18 times in his fourth-century writings), '**Go *and* make disciples of all nations in my name, teaching them to keep all things which I have commanded you**.' The *Ancient Hebrew Matthew* provides a reading very close to the early manuscript *Eusebius* quoted, which reads, 'Go and teach them to carry out all the things that I have commanded you – forever.' Those who had actually heard the instruction from *Yeshua* never baptized in the ***phrase*** (in the name of the Father, Son and Holy Spirit) nor is there any record of any historical group actually following this supposed instruction by speaking the actual *name* of the Father, and the name of the Son, and the ***name*** of the Holy Spirit as part of any baptism ceremony. Both this phrase and the addition of the word 'Amen' at the end of each Gospel appear to be post-*Constantinian* inventions." [2 (page 274)]

Now we know much of what the *talmidim* were instructed to do and not do. They were to make disciples of people of all nations, immerse them, and teach them all *Yeshua* had taught them. The statements in the previous scriptures, combined with all that the *talmidim* had witnessed, practiced, and heard gave them a solid foundation for their own ministries. They would share that the *Kingdom of Heaven* was at hand, and that the people could receive the healing benefits and promises by putting their trust in God and His Messiah.

In the *Book of Acts*, *Luke* sheds light on what was to happen next and how the disciples were empowered by *Ruach Hakodesh*. Both the *Book of Luke* and the *Book of Acts* were written by *Luke* to *Theophilos*. Who was *Theophilos*?

"Until recently, theologians thought that *Theophilos* was a representative member of the *Roman* government, or that the name '*Theophilos*' (meaning 'Dear to God') was a pseudonym for a Gentile official whom *Luke* desired to see the gospel more favorably. Yet, as supported by *Josephus* (*Antiquities* XVII, 78, 164-65) and as seen in archaeological evidence found among the *Herodian Mansions* in the *Jewish* quarter of

Jerusalem, *Theophilos* was the high priest between 37-41c.e. This is significant in that Luke begins and ends this *Gospel* account (of *Luke*) with references to the *Temple* (*Barag and Flusser* 39-44; cf. *Acts* 1:1 note)." [3 (page 1470)]

Luke wrote the letter that holds his name, *Luke*, in about 60 CE., and his narrative letter of *Acts* about 62 CE. This is about thirty-two years after the crucifixion of *Yeshua* and about eight years before the destruction of the *Temple*. "The focus is God's intent for Jews and Gentiles to share in the salvation promised in the *Hebrew Scriptures*. *Acts* explains how the inclusion of Gentiles in the *Yeshua* movement was in accordance with God's plan. It shows that God intended the body of the Messiah to be a place of unity and reconciliation as a part of his restoring creation to wholeness. Multiple retellings of *Sha'ul's* (Paul's) transformation and *Kefa's* (Peter's) message to *Cornelius* underscores the importance of mission and outreach to Gentiles. However, the focus early on was to the *House of Israel* located in various towns and countries. [3 (page 1557)]

Let us back up just a bit, to before the first *Shavu'ot* (Pentecost). This was fifty days after *Passover* and the crucifixion of *Yeshua*, and ten days after *Yeshua's* ascension to the right hand of *Yehovah*. There was a forty-day period where the risen *Yeshua* spent time with his students and others, sharing more information and tying together prophecies given years before and now fulfilled!

Acts [1:3] "After his death, he showed himself to them (his emissaries) and gave many convincing proofs that he was alive. During a period of forty days, they saw him, and he spoke with them about the *Kingdom of God*.

Acts [1:4] "At one of these gatherings, he instructed them not to leave *Yerushalayim* but to
'wait for what the *Father* promised, which you heard about from me. [5] For *Yochanan*
used to immerse people in water; but in a few days, you will be immersed in the *Ruach Hakodesh*!'"

Acts [1:6] "When they were together, they asked him, 'Lord, are you at this time going to
restore self-rule to *Isra'el*?' [7] He answered, 'You don't need to know the dates or times
the *Father* has kept these under his own authority. [8] But you will receive power when the
Ruach Hakodesh comes upon you; you will be my witnesses both in *Yerushalayim* and in
all *Y'hudah* and *Shomron*, indeed to the ends of the earth!' [9] After saying this, he was
taken up before their eyes; and a cloud hid him from their sight. [10] As they were staring
into the sky after him, suddenly they saw two men dressed in white standing next to
them. [11] The men said, 'You *Galileans*! Why are you standing, staring into space? This
Yeshua, who has been taken away from you into heaven, will come back to you in just the
same way you saw him go into heaven.'" [3 (page 1558)]

A note on *Acts* 1:8, in the *Complete Jewish Study Bible,* states, "'To the ends of the earth!' *Yeshua's talmidim* (disciples) are beginning to share the Good News of *Yeshua* where they are, in *Yerushalayim* (Jerusalem), the center of the Jewish world. This phrase 'in *Jerusalem* and in all *Y'hudah* (*Judah*) and *Shomron* (*Samaria*)' is not metaphorical but literal: God is instructing them to share the Good News first to the Jew (*Romans* 1:16) and after that to the ends of the earth (all other nations)." [3 (page 1558)]

The marching orders for their ambassadorships are becoming much clearer, and they will experience more empowerment in just ten days. As we can see in the next part of *Luke's* letter, they return from the *Mount of Olives* to *Yerushalayim,* where they will wait for their next instruction.

Acts [1:12] "Then they returned the *Shabbat*-walk distance from the *Mount of Olives* to *Yerushalayim.* [13] After entering the city, they went to the upstairs room where they were staying. The names of the emissaries were *Kefa*, *Ya'akov*, *Yochanan*, *Andrew*, *Philip*, *T'oma*, *Bar-Talmai*, *Mattityahu*, *Ya'akov Ben-Halfai*, *Shim'on* 'the Zealot,' and *Y'hudah Ben-Ya'akov*. [14] These all devoted themselves single-mindedly to prayer, along with some women, including *Miryam* (*Yeshua's* mother), and his brothers."

Acts [1:15] "During this period, when the group of believers numbered about 120, *Kefa* stood up and addressed his fellow-believers. [16] 'Brothers, the *Ruach HaKodesh* spoke in advance through *David* about *Y'hudah*, and these words of the *Tanakh* had to be fulfilled. He was guide for those who arrested *Yeshua* – [17] he was one of us and had been assigned a part in our work.' [18] (With the money *Y'hudah* received for his evil deed, he bought a field; and there he fell to his death. His body swelled up and burst open, and all his insides spilled out. [19] This became known to everyone in *Yerushalayim*, so they called that field *Hakal-D'ma* – which in their language, *Aramaic*, means '*Field of Blood*.') [20] 'Now," said *Kefa*, 'it is written in the book of *Psalms*, '**Let his estate become desolate, let there be no one to live in it;**' [a] and '**Let someone else take his place as a supervisor.**'" b (a Psalm 69:26 (25), 3 (page 971); b Psalm 109:8, 3 (page 1019); 3 (page 1559)

Acts [1:21] "'Therefore, one of the men who have been with us continuously throughout the time the Lord *Yeshua* traveled around among us, [22] from the time *Yochanan* was immersing people until the day *Yeshua* was taken up from us – one of these must become a witness with us to his resurrection.' [23] They nominated two men – *Yosef Ben Sabba*, surnamed *Justus*, and *Mattityahu*. [24] Then they prayed, 'Lord, you know everyone's heart. Show us which of these two you have chosen [25] to take over the work and the office of emissary that *Y'hudah* abandoned to go where he belongs.' [26] Then they drew lots to decide between the two, and the lot fell to *Mattityahu*. So he was added to the eleven emissaries." 3 (page 1559)

Acts [2:1] "The festival of *Shavu'ot* arrived, and the believers all gathered together in one place. [2] Suddenly there came a sound from the sky like the roar of a violent wind, and it filled the whole house where they were sitting. [3] Then they saw what looked like tongues of fire, which separated and came to rest on each one of them. [4] They were all filled with the *Ruach HaKodesh* and began to talk in different languages, as the *Spirit* enabled them to speak." 3 (page 1559)

With the "Roar of a violent wind and tongues of fire, God emphasizes the connection between the *Torah* and the *Ruach HaKodesh* by giving both with similar miraculous signs. The roar and fire in *Yerushalayim* (Jerusalem) recalled the fire, smoke, and sounds that were experienced at *Mount Sinai*." (Exodus 19:18-19,3 (page 98; Deuteronomy 5: 19(22) –21(24), 3 (page 233); 3 (page 1559)

A note regarding *Acts* 2:4 states, "They were all filled with the *Ruach HaKodesh*. In the *Torah*, certain individuals had the *Ruach* (Holy Spirit) in or with them. In *Numbers* 11:17,

Moshe (Moses) and in *1 Samuel* 10:6, *Sha'ul* (Saul) each had an experience where the Holy Spirit empowered them. Yet in *Acts* 2, God brings to pass what *Moshe* prayed for long ago: that God would put his Spirit on all his people. (*Numbers* 11:29), fulfilling what *Yeshua* promised them (*Luke* 24:29; *John* 16:16, 20:22; *Acts* 1:8). [3 (page 1560)]

Acts [2:5] "Now there were staying in *Yerushalayim* religious Jews from every nation under heaven. [6] When they heard this sound, a crowd gathered; they were confused, because each one heard the believers speaking in his own language. [7] Totally amazed, they asked, 'How is this possible? Aren't all these people who are speaking from the *Galil*? [8] How is it that we hear them speaking in our native languages? [9] We are *Parthian's*, *Medes*, *Elamites*; residents of *Mesopotamia*, *Y'hudah*, *Cappadocia*, *Pontus*, *Asia*, [10] *Phrygia*, *Pamphylia*, *Egypt*, the parts of *Libya* near *Cyrene*; visitors from *Rome*; [11] Jews by birth and proselytes; Jews from *Crete* and from *Arabia*! How is it that we hear them speaking in our own languages about the great things God has done?' [12] Amazed and confused, they all went on asking each other, 'What can this mean?' [13] But others made fun of them and said, 'They've just had too much wine.' [14] Then *Kefa* stood up with the *Eleven* and raised his voice to address them: 'You *Judeans*, and all of you staying here in *Yerushalayim*! Let me tell you what this means! Listen carefully to me! [15] These people aren't drunk, as you suppose – it's only nine in the morning. [16] No, this is what was spoken about through the prophet *Yo'el*:' [17] ***Adonai* says: 'In the Last Days, I will pour out from my *Spirit* upon everyone. Your sons and daughters will prophesy, your young men will see visions, your old men will dream dreams. [18] Even on my slaves, both men and women, will I pour out from my *Spirit* in those days; and they will prophesy. [19] I will perform miracles in the sky above and signs on the earth below – blood, fire, and thick smoke. [20] The sun will become dark and the moon blood before the great and fearful Day of *Adonai* comes. [21] And then, whoever calls on the name of *Adonai* will be saved.'"** [a (a Joel 3:1-5 (2:28-32) page 809-810); 3 (1560)]

Acts [2:22] "'Men of *Isra'el*! Listen to this! *Yeshua* from *Natzeret* was a man demonstrated to you to have been from God by the powerful works, miracles, and signs that God performed through him in your presence. You yourselves know this. [23] This man was arrested in accordance with God's predetermined plan and foreknowledge; and, through the agency of persons not bound by the *Torah*, you nailed him up on a stake and killed him! [24] But God has raised him up and freed him from the suffering of death; it was impossible that death could keep its hold on him. [25] For David says this about him: '**I saw *Adonai* always before me, for he is at my right hand, so that I will not be shaken. [26] For this reason, my heart was glad; and my tongue rejoiced; and now my body too will live on in the certain hope [27] that you will not abandon me to *Sh'ol* or let your Holy One see decay. [28] You have made known to me the ways of life; you will fill me with joy by your presence.'''** [b (b Psalm 16:8-11, 3 (page 911-912), 3 (page 1561)]

Acts [2:29] "'Brothers, I know I can say to you frankly that the patriarch David died and was buried – his tomb is with us to this day. [30] Therefore, since he was a prophet and knew that God had sworn an oath to him that one of his descendants would sit on his throne, [31] he was speaking in advance about the resurrection of the Messiah, that it was he who was abandoned in *Sh'ol* and whose flesh did not see decay. [32] God raised up this *Yeshua*! And we are all witnesses of it! [33] Moreover, he has been exalted to the right hand of God; has received from the *Father* what he promised, namely, the *Ruach HaKodesh*; and has poured out this gift, which you are both seeing and hearing. [34] For David did not ascend into heaven. But he says, [35] **'ADONAI said to my Lord, 'Sit at my right hand until I make your enemies a footstool for your feet.'''** c (c Psalm 110:1, 3-page 1021) 3 (page 1561)

Acts 2:36 "'Therefore, let the whole house of *Isra'el* know beyond doubt that God has made him both Lord and Messiah – this *Yeshua*, whom you executed on a stake!'

Acts 2:37 "On hearing this, they were stung in their hearts; and they said to *Kefa* and the other emissaries, 'Brothers, what should we do?' [38] *Kefa* answered them, '*Turn from sin, return to God, and each of you be immersed in the authority of Yeshua the Messiah into forgiveness of your sins, and you will receive the gift of the Ruach HaKodesh!* [39] *For the promise is for you, for your children, and for those far away – as many as ADONAI our God may call!*' [40] He pressed his case with many other arguments and kept pleading with them, 'Save yourselves from this perverse generation!' [41] So those who accepted what he said were immersed, and there were added to the group that day about three thousand people. [42] *They continued faithfully in the teaching of the emissaries, in fellowship, in breaking bread and in prayers.*" 3 (page 1562)

The scripture speaks of *teaching of the emissaries*. "This means either the act of teaching or the content taught, here more likely the latter. Since in Hebrew, *Torah* means 'teaching or instruction,' this phrase can be translated 'the *Torah* of the emissaries.' In fellowship, in breaking bread and in the prayers, 'Fellowship' means community, commonness or fellowship. It was customary to begin a meal by breaking bread over which a special blessing is said. The prayers imply the traditional synagogue prayers, common in this day." 3 (page 1562)

Kefa and the others were speaking to fellow Jews who had come to *Yerushalayim* for one of the three festivals required of them – *Shavu'ot*. Therefore, all were intimately familiar with the *Torah* and the *Tanakh*, as well as the other teachings added by the rabbis. Even though they spoke in various languages and came from many different countries, the teachings they heard weekly in their synagogues were the same. Each week in every synagogue, the scriptures from *Torah* and *Tanakh* were read. A specific section was read each week, so all were learning the same thing, no matter where they lived. They knew their history and the *Word of God*. They had heard the prophecies and now they could understand that many were fulfilled in *Yeshua*.

From these scriptures, we see the foundation laid by *Yeshua* and the empowerment his followers experienced through the infilling of the *Ruach HaKodesh*. He also warned them of events that would take place in the future, both near and far.

In *John* 16:1, *Yeshua* warns, "'I have told you these things so that you won't be caught by surprise. [2] They will ban you from the synagogue; in fact, the time will come when anyone who kills you will think he is serving God! [3] They will do these things because they have understood neither the *Father* nor me. [4] But I have told you this, so that when the time comes for it to happen, you will remember that I told you. I didn't tell you this at first, because I was with you. [5] But now I am going to the *One* who sent me.'" 3 (page 1547)

He continues his warning in *John* [16: 35] "'I have said these things to you so that, united with me, you may have *shalom*. In the world you have troubles. But be brave! I have conquered the world! [3 (page 1548)]

Just as *Yeshua* had warned, within a brief time, persecution came to the *Messianic* community in Jerusalem. They had worshipped and studied in the synagogues, but the time had come that they were no longer welcome. Believers began to meet in homes for the breaking of bread, as well as worshipping, healing, and teaching.

"At the beginning of the Christian era, churches began in believers' homes, as this was a safer place to meet and worship without the threat from religious leaders of the synagogues or persecution from certain Pharisees, Sadducees, and priests at the temple. In their home groups, believers would study, pray, and sing hymns (*Ephesians* 5:19). [5 (page 27)]

"Believers would meet together on the first day of the week (*Acts* 20:7; 1 *Corinthians* 16:2) during which time they would break bread. The first day of the week on the Jewish calendar is Sunday." [5 (page 27)]

A note in *The Complete Jewish Study Bible* gives us more information regarding this first day of the week. In *Hebrew*, it reads, "Every week, on *Motza'ei-Shabbat*. The Hebrew expression literally means '*Departure of the Sabbath*,' signifying Saturday night. This is also when the first day of the week begins." [3 (page 1652)]

"Scripture indicated the practice of *breaking bread* was a central part of the early activity among believers in their homes. …According to numerous Christian commentaries, the daily breaking of bread referred to having the *Lord's Supper* (Communion) in the believer's house! Remember, the original *Passover* supper was in the homes of the Hebrews in Egypt, and the Lord's Supper was initially instituted by Christ from a home." [5 (pages 28)]

Yeshua's crucifixion took place on "*Passover Day*, *Nissan* 14, April 5th, the year 30 AD. Christ was resurrected toward the end of the weekly *Sabbath*, *Nissan* 17. He then appeared to disciples for forty days from *Nissan* 18 to His ascension *Iyar* 27, May 18th, 30AD. The Holy Spirit poured out on Pentecost, *Shavuot*, Sunday, May 28th, 30 AD, and the *Gospel* was preached in Jerusalem that same year. (*Acts* 3-5) [4]

In 31AD, the *Gospel* continued to be preached in Jerusalem, and the Apostles compiled the teachings of Jesus. (*Acts* 5 and 6) [4]

The persecution of the church was getting worse, and Stephen was martyred in 32 AD. (*Acts* 6,7). *Acts* 8:1-4 describe more persecution against the early church. "Because of the persecutions, brethren scatter and preach the *Word* everywhere (*Acts* 8:4). Philip goes to *Samaria*; *Simon Magnus* becomes a believer and follows Philip (*Acts* 8:5-13); Peter and John were sent to *Samaria* (*Acts* 8:14-25)." [4]

Sha'ul, also called Saul and/or Paul, continues to persecute the church until the Spring of 33AD (*Acts* 9:3-18) at which time he meets the Lord Jesus on his trip to *Damascus*. A plot to kill *Sha'ul* is discovered, and he escapes to *Arabia*. (*Acts* 9:24-25). *Galatians* 1:15-18 relates that *Sha'ul* was taught by the resurrected *Yeshua* for three years. [4]

With this foundation, we now can look at several scriptures and incidents about Peter, James, and Paul that have been misunderstood or mistranslated. We will visit *Cornelius* with Peter, as told in *Acts* 10:1-48. This event took place approximately eight years after *Yeshua's* resurrection and the infilling of the *Ruach HaKodesh*. It is now 38 AD.[4]

Acts 9:32 through Acts 9:43 tells of *Kefa's* (Peter) avoiding persecution as he visited the "saints who dwelt at *Lydda*." There, he continued teaching and healing. One who was healed was *Aeneas*, a man bedridden for eight years. Then he, *Kefa*, went to *Yaffo*, where he heard that a woman named *Tabitha* became sick and died. *Kefa* accompanied the people that brought the news of her death to where she was and sent everyone out of the room. He prayed and then spoke directly to her body saying, "'*Tabitha*, arise!' She opened her eyes, and when she saw *Kefa*, she sat up. He gave her *his* hand and lifted her up, and when he had called the saints and widows, he presented her alive. This became known throughout all *Yaffo*, and many believed in Messiah. Then *Kefa* stayed in *Yaffo* for many days with *Shimon*, a tanner." *Acts* 9:32 – 43. [2 (page 294)]

Acts 10:1 "There was a certain man in *Caesarea* called *Cornelius*, a centurion of the famed *Italian* detachment. 2 He was a devout man who feared *YHWH* with all his house, gave alms generously to the people, and prayed to *YHWH* continually. 3 At about the ninth hour of the day, he saw clearly in a vision an angel of *YHWH* coming to him, saying, '*Cornelius*.' 4 And when he looked at him, he was afraid, and said, 'What is it, *Adonai*?' And he said to him, 'Your prayers and your alms have come up for a memorial before *YHWH*. 5 Now send men to *Yaffo* and call for *Shimon*, whose surname is *Kefa*. 6 He is staying with a man called *Shimon*, a tanner, whose house is by the seaside. He shall tell you what you need to do.' 7 When the angel departed, *Cornelius* called two of his household servants and one of the devoted soldiers who waited on him continually. 8 When he had told them all these things, he sent them to *Yaffo*." [2 (page 294)]

Acts 10:9 "The next day, as the *emissaries of Cornelius* went on their journey and drew near to the city, *Kefa* went up on the housetop to pray at about the sixth hour. 10 He became very hungry and would have eaten, but while they were preparing *the meal*, he received an open vision. 11 He saw heaven opened and something like a great sheet gathered at the four corners descended on the earth. 12 In *the sheet* were all kinds of rodents and carnivorous animals, and crawling insects, and carrion eaters, and birds of prey. 13 He heard a voice say to him, 'Rise, *Kefa*. Kill and eat!' 14 But *Kefa* refused, 'Not so, *Adonai*, for I have never eaten anything that is defiled or unclean.' 15 Then the voice *spoke* to him again the second time, 'What *YHWH* has cleansed, do not call defiled.' 16 This was done three times, and the sheet returned again into heaven." [2 (page 295)]

Keep in mind that *Kefa* would soon understand this vision was about people - not food. He knew that God created all animals as "good". But not all were created for food. In *Kefa's* vision, all kinds of animals are in the sheet. Again, they were all created "good", but only a select few were for food or for sacrifices. Although many people see the dietary rules in Leviticus 11 as only for the Israelites, actually, they are for all God's people. The Israelites were to teach the nations how to live as *YHWH* intended, and through *Kefa* and *Shaul*, that was about to happen.

On its face, this does seem like a conundrum! It has been eight years since *Kefa* was with *Yeshua,* and he has been filled with *Ruach HaKodesh*. Over the years, *Kefa* shared the teachings of *Yeshua* and clarified *Torah* and *Tanakh* to new followers of *Yeshua's* Way. The followers up to that time have all been *Hebrew* themselves. They were all familiar with the *Torah*, the *Tanakh*, and lived an observant lifestyle in the *Way of Yeshua*. As we have learned, *Yeshua* was not doing away with *Torah*; he was clarifying and separating *Torah* from the false teachings and traditions of men. It is obvious from *Kefa's* response to the vision, he had not strayed from *Torah*, nor the dietary teachings. So, what did this vision mean?

Acts [10:17] "Now while *Kefa* pondered what this vision meant, the men who were sent from *Cornelius* had asked where *Shimon's* house was and were standing outside the gate. [18]
They called out, asking whether *Shimon*, who was surnamed *Kefa*, was lodging there. [19]
While *Kefa* pondered the meaning of the vision, the *Ruach* said to him, '**Behold, three men are looking for you.** [20] **Arise and go down. Go with them, doubting nothing, for I have sent them.'** [21] Then *Kefa* went down to the men *Cornelius* had sent to him and said, 'Behold, I am he whom you seek. Why have you come?' [22] They said, 'The centurion *Cornelius*, a just man who fears *YHWH* and is well spoken of among the whole Jewish nation, was instructed by a holy angel to send for you to come to his house and hear what you have to say.' [23] So *Kefa* invited them in, and they *stayed the night with him*. The next day *Kefa* went with them, and some of the brothers from *Yaffo* accompanied him." [2 (page 295)]

Acts [10:24] "The next day they entered *Caesarea*. *Cornelius* had called together his family and close friends, and they were waiting for them. [25] As *Kefa* was coming in, *Cornelius* met him, fell down at his feet, and worshiped *him*. [26] But *Kefa* made him get up, saying, 'Stand up. I myself am just a man.' [27] As he talked with *Cornelius*, *Kefa* went into the house and found many people gathered together. [28] *Kefa* said to them, 'You know that it is unlawful for a *Yehudi* to keep company with or visit someone of another nation, **but *YHWH* has shown me that I should not call any man defiled or unclean**. [29] So I came *to you* without argument as soon as I was sent for. Therefore, I ask *you*, why have you sent for me?'" [2 (page 295)]

"*Kefa* was a follower of the Messiah and kept the commandments concerning not eating abominable flesh. Nothing that *Yeshua* did or said could add to or diminish from the commandments that the Almighty gave us at *Sinai* (*Deuteronomy* 4:2, 12:32). *Kefa* pondered the meaning of this strange vision, yet he did not go down to the street, kill a cat, and roast it on the rooftop. The Holy Spirit gave him direction concerning the vision (that occurred three times) and told him to go with three men, doubting nothing that they were about to tell him. *Kefa* fully understood the vision and plainly said, '***YHWH* has shown me that I should not call any man defiled or unclean**.' Only those who refuse to hear what *Kefa* confessed to his unexpected gentile guests can construe that this vision is about eating pigs, spiders, monkey brains, or sewer rats – if that is 'what is set before you.'" [2 (page 295)]

The vision was about humankind – PEOPLE! Specifically, GENTILE PEOPLE! This was the first time any of the apostles had met with Gentiles to invite them into *Yeshua's* family! The *talmidim* had been instructed to go to the *Hebrew* communities in Jerusalem, Judea, and Samaria and then to the ends of the earth! That is what they had been doing and now, the family circle of *Yeshua* was growing even more!

Acts [10:30] "*Cornelius* related to *Kefa*, 'Four days ago I was fasting until this time, and at the ninth hour, as I prayed in my house, I beheld a man standing before me in bright clothing. [31] He said, '*Cornelius*, your prayer is heard, and your alms are remembered in the sight of *YHWH*. [32] Therefore, send to *Yaffo* and call for *Shimon*, whose surname is *Kefa*. He lodges in the house of *Shimon*, a tanner, who lives by the seaside. When he comes, he shall speak to you.' [33] 'So I immediately sent for you, and it is good that you have come. This is why we are all present here before *YHWH* to hear all the things he has commanded you.'" [2 (page 295-296)]

Acts [10:34] "Then *Kefa* opened his mouth and said, '**Truth, I perceive that *YHWH* is no respecter of persons, [35] but in every nation he who fears him and works righteousness is accepted by him.** [36] The word which *YHWH* sent to the children of *Israel* – preaching peace by *Yeshua Messiah* (who is master of all) – [37] that word, as you already know, began in the *Galilee* with the *mikveh* which *Yochanan* preached, and was later published throughout all *Yedudah*. [38] "*YHWH* anointed *Yeshua* of *Natzeret* with the *Ruach Kodesh* and with power, and he went about doing good and healing all that were oppressed of *hasatan*, for *YHWH* was with him. [39] We are witnesses of all the things which he did both in the land of *Yehudim* and in *Yerushalayim*. They put him to death by hanging him on a tree, [40] but *YHWH* raised him on the third day and revealed him openly – [41] not to all the people but to witnesses chosen before by *YHWH*, *even* to us, who ate and drank with him after he rose from the dead. [42] Then he commanded us to preach to the people and to testify that it is he who was ordained of *YHWH to be* the Judge of the living and the dead. [43] Concerning him all the prophets testify that through his name, whoever believes in him shall receive remission of sins.'" [2 (page 296)]

Acts [10:44] "While *Kefa* spoke these words, the *Ruach Kodesh* fell on *all* of them who heard the word. [45] They of the circumcision who believed were astonished, as many as came with *Kefa*, because the *Gift* of the *Ruach Kodesh* was also poured out on the gentiles, [46] for they heard them speak with tongues and magnify *YHWH*. Then *Kefa* answered, [47] 'Can anyone forbid water that these should not be *mikveh-ed* who have received the *Ruach Kodesh* just as we have?' [48] So *Kefa* commanded them to be *mikveh-ed* in the name of *Yeshua Messiah*. Then they asked him to remain for some days." [2 (page 296)]

Cornelius and his household had received the *Gift* of the *Ruach Kodesh* of speaking in another tongue; and *Kefa* made sure they were also immersed (*mikveh-ed*) in the *Name of Yeshua* the *Messiah*. Those were the two signs required for becoming part of the family of *YHWH*!

After a time, *Kefa* returned to *Yerushalayim*. He remained in *Yerushalayim* from 38 AD to 44 AD. When he first returned, there was a bit of a backlash from the other apostles and brothers – "they that were of the circumcision." [4, 2 (page 297)]

Acts [11:1] "The apostles and brothers that were in *Yehudah* heard that the gentiles had also received the word of *YHWH*. [2] So, when *Kefa* came up to *Yerushalayim*, they that were of the circumcision contended with him, [3] charging, 'You went into *the home of uncircumcised gentiles* and ate with them?' [4] So *Kefa* rehearsed *the matter* from the beginning and expounded *it* to them in order, saying, [5] 'I was in the city of *Yaffo* praying and I saw an open vision. Something like a great sheet was let down from heaven by *its* four corners directly in front of me. [6] When I had fastened my eyes on it, I saw rodents,

and carnivorous animals, and crawling insects, and carrion eaters, and birds of prey.' 7
And I heard a voice saying to me, 'Arise, *Kefa*. Kill and eat!' 8 But I said, 'Not so,
Adonai, for no defiled, unclean *abomination* has at any time entered into my mouth.' 9
But the voice spoke to me again from heaven, 'What *YHWH* has cleansed, do not call
defiled.' 10 This was done three times, and everything was drawn up again into heaven. 11
Immediately there were three men, sent to me from *Caesarea*, who had already arrived at
the home. 12 The *Ruach* again spoke to me and told me to go with them, doubting
nothing. Even these six brothers also accompanied me to *Caesarea*, and we all entered
into the man's house. 13 He told us how he had seen an angel, who stood in his house and
said to him, 'Send men to *Yaffo*, and call for *Shimon*, whose surname is *Kefa*. 14 He will
give you a message, by which you and all your household shall be saved.' 15 'As I began
to speak to them, the *Ruach Kodesh* fell on them, as it did on us at the beginning. 16 Then
I remembered the word of the master, who said, '*Yochanan* indeed *mikveh-ed* with water,
but you shall be *mikveh-ed* with the *Ruach Kodesh*.' 17 'Therefore, if *YHWH* gave them
the same gift he gave to us, who also believed on the master *Yeshua Messiah*, who was I
that could hinder *YHWH*? [And that is when I commanded that these should be *mikveh-ed*
in water in obedience to the master's command.]' 18 When they heard these things, they
held their peace and glorified *YHWH*, saying, 'Then *YHWH* has also granted to the
gentiles' repentance unto life.'" [2 (page 296-297)]

"These 'of the circumcision' were those who were raised as *Pharisees* and became believers (*Acts* 15:5; *Galatians* 2:4, 11-13), They had been taught the false authority of the fictitious oral torah – all the innovations and man-made laws (*takanot*) enacted by the Pharisee rabbis that defined first-century Judaism. This incident is the first of many which first-century believers had to deal with in the religious predisposition of those who were raised as Pharisees – just as *Yeshua* did." [2 (page 297)]

One additional thought on *Cornelius* and his household. In *Acts* 10:2, Cornelius is described as a devout man, a 'God fearer.' "According to most scholars, 'God-fearer' is a technical term describing a Gentile who attached himself or herself to Judaism but chose not to undergo formal conversion, which included circumcision (for males) and public immersion (for females). They were attracted to the nobility and reality of Judaism, but for various reasons chose not to become Jews (Shulam 548)." [3 (page 1574)]

If that is the case, *Cornelius* was a follower of *Torah*, including dietary teachings. Therefore, *Kefa* was under no obligation to refuse foods not acceptable or politely excuse himself from eating an abomination! *Cornelius* already was eating according to the *Torah*.

As we can see, eight years after the resurrection of *Yeshua* the Messiah, *Kefa* and the other *talmidim* were still following all aspects of *Torah*. Next, we will take a look at the meeting of *Sha'ul*, *Ya'akov* (the half-brother of *Yeshua*), and *Kefa* in Jerusalem about ten years later – 49 AD. This is nineteen years after the resurrection. Much had taken place, and many people, both Jew and Gentile, had been added to the family of God.

"*Ya'akov* (James) served as the chief rabbi of the early Messianic Jewish community centered in *Yerushalayim*. He was a *Torah* teacher par excellence, spokesman for the entire community, and chief *halakhic* judge and authority (*halakhic* refers to Jewish religious law, which means that *Ya'akov* interpreted and applied community practices based on his understanding of the *Torah*. cf. *Acts* 15). He was respected in the non-Messianic Jewish world, where he was referred to as a *tzaddik*, a wise man. Understanding *Ya'akov* in these contexts can help us better understand the purpose of his book. Behind the *Koine Greek* are thoroughly *Torah*-based concepts, and the textual sources for the subjects he addresses are all from the five books of *Moshe*. He does not present new teaching but a uniquely Messianic Jewish view of *Torah* – based as seen in his encouraging *asiyat hatorah* (the practical application of the *Torah's* teachings). [3 (page 1750)]

"It is crucial to see the continuity between the teachings of *Ya'akov* and *Sha'ul* (Paul). Too often, incorrect understanding of *Ya'akov's* writings on 'faith and actions' leads the reader to view them as holding diametrically opposed views about the role of faith and the function of 'actions.' Here we should think of 'actions' as *mitzvot* (the faithful performance of the biblical commandments). This is how the first-century Jewish world defined this concept of 'actions.' All first-century Jews, including Messianic Jews, saw the performance of the biblical commandments as stemming *from* one's faith in God, *never* in opposition to it. Keeping the *mitzvot* was a result of their relationship with God, not to earn a relationship. In Jewish thought, the purpose of fulfilling the biblical commandments was *never* to earn entrance into the 'world to come.'" [3 (page 1750)]

"If we understand *Ya'akov's* belief that faith in God and in his Messiah is the basis for correctly fulfilling the biblical commandments, then his book makes more sense. The letter was likely among the first books written in the *B'rit Hadashah* (*New Testament*) between 46 and 69 C.E. According to Jewish historian *Josephus*, *Ya'akov* was martyred in 62 C.E" [3 (page 1750)]

Dr. Miles Jones, in his book *The Epistle of James (Ya'akov),* says, "The walk of truth with *Yehovah* is the important theme of the *Epistle* written by *Ya'akov* (James), the brother of *Yeshua*, who suddenly appears in Scripture in the book of *Acts* as a leader of the *Nazarenes*! Does this seem strange to you? Someone we have not even heard of in the *Gospels* becomes the leader of the *Nazarenes* – the early church – immediately after the resurrection, apparently with unanimous support of the Apostles. Remember that *Yeshua* was led to each of these men by the direct vision of *Yehovah*. So, the Apostles are God's chosen ones. Who is this new guy? How did he get there? Something is missing in the story! Indeed, it is." [6 (page 2)]

"There is no explanation of this in the *Greek* gospels. In *The Hebrew Gospels*, however, it says that *Yeshua* appeared to James after his resurrection and anointed him as leader of the *Nazarenes*. Paul said, '**He [*Yeshua*] was seen by 500 of the brethren at once… After that, he was seen of James**, then of all the apostles. And last of all, he was seen of me' (*1 Corinthians* 15:6-7). Paul says *Yeshua* was seen by James even before the apostles – which would make sense if James was being anointed to lead them. In *Acts* 10:40, *Yeshua* returns from the dead and appears to two of his family members on the road to *Emmaus*. The Greek gospels specify only one of them, *Cleophas* – *Yeshua's* uncle, also known as *Alphaeus*, who was the brother of Joseph, *Yeshua's* father. It is likely that the second was *Yeshua's* brother *Ya-akov* (James), at least according to Paul and *The Hebrew Gospels*. Why is there no mention of this in the Greek *Gospels*? **The Greek Church did not want to sanctify a Hebrew dynasty!**" [6 (page 2)]

"The Greeks did not want a Hebrew dynasty of the Church to challenge their authority. They wanted a Greek church. To establish this new Greek church, they needed a Greek Scripture, a Greek doctrine, a Greek God, and a *Greek Jesus*. From this basic fact spring all the '*adjustments*' that Greek editors have made to the *Bible*! For this reason, the *Yeshua* dynasty has been ignored." [6 (page 4)]

"*James the Just* (*Ya'akov* – the brother of *Yeshua*) was a dynamic leader of the *Messianic Church* for thirty years through a period of persecution that could easily have wiped it from history. *Clement of Rome* later calls James the '*bishop of bishops, who rules Jerusalem, the Holy Church of the Hebrews, and all the churches everywhere!*' *Clement* cites the anointment of James by *Yeshua* to lead the Church as coming from *The Hebrew Gospels*. That anointment is also verified by *Jerome* in chapter two of *Illustrious Men*, and in the *Gospel of Thomas*. '*James the Just was so righteous and revered among both Messianics and Jews that the sect of the Nazarenes almost took over Judaism. It was this threat to the power structure that led to James' martyrdom!*'" [6 (page 4)]

With that information, we will look at one of the scriptures from *James* that has been an area of confusion and see if we can learn something from the *Hebrew* translation.

James [1:21] "Therefore, remove from among you all uncleanness and predominant evil, and
receive with humility the Word planted in your inner parts that will save your souls. [22]
Please, be doers of the Word, and not hearers alone, deceiving yourselves (leading
yourselves astray). [23] For he who will hear The Word, and will not do, he seems to expect
a vision of his generations in a looking glass. [24] So, he observes his own essence, and
will he excuse himself (pass over) and immediately forget who he is? [25] But anyone who
observes himself by the whole *Torah*, which is the instruction of *The Examiner*, and stands in *Torah*, not hearing [*the Torah*] in forgetfulness, for if he works the work, his happiness is in his actions." [6 (page 24-25)]

The *Torah* is the standard and "the perfect *Torah*, which gives freedom, is literally 'a perfect [or complete] law of liberty." [3 (page 1752)]

With this in mind, let us now take a look at the meeting of the Jerusalem council in the autumn of 49 AD. The Pharisaic *Judaizers* came to *Antioch* (*Acts* 15:1, 5) in the summer of 49 AD. They were teaching mandatory circumcision in order for disciples to be saved. Keep in mind, this is almost twenty years after the resurrection of *Yeshua*; and ten years after *Kefa* met with *Cornelius*. Still, the issue of legalism was surrounding *Torah* and Gentile believers. *Sha'ul* (Paul), *bar Nava* (Barnabas), and certain others sent word to the apostles and elders in Jerusalem about this question. It was now autumn of 49 AD, and the *Feast of Tabernacles* was to take place. (*Acts* 15:2) [4]

The *Feast of Tabernacles* was one of three feasts *Yehovah* implemented requiring the Israelites and other followers of *Yehovah,* attend yearly in the Fall. The requirement was primarily for the men, but families and other people came too. *Sha'ul* (Paul) and *bar Nava* (Barnabas) would have a private meeting with the apostles *Ya'akov* (James), *Kefa* (Peter), and *Yochanan* (John) about the question of the circumcision requirement and the gentiles. The apostles' agreement was stated by *Ya'akov* that Gentiles were **not** required to be circumcised. Thus, *Titus* was not required to be circumcised as mentioned in *Galatians* 2:2-3. [4]

Although this meeting was regarding circumcision, a decision of the requirements for Gentile followers was determined and a letter was written by *Ya'akov* to the various churches.

Acts 15:1 "Certain men who came down from *Yehudah* taught the brothers, saying, 'Unless you are circumcised after the manner of *Moshe*, you cannot be saved.' [2] After *Sha'ul* and *bar Nava* had *great* dissension and debate with them, they decided that *Sha'ul*, *bar Nava*, and certain others from amongst them should go up to *Yerushalayim* to the apostles and elders concerning this question. [3] Being sent off by the *kehilah*, they passed through *Phenice* and *Shomron*, declaring the conversion of the gentiles and causing great joy among all the brothers. [4] And when they came to *Yerushalayim*, they were received by the *kehilah* and the apostles and elders, and they reported all the things *YHWH* had done with them. [5] But **certain *spokesmen* of the sect of the Pharisees who believed** stood up and said that it was necessary to circumcise the gentiles and command them to keep the law of *Moshe*. [6] So the apostles and elders came together to consider this matter. [7] When there had been much discussion, *Kefa* rose up and said to them, 'Brothers, you know how a good while ago *YHWH* chose me from among us to preach to the gentiles so that they would hear the word of the gospel and believe. [8] *YHWH*, who knows the hearts, bore them witness, giving them the *Gift of the Ruach Kodesh*, even as *he did* to us; [9] and made no difference between us and them, purifying their hearts by faith. [10] Therefore, why do you tempt *YHWH* by putting upon the necks of the disciples a yoke which neither our fathers nor we were able to bear? [11] We believe that we also are saved through the grace of the master *Yeshua Messiah*, even as the gentiles evidently are.'" [2 (page 303)]

"This 'sect of Pharisees which believed' may have confessed that *Yeshua* is the Messiah, but they wanted everyone to continue to submit to their rules 'which neither we nor our fathers were able to bear.' (v 10). It is not the eternal commandments in the *Torah* that are 'grievous to be borne' but rather the manipulative man-made rules of religious sects, which are impossible to fulfill (*Luke* 1:6; *1 John* 5:3). Gentiles are not required to be circumcised; it is the physical token of the *Abrahamic* land covenant. Gentiles may decide to become circumcised, but it is not required for them to become a believer in the Messiah." [2 (page 303)]

Now back to the story.

Acts [15:12] "Then all the multitude kept silent and gave audience to *bar Nava* and *Sha'ul*, who declared what miracles and wonders *YHWH* had done among the gentiles through them. [13] After they had finished, *Ya'akov* spoke up, 'Brothers, listen to me. [14] *Shimon Kefa* was the first to declare how *YHWH* visited the gentiles to separate from among them a people for himself. [15] The words of the prophets agree with this, as it is written. [16] After this, I will return and rebuild the tabernacle of David which has fallen down. I will rebuild the ruins, and I will set it up [17] so that the remnant of men might seek after the Almighty – and all the gentiles upon whom my name is called.' Thus says *YHWH*, who does all these things, [18] 'Known to *YHWH* are all his works from the beginning of the world.'" [2 (page 303)]

Note: "{*Acts* 15:18.1} This is not being cited as a fulfillment of *Amos* 9: 11-12, but as a proof text that the heathen, i.e., the gentiles, have a certain and prophetic place in the household of Israel if they take hold of the covenant, love his name, and learn his ways." [2 (page 304)]

Ya'akov continues in *Acts* [15:19] "Therefore my verdict is that we do not trouble those from among the gentiles who are turning to *YHWH*, [20] rather, let us write unto them that they should abstain from the abominations of idolatry, *from ervah* sexual behavior, *from* strangled flesh, and *from* blood, [21] because in every city *Moshe* has been preached for generations, and he is read in the synagogues every Sabbath day." [2 (page 304)]

Acts [15:22] "Then it pleased the apostles and elders, as well as the whole *kehilah*, to send chosen men of their own company to *Antioch* with *Shaul* and *bar Nava*, namely *Yehudah* surnamed *bar Saba*, and *Silas*, who were honored men among the brothers. [23] They wrote *a letter and sent it* with them. [2 (page 304)]

A note on *Acts* 15:21. "The Pharisee synagogue was the one place in the ancient world where one could go to hear the *Torah* read and taught. The apostles in Jerusalem were reiterating minimal requirements for the gentiles to be allowed into the synagogue and to join in the study of the *Torah* of Moses, those whose heart upon which the *Torah* was written would then come naturally into full obedience to *YHWH's* commandments. Keeping the *Torah* commandments is an appropriate heartfelt response from one who has been redeemed by *Yeshua's* blood. The wages of sin is death (*Romans* 6:23) – but the gift of life eternal is given to all who call upon his name in faith. If one is not taught to have enmity against the *Torah*, the response of the new creation is to live in complete obedience to the instructions of our Creator – and then learn to listen to his voice so that we can walk by the Spirit, as we see exemplified in the book of *Acts*. Those who have enmity against, and deliberately break the commandments of *YHWH*, do not have the Holy Spirit living in them – no matter how religious they may appear to be in their flesh. (*1 John* 2:4). [2 (page 304)]

"There was no requirement for a gentile to be circumcised to enter the synagogue on the Sabbath to learn the *Torah* of Moses. Circumcision is the sign of the covenant between *YHWH* and *Abraham*: that all of the land from the *Euphrates* to the *Nile* belongs to his offspring, the sons of *Israel*. Gentiles are not a part of the *Abrahamic* covenant, but they can elect to become so." [2 (page 304)]

"Those who desired to enter into the *kehilah* of *Israel* to learn the *Torah* had to at least be in compliance with the four basic things that James quoted from the *Torah* and were again reiterated at *Shaul's* last Feast in Jerusalem. They did **not**, however, have to follow the man-made rules (*takanot*) of the Pharisees. *Yeshua* broke them, he taught his disciples to break them, he demanded those he healed to break them – yet the Pharisees who became followers of Messiah wanted to bring their *eruv* (Sabbath boundary), their *kippot* (submissive headcover), and their *negel vasser* (handwashing vessel) with them; they wanted to require the gentiles to follow the *takanot* that *Yeshua* absolutely forbade. On the other hand, Gentiles in pagan cultures tended to bring their idolatry and abominations into the fellowship of the saints. Some refused to observe even the minimum requirements repeatedly detailed by the apostles, and *Shaul* had to deal with such perversion among the *Corinthian* believers (*1 Corinthians* 5:1). Both groups – the legalists and the licentious – will be thinned from the fold on the day that *Yeshua* sentences, 'Depart from me, you *anomians – you* violators of the *Torah*!'" [2 (page 304)]

Ya'akov continues:

Acts 15:23 "'To: the gentile brothers in *Antioch* and *Syria* and *Cilicia*

From: the apostles and elders and brothers in *Yerushalayim*

Greetings,

24 We heard that certain brothers, to whom we had given no *authority*, went out from among us and troubled you with their teaching, unsettling your souls and saying, 'You *must* be circumcised and keep the law.' 25 It seemed good to us, being of one mind, to send chosen men to you with our beloved *bar Nava* and *Shaul*, 26 men who have risked their lives for the name of the master *Yeshua Messiah.* 27 Therefore, we have sent *Yehudah* and *Silas*, who shall tell *you* the same things *in person.*'" [2 (page 305)]

Acts 15:28 "'It seems good to the *Ruach Kodesh* and to us to lay upon you no greater burden than these fundamental *Torah* instructions: 29 that you abstain from food *offered to idols*, and from blood, and from things strangled, and from sexual immorality. If you restrain yourselves from these things, you shall do well. Farewell.'" [2 (page 305)]

Acts 15:30 "When they were dismissed, they came to *Antioch*, and after they had gathered the multitude together, they delivered the letter. 31 After they had read *it*, they rejoiced for its encouragement." [2 (page 305)]

"The four principles laid out in *Acts* 15:19-20 are often seen as a subset of Jewish precepts taken from what is called the *Seven Noachide Laws*: no idolatry, no blasphemy of the name of God, no murder, no fornication, no stealing, no eating the flesh of live animals, and court of justice established. Based on *Genesis* 2:16 and 9:4-6, the *Talmud* says that these seven laws were given to the surviving families of the earth, the families of *Noach* (Noah). Therefore, they are called the *Noachide Laws*. [3 (page 1584)]

"Although it is possible that *Ya'akov* (James) and the apostles may have gleaned from the principles of the *Noachide Laws*, a general reading of the *Epistles* shows that the commands they placed upon *Gentile* followers of *Yeshua* extended beyond the four principles set in place at the *Jerusalem Council.* Based on this observation, the four principles given should not be seen as the only commandments expected for the non-Jewish followers of *Yeshua* to keep, but they were necessary commands to peacefully coexist with Jews. There were no Catholic or Protestant churches down the street for these *Gentiles* to attend, so the natural understanding was that they would worship in the synagogue. This would explain *Ya'akov's* (James) exhortation in verse 21: 'For from earliest times, *Moshe* has had in every city those who proclaim him, with his words being read in the synagogues every *Shabbat*.'" [3 (page 1584)]

In Section One of this book, we looked in *Genesis* 2:16 at the *Noachide Covenant*. As noted in Section One, these teachings were already in place, with the exception of those that dealt with consuming animals. The animal and blood commandments were added after the *Flood* due to the lack of plants, herbs, fruit trees, and grasses.

The note that these were commands "to peacefully coexist with Jews" would extend to the eating habits and choices of the Jews. There is no mention of eating something different, or the Jews changing their eating habits to match those of other people groups.

As *Moses* would be taught every *Shabbat* in the synagogues, if the new believers, *Gentiles*, had been eating something different from the Jews, they would certainly learn of proper foods and experience new and better food choices.

The third Apostle is the apostle called *Paul* in the Greek and English translations. However, in the *Hebrew* language and *Hebrew* manuscripts, the apostle's name is *Sha'ul*, or sometimes written *Saul*.

After *Yeshua's* resurrection in 30AD, *Yeshua* appeared to His disciples for forty days, and then He ascended to "the right hand of the Father". Ten days later, the Holy Spirit, *Ruach HaKodesh*, fell on the Messianic followers. This happened on *Shavuot*, or Pentecost. From that time forward, the *Gospel* was preached. However, persecution against the Messianic communities, followers of *Yeshua*, began too! [4]

In 32AD, as told in the *Book of Acts* chapters 6 and 7, *Stephen*, a Hebrew follower of *Yeshua*, was martyred after reciting Israel's history and pattern of rejecting God's messengers to the *Sanhedrin.* He was accused of "speaking blasphemously against *Moshe* and against God." [3 (page 1567)] His speech included many various scriptures from the *Tanakh* and the *Prophets,* quoting the words of God.

Acts [7:49] "'**Heaven is my throne,' says *ADONAI*, 'and the earth is my footstool. What kind of house could you build for me? What kind of place could you devise for my rest?** [50] **Didn't I myself make all things?'"** [a Isaiah 66:1-2; 3(page 1570)]

Acts [7:51] "'**Stiffnecked people,** [b] with **uncircumcised hearts and ears!** [c] You continually oppose the *Ruach HaKodesh*! [d] You do the same things your fathers did! [52] Which of the prophets did your fathers not persecute? They killed those who told in advance about the coming of the *Tzaddik*, and now you have become his betrayers and murderers! – [53] you! – who receive the *Torah* as having been delivered by angels – but do not keep it!'" [b-Exodus 32:9, 33:3,5; c-Leviticus 26:41; Jeremiah 6:10; 9:25 (26); d-Isaiah 63:10; 3 (page 1570)]

Acts [7:54] "On hearing these things, they were cut to their hearts and ground their teeth at him. [55] But he, full of the *Ruach HaKodesh*, looked up to heaven and saw God's *Sh'khinah*, with *Yeshua* standing **at the right hand of God.** [56] 'Look!' he exclaimed, 'I see heaven opened and the Son of Man standing **at the right hand of God!'"** [e-Psalm 110:1; 3 (page 1570)]

Acts [7:57] "At this, they began yelling at the top of their voices, so that they wouldn't have to hear him; and with one accord, they rushed at him, [58] threw him outside the city and began stoning him. And the witnesses laid down their coats at the feet of a young man named *Sha'ul.* [59] As they were stoning him, Stephen called out to God, 'Lord *Yeshua*! Receive my spirit!' [60] Then he kneeled down and shouted out, 'Lord! Don't hold this sin against them!' With that, he died;" *Acts* [8:1] "and *Sha'ul* gave his approval to his murder. Starting with that day, there arose intense persecution against the Messianic Community in *Yerushalayim*; all but the emissaries were scattered throughout the regions of *Y'hudah* and *Shromron.* [2] Some godly men buried Stephen and mourned him deeply. [3] But *Sha'ul* set out to destroy the Messianic Community – entering house after house, he dragged off both men and women and handed them over to be put in prison. [4] However, those who were scattered announced the Good News of the Word wherever they went." [3 (page 1570)]

In the spring of 33AD, *Sha'ul* was heading to *Damascus* to continue his persecutions, carrying with him letters from the high priest approving the persecution. (*Acts* 9:19-23) and the "arrest of any people he might find, whether man or women, who belonged to '*the Way*,' and bring them back to *Yerushalayim*" for trial and punishment. [3 (page 1572)]

As I once heard motivational speaker, *Jim Rohn*, say regarding Paul (*Sha'ul*), "God used recruiting methods only He has!" And with that, *Sha'ul's* life was radically changed in a moment!

Acts [9:3] "Suddenly a light from heaven flashed all around him. [4] Falling to the ground, he heard a voice saying to him, '*Sha'ul*! *Sha'ul*! Why do you keep persecuting me?' [5] 'Sir, who are you?' he asked. 'I am *Yeshua*, and you are persecuting me. [6] But get up, and go into the city, and you will be told what you have to do.'" [3 (page 1572)]

"*Sha'ul* was persecuting *Yeshua* by persecuting the Messianic Jews. This demonstrated how closely the Messiah identifies with his people (*Acts* 8:32-33; John 17). *Yeshua* is the 'head' of the 'Body of the Messiah;' when the body is pained, the head responds." [Note Acts 9:5, 3 (page 1572)]

Chronologically, *Sha'ul* meets *Yeshua* on the way to *Damascus* in the spring of 33AD. As a result, he preached *Christ* in *Damascus* as seen in *Acts* 9:19-23. [4]

Acts [9:18] "In that moment, something like scales fell away from *Sha'ul's* eyes; and he could see again. He got up and was *immersed*; [19] then he ate some food and regained his strength. *Sha'ul* spent some days with the *talmidim* in *Dammesek,* [20] and immediately he began proclaiming in the synagogues that *Yeshua* is the *Son of God.* [21] All who heard him were amazed. They asked, 'Isn't that why he came here, to arrest them and bring them back to the head *cohanim*?' [22] But *Sha'ul* was being filled with more and more power and was creating an uproar among the Jews living in *Dammesek* with his proofs that *Yeshua* is the Messiah. [23] Quite some time later, the non-believing Jews gathered together and made plans to kill him; [24] but their plot became known to *Sha'ul*. They were watching the gates day and night in order to do away with him; [25] but under cover of night, his *talmidim* took him and let him down over the city wall, lowering him in a large basket." [3 (page 1572)]

Thus, a plot to kill *Sha'ul* was discovered and *Sha'ul* escaped by night to *Arabia,* where he was taught by *Yeshua* for three years, as he reveals in his letter to the *Galatians*.

"*Galatians* is a letter about faith and the *Torah* directed to *Gentile* disciples in *Galatia* (written between 53 and 56c.e. or as early as 49c.e.)." [3 (page 1668)]

Galatians [1:11] "Furthermore, let me make clear to you, brothers, that the *Good News* as I proclaim it is not a human product; [12] because neither did I receive it from someone else nor was I taught it – it came through a direct revelation from *Yeshua* the Messiah. [13] For you have heard about my former way of life in [traditional] *Judaism* – how I did my best to persecute God's *Messianic Community* and destroy it; [14] and how, since I was more of a zealot for the traditions handed down by my forefathers than most Jews my age, I advanced in [traditional] *Judaism* more rapidly than they did." [3 (page 1669-1670)]

Galatians [1:15] "But when God, who picked me out before I was born and called me by his grace, chose [16] to reveal his *Son* to me, so that I might announce him to the *Gentiles*, I did not consult anyone; [17] and I did not go up to *Yerushalayim* to see those who were emissaries before me. Instead, I immediately went off to *Arabia* and afterwards returned to *Dammesek.* [18] Not until three years later did I go up to *Yerushalayim* to make *Kefa's* acquaintance, and I stayed with him for two weeks, [19] but I did not see any of the other emissaries except *Ya'akov*, the Lord's brother. [20] (Concerning these matters, I am writing you about, I declare before God that I am not lying!)" [3 (page 1670)]

In *Acts* 9:26-30, we hear about the meeting *Sha'ul* mentions with *Kefa* in *Yerushalayim.* The meeting lasted fifteen days and was *Sha'ul's* first trip to *Yerushalayim* after his conversion. [4]

Acts [9:26] "On reaching *Yerushalayim*, he tried to join the *talmidim*; but they were all afraid of him – they didn't believe he was a *talmid.* [27] However, *Bar-Nabba* got hold of him and took him to the emissaries. He told them how *Sha'ul* had seen the Lord while traveling, that the Lord had spoken to him, and how in *Dammesek Sha'ul* had spoken out boldly in the name of *Yeshua.* [28] So he remained with them and went all over *Yerushalayim,* continuing to speak out boldly in the name of the Lord. [29] He talked and debated with the Greek-speaking Jews, but they began making attempts to kill him. [30] When the brothers learned of it, they brought him down to *Caesarea* and sent him away to *Tarsus.*" [3 (page 1573)]

As we see in *Acts* 9:30, *Sha'ul* goes to *Tarsus* where he remains for four years from the summer of 36AD to summer of 40 AD. At that time, *Barnabas* goes from Jerusalem to *Tarsus* to find *Sha'ul* and bring him back to *Antioch* to help teach *Gentiles*. (*Acts* 11:25) [4]

Acts [11:25] "Then *Bar-Naba* went off to *Tarsus* to look for *Sha'ul*; [26] and when he found him, he brought him to *Antioch.* They met with the congregation there for a whole year and taught a sizable crowd. Also, it was in *Antioch* that the *talmidim* for the first time were called '*Messianic.*'" [3 (page 1577)]

The ministry of *Sha'ul* started in 33AD and continued until he was martyred in 67AD. His ministry involved so much more than we can ever know. The apostle *Luke* began writing the *Gospel of Luke* and the *Book of Acts* under *Sha'ul's* supervision during *Sha'ul's* imprisonment in *Yerushalayim* in 58AD. By 63AD, *Luke* finishes his gospel and up to *Acts* 28:31. It is thought he had intentions of adding more to *Acts* later but was unable to do so. [4]

Who was this man called *Sha'ul*? Did people refer to him as *Paul*? *Sha'ul* was a Hebrew from the tribe of Benjamin. He was a Pharisee, born in *Tarsus* and trained in Israel. Throughout his life and ministry, he stayed true to his *Hebrew* culture and teachings of the God of Israel and the Messiah. He most likely never changed his name to 'Paul the Christian.' Instead, *Sha'ul* held fast to his culture and the teachings of the God he had always followed. When speaking with Hebrews, he used the name *Sha'ul,* and with Greek-speaking Gentiles, used the Greek form, which was *Paulos* or *Paulus*. In English, this was shortened to Paul. In speaking the languages common to the people, he was meeting them where they were, in a way they could understand. "*Sha'ul* called himself a *Hebrew* and a *Pharisee* long after he began following Messiah *Yeshua.* [10]

Brad Young, in his book *Paul, the Jewish Theologian: A Pharisee Among Christians, Jews, and Gentiles*, gives more insight into the apostle Paul.

"The *New Testament* describes the *Apostle Paul* as a *Pharisee* who comes to faith in Jesus as the *Messiah*, boldly proclaiming the gospel as the power of the *God of Israel* unto salvation, to the diverse peoples in distant parts of a *Gentile* world. Working in a largely pagan environment, the one who is referred to in the book of *Acts* as *Saul of Tarsus* established churches as the *Apostle Paul*. Paul has been referred to as the 'second founder of Christianity'. He has been called a 'mystic.' Now he is referred to as a '*Gnostic*'. The consensus of scholarship has come to view him as a *Hellenistic Jew* who departed radically from his *Judaism*. Scholars view him as being influenced by his upbringing in the Stoic environs of *Tarsus* and various streams of thought flowing forth from paganism, *Greco-Roman* culture, popular *Hellenistic* philosophy, mystery religious cults, and *Gnostic* systems. Seldom is the origin of Paul's faith seen as rooted in *Pharisaism*." [7 (page 1)]

"What if we begin with a different set of presuppositions?" What does Paul say about himself?

"Paul calls himself a *Pharisee*. We should listen to what Paul tells us about himself. In fact, there is no evidence anywhere in the *New Testament* that he departed from his firm convictions as a *Pharisee*. Paul is a *Jewish* theologian who anchored his beliefs in the *Hebrew Bible* and the teachings of his eminent mentors in Jerusalem. He is a *Hebrew of Hebrews* rather than a *Hellenist of the Greeks*. Fresh evidence from the literary discoveries of the *Dead Sea Scrolls,* as well as renewed interest in the analysis of rabbinic literature place the Apostle Paul squarely within the Judaism of the land of *Israel* and not *Hellenism* of *Asia Minor*, although surely there was much interaction between *Hellenism* and *Judaism* in the first century, and this influenced *Pharisaism*." [7 (page 1-2)]

"Paul is a *Pharisee* who has been rejected by the synagogue and misunderstood by the church." "The synagogue could not accept the profile of Paul's style of *Pharisaism*. For one thing, under the direction of the *Sadducean* high priests, he persecuted the early church. The leader of the *Pharisees* in those days, *Rabban Gamaliel*, fought hard against this type of religious persecution."

"The early church, on the other hand, largely rejected the *Jewish* heritage of Paul, denying his *Pharisaism*. For the church, Paul is a *former* Pharisee. When he stopped persecuting the church, he departed from his *Pharisaism*. As a Pharisee, he was evil. As a Christian, he parted ways with his *Judaic* heritage to become a Christian." [7 (page 2)]

"Paul, however, considered himself a Pharisee throughout his entire life. He was proud of his *Judaic* heritage and his upbringing in Jerusalem." "He practiced the life of *Pharisaism* in accordance with his family background and his training in the land of Israel." [7 (page 2)]

"For him, faith in Jesus as Messiah brought deeper conviction and enrichment. Above all, his energies were redirected toward the Gentile's world. The *Jewish* apostle sought to call the pagan nations to a faith in the *one God* of Israel by preaching the message of

Jesus the Messiah. For, everyone who calls upon the name of the Lord will be saved." (*Romans* 10:13) [7 (page 2-3)]

"The time has come for a reevaluation of the foundation pillars of Paul's thoughts. His theology is rooted in *Torah* – true *Judaism*." [7 (page 3)]

"When Paul is viewed as a *Pharisee*, many aspects of his teachings concerning grace and law are better understood. This is especially true when one realizes that the apostle was solving problems in congregations made up of both *Jews* and *Gentiles*." "He is a bridge builder." [7 (page 4)]

"Clearly Paul's work among the *Gentiles* and our unfamiliarity with ancient *Judaism* make understanding his *Jewish* theology difficult. In spite of this, his mission to the Gentiles is deeply rooted in the *Jewish* way of thinking. His upbringing as a *Pharisee* molded his character and guided his teachings." [7 (page 7)]

"Often, we misunderstand Paul: first because we do not know the problems he was trying to solve, and second, perhaps even more significantly, because we do not know very much about his *Jewish* faith and culture." "The *Judaism* of Paul must be the starting point for any serious analysis of his writings." [7 (page 7)]

"By the way of comparison, studying Paul's correspondence is like reading answers without the questions. The student of Paul's writing is forced to guess what the original questions surrounding his correspondence really were." [7 (page 7)]

"This Paul's theology was rooted in *Judaism* from late antiquity of his family heritage as *Jewish* stock. He was from the *Middle East*. His mentality was quite different from that of the West." "To make peace with Paul, we must listen carefully to the apostle's message in his original cultural context. The starting point is crucial." [7 (page 10)]

"Paul's theology is more a product of *Jerusalem* than of his birthplace, *Tarsus*." "He taught that Gentiles were grafted into the olive tree Israel, and he never intended for a replacement theology to take root in the Christian church." "Paul upheld the teachings of Jesus as well as the authority of the law and the prophets." "At least in Paul's view, the Holy Spirit empowered him to live a life pleasing to God. By dying to himself and experiencing the Messiah's resurrection through faith, the apostle could obey God." [7 (page 10)]

"Paul's theology begins with an unshakable faith in the one *God of Israel*. Paul possesses a great love derived from his rich *Hebrew* heritage for all humanity." "Because of his belief in the goodness of God, Paul, like other *Pharisees*, had looked for a future redeemer who would resemble *Moses* and bring help to people in need." "[He] focused upon Jesus as the anointed one designated to bring God's goodness to all humanity, including the pagan Gentiles. He struggled with the seeming contradiction of a *suffering* Messiah and a future redeemer." [7 (page 11)]

"Indeed, he talked about *Torah* constantly. His incessant occupation with the biblical foundation of his beliefs and his conceptual approach to his interactive theology might even be described as a passion." "Paul was a *Jewish* theologian. He was a *Pharisee* who sought the wisdom of *Torah* for guidance and direction." [7 (page 11)]

"In his zeal for God, he had once felt that it was his duty to persecute the early church. Paul's sincere '*no*' to Jesus and his followers was his '*yes*' to God, although it seemed greatly misguided in the eyes of the Christians." [7 (page 16)]

"According to the teachings of the *Pharisees*, God's great compassion is revealed when people ask for forgiveness. No one could live a life without sin, but each individual could be blameless before God as he or she asked for forgiveness and lived an observant life. (He was observant) Paul celebrated Jewish festivals." [7 (page 17)]

"The *Torah*, *Prophets*, and *Writings* are not merely a reservoir of proof texts from which Paul draws to inculcate would-be converts. On the contrary, Paul employs the *Bible* as his primary source of faith and practice." "The *Hebrew Scriptures* are the foundation of his teachings. In *Galatians* 5:3, he writes, 'I testify again to every man who receives circumcision that he is bound to keep the whole law." This verse "suggests that Paul continued to live an observant life even after his experience on the road to *Damascus*. Though he became all things to all people so that he might win them for the Lord (*1 Corinthians* 9:19-23), this does not mean that he stopped living an observant life…Paul was a man of integrity." [7 (page 19-20)]

"Even in *Galatians*, he affirms that the whole law is fulfilled in the commandment 'Love thy neighbor as thyself.' (*Leviticus* 9:18). By strictly observing the principle of love, a person is able to fulfill all the requirements of *Torah* regarding interpersonal relationships." [7 (page 20)]

Circumcision continued to be an issue throughout *Sha'ul's* ministry. We took a look at the *Jerusalem Counsel* meeting with *Ya'akov* and *Kefa*. As noted, this meeting took place in 49AD. Troubles continued even after the decision was made and the letter written.

"The proselytes who believed in Jesus were the strongest opponents of Paul's gospel of grace, which allowed Gentiles to enter the community without circumcision. *Alan Segal* notes the irony of the situation: 'Paul's preaching would have offended the circumcised, ex-Gentile Christians. After all, the ex-Gentile believers had become proselytes to *Judaism* first. They had already become circumcised and had accepted the difficult challenge of living everyday life as religious Jews.'" [7 (page 20-21)]

"Thus, we have a double irony. Circumcision was *defended* by Gentiles who had undergone circumcision to become *Jews*, and the gospel of the uncircumcised was defended by a former Pharisee. Paul did not cancel the law. In *Galatians,* he is not opposed to the observance of *Torah*. But in *Jewish* theology, the teachings of *Torah* have a different application for *Jews* who are from the circumcision, and thus part of the covenant relationship, than they have for non-*Jews*, who have not entered fully into God's covenant with the people of *Israel*." [7 (page 21)]
"Paul viewed *Torah* as giving divine revelation for holy living. Paul learned the teachings of *Torah* in order to understand the mystery of God and to revere him by entering into a life of obedience. The apostle loved the *Hebrew* scriptures and lived his life in accordance with the moral and spiritual values expressed in them." [7 (page 22)]

Like *Yeshua*, "When Paul used *nomos* (the *Greek* term), he was referring to *Torah* within the context of *Judaism*. Paul does not mean natural law, as distinct from spiritual law, or the various other suggestions for the meaning of *nomos*. The *Hebrew* concept of *Torah* is Paul's intended meaning. *Law* is a poor translation of *nomos* in Paul's writing. This translation stems from the *Latin Vulgate*. In it, *nomos* is translated by the *Latin* word *lex*, which means '*law*.' Although in his letters Paul quotes the *Bible* according to the *Septuagint* as the accepted translation for his *Greek*-speaking congregations, his theology is thoroughly *Hebraic*. He is thinking *Torah*, not *law*." [7 (page 23)]

"When the translation of *nomos* as '*law*' becomes normative in *English* discussions of *Pauline* thought, a great deal of the apostle's *Hebrew* heritage is eradicated from his life experience. He could only see the world through his understanding of *Torah*." [7 (page 23)]

"*Torah* for Paul, as it was for *Israel's* sages, is as vast as God himself. *Torah* teaches God's higher purposes and reaches far beyond a simple enumeration of the five books of *Moses*. *Torah* is spiritual. When Paul writes, 'The *law of the Spirit of life*,' in *Romans* 8:2, he is referring to the higher meaning of the *Torah*. It is a spiritual force. The same *Torah* that gives life through Jesus the Messiah, in Paul's thought, also exposes human need and moral failure. *Torah* is both the '*Law of the Spirit'* and the '*Law of sin and death'* (*Romans* 8:2). All depends upon the human response to the divine initiative. In Paul's thinking, *Torah* is good. The apostle declares, 'So the law is holy, and the commandment is holy and just and good' (*Romans* 7:12). The problem is human weakness. In his weakness, Paul had failed to live by the higher principle of God's reign, and in this respect, *Torah* had shown his own shortcoming. Only because of human weakness can *Torah* be spoken of within the framework of sin and death. But because of God's mercy, it is spirit and life. Hence, *Torah* means both the '*law of the Spirit'* and the '*law of sin and death*.' Holding *Torah* in high esteem, he applied it in every aspect of life. Paul revealed an intense passion for the higher meaning of *Torah*." [7 (page 23)]

"In Paul's day, the essence of *Jewish* faith had little to do with an *earn-your-salvation* religious system, *Jewish* faith begins with the nature of God. He is one. He is compassionate and full of grace. In *Exodus* 34:6, this high, lofty *Hebrew* idea of God is expressed. 'The LORD, The LORD God, merciful and gracious, long-suffering and abundant in goodness and truth.' The *Hebrew* mind viewed God quite differently from the systematic theological thinking of the *West*, which defines God and his work with creation in a linear manner. The Western style treatment of the divine character attempts to explain inconsistencies and harmonize contradictions systematically. The *Hebrew* mind was filled with wonder at the mystery of God. The vastness of God and his inscrutable ways left them awestruck. Inconsistencies and contradictions are intimately related to human, finite understandings of the infinite God. He is beyond human comprehension. First-century Jews approached God through an interactive associative mentality. The fact that God is incomprehensible is very much a part of *Jewish* thought processes. The *Western* mind, however, explains everything, but understands so little of the divine nature. The *Hebrew* mind, on the other hand, is overpowered by a sense of wonder and amazement. It thrives on the inconsistencies and contradictions of the one awe-inspiring God." [7 (Page 23, 25)]

"On one hand, Paul views history as moving toward the goal of God's final redemptive plan, which will culminate in the *Parousia* (the second coming of Messiah) and the eschatological judgement; on the other, he views God through the prism of perplexing curiosity, which inspires wonder. In his contemplation of the mystery of God, like other *Jewish* theologians of his day, the apostle is content to leave questions unanswered and inconsistencies unresolved. He views theology as a conceptual whole." [7 (page 25)]

"'*Torah* encompasses so much of what can be known about God in the conceptual worldview…Paul focuses on the sum of the whole instead of dissecting the individual parts,' suggests *Max Kadushin*. *Kadushin* points out, the rabbis could not speak about the kingdom of heaven without a myriad of verses coming into their minds. Not only did they realize that these *Bible* passages possess a literal meaning, but they pushed beyond to deepen realms of *Torah* learning. It is a conceptual approach. The mere mention of the term 'kingdom of heaven' brought to their mind verses such as 'The LORD reigns forever and ever' (*Exodus* 15:18) and 'The LORD reigns' (*Psalm* 93:1). Although these passages mentioned only that the Lord reigns, for the rabbis they refer to the conceptual approach of the *Rabbinic* mind, many other meanings were associated with God's reign. The kingdom conveys a cluster of theological ideas. In the higher view of *Torah*, God's reign means affirming who God is by praying, 'Hear O Israel, the LORD our God, the LORD is One!'[a] The kingdom of heaven means obedience to the commandments. It refers to the deliverance of the people from the yoke of bondage in *Egypt* and their great liberty when they entered the promised land. It is divine protection and God's salvation. In *Jewish* thought, one discovers a rich associative method. The theological ideas come in clusters. So, it is with Paul. His theology is not systematic; rather, it compares clusters of associated concepts." [a: Deuteronomy 6:4; 7 (page 26)]

"*Torah* for Paul cannot be defined simply by the term *Law* in English. The term *Torah* expresses the highest dimension of *Jewish* experience because it reveals the nature of God to his people. *Torah* encompasses all that is known about God and his love for each individual created in the divine image. Paul possesses a passion for *Torah* as the quintessential self-disclosure of God and the divine will. Its preeminent purpose is found in Jesus the Messiah because, as Paul declares, now the Gentiles have been grafted into the olive tree (*Romans* 10:4). As a *Pharisee*, the focal point of Paul's thought was *Torah*. After his experience on the road to Damascus, *Torah* for Paul took a deeper meaning in the coming of Jesus. Paul's *Torah*-centered theology was eclipsed with an understanding of the Messiah as the higher purpose of *Torah*. The great vision of the *Hebrew* prophets is realized when the Gentile comes into a relationship with the one *God of Israel*." [7 (page 27)]

"God has not rejected his people. The *Jewish* people are the true *Israel,* according to Paul. God's call cannot be lifted. Traditionally, Christians have tended to divide people into two groups, believers and non-believers. The *Jewish* people were placed in the second group. But Paul would never feel comfortable with such a neat category for the *Israelites* according to the flesh. In Paul's metaphorical way of thinking in *Romans* 11:17, they represent the olive tree. He does not speak of replacement. Instead, he describes engraftment, which joins the wild olive shoot to the tree. Clearly, the church has not replaced *Israel*. On the contrary, for Paul, the destiny of the church and the synagogue is interrelated in the incomprehensible mystery of the divine purpose. In perspective, however, the *Jewish* '*no*' to *Jesus* is in reality a '*yes*' to the *God of Israel*. Christians cannot hate Jews who seek to serve the God of the *Bible* in good conscience." [7 (page 28)]

"*Engraftment* is not the same as *replacement*. Paul cannot accept God's rejection of his people *Israel*. On the one hand, the apostle affirms his strong belief in Jesus as Messiah. On the other, he declares that God did not and will not violate his word to the *Jewish* people." [7 (page 29)]

"Not everyone embraced the preaching of Paul, and the apostle could accept this. Paul recognized that when some of the *Jewish* people rejected his preaching of Jesus, they were really only reaffirming their own strong faith in God. Their '*no*' to Paul's preaching was not synonymous with a '*no*' to *God Almighty*. In their minds, they were saying '*yes*' to *God*. Paul was willing to sacrifice a part of his theological integrity in order to achieve the higher goal of unrestricted love." [7 (page 30)]

"Often *Romans* 10:4 has been translated improperly, 'For Christ is the end of the law…' The *Greek* word *telos*, which is translated as '*end*' in the verse, is better understood in its wider meaning, '*goal*' or '*purpose*.' Paul viewed the coming of the Messiah as the climax of salvation history…On the contrary, through Jesus, Paul argued, *Torah* had reached its objective by bringing the *Gentiles* into a right relationship with God. Paul is a *Jewish* apostle to the Gentiles, and the higher purpose of *Torah* is achieved as the pagan nations reject idolatrous practices and accept Jesus… In the mind of Paul, Jesus the *Jewish* Messiah makes this possible. [7 (page 31)]

"Do we then overthrow the law by this faith? By no means! On the contrary, we uphold the law (*Romans* 3:31; cf. *Matthew* 5:17). Paul upholds the goal of *Torah*." [7 (page 32)]

"A convert to *Judaism* had three requirements: he was first required to be circumcised, then undergo ritual immersion in baptism, and finally to offer a sacrifice in the temple." [7 (page 37)]

As we learned when looking at the *Jerusalem Council*, "in essence, the council came to a compromise. The decision had roots in *Jewish* legal discussion. The non-Jews from a pagan background would be viewed more like *God fearers* than like converts to *Judaism*. 'For it has seemed good to the Holy Spirit and to us to lay upon you no greater burden than these necessary things: that you abstain from what has been sacrificed to idols and from blood and from what is strangled and from unchastity. If you keep yourselves from these, you will do well. Farwell!' (*Acts* 15:28-29) The strongest point of the letter is the reference to avoid idolatrous worship… People who feared God would obey these fundamental ethical requirements." [7 (page 38)]

"The misconception that *Judaism* preaches a message of salvation by works has undermined the rich heritage of the *Hebrew Scriptures*, which both Christians and Jew hold sacred. The Christian faith rests upon its concept of the nature of God. *Faith in Jesus* should not contradict the *faith of Jesus*. Indeed, the all-pervasive root of *Jewish* belief, 'Hear, O Israel, the LORD our God, the LORD is One,' is taught throughout the *New Testament* itself." [7 (page 115)]

With this information in mind, we now turn to various scriptures in question regarding doctrine of *Torah* and Paul's responses to the various people and congregations. Did he indeed move away from *Torah* or decide it was no longer a valuable tool in relationship with the God of Israel? Let's see!

As we covered previously, the Jerusalem Council determined four rules for new Gentile converts to follow the Way of Messiah *Yeshua*. Of those rules, three directly relate to the dietary rules of the *Torah*.

Acts [15:19] "Therefore my verdict is that we do not trouble those from among the Gentiles who are turning to *YHWH*, [20] rather, let us write unto them that they should abstain from the abominations of idolatry, [1] from *ervah* sexual behavior, [2] *from* strangled *flesh*, [3] and *from* blood, [4] [21] because in every city *Moshe* has been preached for generations and he is read in the synagogue every Sabbath day." [2 (page 304)]

These conditions are based on the following scriptures: {Acts 15:20.1} *Deuteronomy* 12:29-32; {Acts 15:20.2} *Leviticus* 18:1-30; {Acts 5:20.3} *Leviticus* 11:1-47; and {Acts15:20.4} *Genesis* 9:34. *Leviticus* 17:10-14. [2 (page 304)]

[1] *Deuteronomy* 12:29-32 Don't serve the gods of other nations, nor the abomination that God hates! That included burnt offerings using their children as sacrifices. [3 (page 245)]

[2] *Leviticus* 18:1-30 is about sexual behavior. God tells the people "not to engage in the activities found in the land of Egypt, where you used to live; and not to engage in the activities found in the land of *Kena'an,* where I am bringing you; nor are you to live by their laws." [:4] "You are to obey my (*ADONAI*) rulings and laws and live accordingly, I am *ADONAI* your God. [5] You are to observe my laws and rulings; if a person does them, he will have life through them; I am *ADONAI*." [3 (page 153)]

The issues they were warned about in *Leviticus* 18 all dealt with sexual behavior especially in situations of adultery and incest with anyone of a persons close or extended family.

The note regarding *Leviticus* 18:5 states, "'You are to observe' is one word in Hebrew, *she'martem*; which describes a soldier's service as a watchman. Just as an armed guard will pay attention to every detail in order to protect his company, so *Isra'el* is to keep the *Torah* continually, with seriousness, resolve, and nonstop effort and attention." The *Torah* is still upheld! [3 (page 153)]

[3] *Leviticus* 11:1-47 – Dietary Laws. *Leviticus* 11 gives a thorough overview of those animals considered fit for eating and situations that would be considered *unclean*. Verses 46 and 47 explain these rules.

Leviticus [11: 46] "Such, then, is the law concerning animals, flying creatures, all living creatures that move about in the water, and all creatures that swarm on the ground. [47] Its purpose is to distinguish between the unclean and the clean, and between the creatures that may be eaten and those that may not be eaten.'" [3 (page 143)]

[4] *Genesis* 9:3-4 God is speaking to *Noach*. [3]"Every moving thing that lives will be food for you; just as I gave you green plants before, so now I give you everything – [4] only flesh with its life, which is the blood, you are not to eat.'" [3 (page 13)]

Leviticus [17:10] "'When someone from the community of *Isra'el* or one of the foreigners living with you eats any kind of blood, I will set myself against that person who eats blood and cut him off from his people. [11] For the life of a creature is in the blood, and I have given it to you on the altar to make atonement for yourselves; for it is the blood that makes atonement because of the life. [12] This is why I told the people of *Isra'el*, 'None of you is to eat blood, nor is any foreigner living with you to eat blood.' [13] When someone from the community of *Isra'el* or one of the foreigners living with you hunts and catches game, whether animal or bird *that may be eaten*, he is to pour out its blood and cover it with earth. [14] For the life of every creature – its blood is its life. Therefore, I said to the people of *Isra'el*, 'You are not to eat the blood of any creature, because the life of every creature is its blood. Whoever eats it will be cut off.'" [3 (page 153)]

Leviticus [17:11] states, "'For the life of a creature is in the blood.' The bloodshed was sacred, as it represented the life of the sacrificed victim. Since life was sacred, blood, as the symbol of life, was treated with respect (cf. *Gen.* 9:5-6), and so according to the *Torah*, eating blood is strictly forbidden. Kosher laws to this day forbid the eating of blood." [3 (page 153)]

A note about *Leviticus* 17:14 states, "Whoever eats it will be cut off." "The Hebrew expression translated 'cut off' is the same used in other verses to express the idea that a person was to be exiled from his community and left alone for God to judge. Most often, that was thought to occur by sudden death." [3 (page 153)]

These scriptures provide background for the four rules *Ya'akov*, *Kefa*, and *Sha'ul* settled on for new converts following *Yeshua,* their Messiah. They were aware there was more for them to learn, and those things would be learned in weekly teachings of *Torah* portions (called *Parasha*) in the various synagogues. For now, three of the rules dealt with foundational teachings for foods. Instead of deleting dietary laws, it seems they are definitely upheld.

"Some people have misinterpreted these recommendations as abolishing the rest of the law. But, by that logic, the Gentile converts would be free to steal or kill or blaspheme, but the Jewish believers could not. The same could be said for incest, witchcraft, child sacrifice, and a host of other prohibitions. That would be absurd, and a faulty "*argument from silence*." [11 (page 23-24)]

"It is interesting to note that of all things the Council could have said, they restricted their recommendations to just four requirements, and THREE of these are DIETARY. Some have said that this is just because the Gentile practice of eating forbidden foods was so repulsive to the Jews. But surely murder, rape, blasphemy, or theft were much more abhorrent. The meaning is not hard to see. These dietary rules were for their own good, not just because they offended someone. As fornication is sin against one's own body (*1 Corinthians* 6:18), so also is eating forbidden foods (*Leviticus* 11:43-44). It was a place for the Gentile believers to begin on their road to personal sanctification." [11 (page 23-24)]

In 53AD [4], *Judaizers* were troubling the church in *Galatia*. *Sha'ul* addressed their concerns in his letter to the church. The next scripture we will look at is *Galatians* 2:11-21. This scripture speaks of *Sha'ul's* disapproval of *Kefa's* behavior in *Antioch* when followers of *Yeshua* from *Yerushalayim* arrived.

Galatians 2:11 "Furthermore, when *Kefa* came to *Antioch*, I opposed him publicly, because he was clearly in the wrong. 12 For prior to the arrival of certain people from [the community headed by] *Ya'akov*, he had been eating *with* the Gentile believers; but when they came, he *withdrew* and *separated* himself, because he was afraid of the faction who favored circumcising Gentile believers. 13 And the other Jewish believers became hypocrites along with him, so that even *Bar-Nabba* was led astray by their hypocrisy. 14 But when I saw that they were not walking a straight path, keeping in line with the truth of the Good News, I said to *Kefa*, right in front of everyone, 'If you, who are a Jew, live like a Gentile and not like a Jew, why are you forcing the Gentiles to live like Jews?' 15 We are Jews by birth, not so-called 'Gentile sinners'; 16 even so, we have come to realize that a person is not declared righteous by God on the ground of his *legalistic* observance of *Torah* commands, but through the Messiah *Yeshua's* trusting faithfulness. Therefore, we too have put our trust in Messiah *Yeshua* and become faithful to him, in order that we might be declared righteous on the ground of the Messiah's trusting faithfulness and not the ground of our *legalistic* observance of *Torah* commands. For on the ground of *legalistic* observance of *Torah* commands, **no one will be declared righteous.** [a]"

"17 But if, in seeking to be declared righteous by God through our union with the Messiah, we ourselves are indeed found to be sinners, then is the Messiah an aider and abettor of sin? Heaven forbid! 18 Indeed, if I build up again the *legalistic bondage* which I destroyed, I really do make myself a transgressor. 19 For it was through letting the *Torah* speak for itself that I died to its *traditional legalistic misinterpretation*, so that I might live in direct relationship with God. 20 When the Messiah was executed on the stake as a criminal, I was too; so that my proud ego no longer lives. But the Messiah lives in me, and this life I now live in my body I live by the same trusting faithfulness that the Son of God had, who loved me and gave himself up for me. 21 I do not reject God's gracious gift; for if the way in which one attains righteousness is through *legalism*, then the Messiah's death was pointless." [a Psalm 143.2; 3 (page 1671)]

In *Galatians* 3:1, *Sha'ul* continues in very strong language! "You stupid *Galatians*! Who has put you under a spell? Before your very eyes, *Yeshua,* the Messiah, was clearly portrayed as having been put to death as a criminal! 2 I want to know from you just one thing: did you receive the Spirit by *legalistic* observance of *Torah* commands or by trusting in what you heard and being faithful to it? 3 Are you that stupid?" [3 (page 1671)]

Once again, we are looking at a letter written in response to a question we don't have. However, we do have some information and need a bit of clarification. Is *Sha'ul* doing away with *Torah*? Did *Kefa* actually eat something not allowed? What really happened here? Let's look at some references for these scriptures.

First, a note regarding *Galatians* 2:14. "'Why are you forcing the Gentiles to live like Jews?" *Galatians* speak of three general types (of people) based on emphases. The *Circumcision* faction insisted that Gentile believers must be circumcised to be part of God's family. *Assimilationists* insisted that Gentiles adopt Jewish customs and assimilate into the Jewish community. *Legalizers* taught that doing what God demands earned them greater status with God. To this, *Sha'ul* questions why *Shim'on Kefa* (Simon Peter) was forcing the Gentiles in Antioch to live as Jews." [3 (page 1671)]

Second, we look at the notes for *Galatians* 2:15-16. "'A person is not declared righteous by God on the ground of his legalistic observance of *Torah* commands.' Here, *Sha'ul* pivots from defending the authority behind his presentation of the Good News to explaining why under this *Renewed* covenant it is wrong to force Gentile believers into a legalistic observance of *Torah* through the act of *brit-milah* (circumcision). From this verse to the end of *Galatians*, *Sha'ul* attacks the Circumcision faction, while defending the true *Gospel*, in which Gentiles need not become Jews in order to follow *Yeshua* the Messiah." [3 (page 1671)]

The note for *Galatians* 2:19 reads: "'For it was through letting the *Torah* speak for itself that I died to its traditional legalistic misinterpretation.' *Sha'ul* dies to the traditional legalistic misinterpretation so that he might live in direct relationship with God, instead of being shut off from God by a legalistic misinterpretation of the *Torah*." [3 (page 1671)]

The last note we look at for this section is for *Galatians* 2:21. "'If the way in which one attains righteousness is through legalism, then the Messiah's death was pointless.' If someone tries to attain righteousness through any form of self-generated effort, and specifically through legalistic following of *Torah* commands, then the Messiah's death was pointless, and so is his ongoing resurrected life." [3 (page 1671)]

We can see from this portion of *Sha'ul's* letter, the problem isn't the *Torah*, it is legalistic observance of *Torah* and not trusting faithfully in the atonement *Yeshua* attained through his obedience to the Father through scourging and crucifixion. It wasn't that *Kefa* had eaten something 'unclean,' but his separation to only the Jews when they arrived on the scene instead of inviting the others to join together with them. This issue of legalism is a frequent topic in *Shaul's* letter.

Sha'ul continues his discussion of *Torah* and legalism as he looks back to *Avraham*, who followed God prior to the written *Torah* of *Moshe*.

Galatians 3:15 "Brothers, let me make an analogy from everyday life: when someone
swears an oath, no one else can set it aside or add to it. 16 Now promises were made to
Avraham and to his seed. It doesn't say, 'and to seeds,' as if to many; on the contrary, it
speaks of one – '**and to your seed**' [a] – and this 'one' is the Messiah. 17 Here is what I am
saying: the legal part of the *Torah*, which came into being 430 years later, does not nullify
an oath sworn by God, so as to abolish the promise. 18 For if the inheritance comes from
the legal part of the *Torah*, it no longer comes from a promise. But God gave it to
Avraham through a promise.

19 "So then, why the legal part of the *Torah*? It was added to create transgressions, until
the coming of the seed about whom the promise had been made. Moreover, it was
handed down through angels and a mediator. 20 Now a mediator implies more than one,
but God is one.

21 "Does this mean the legal part of the *Torah* stands in opposition to God's promise?
Heaven forbid! For if the legal part of *Torah,* which God gave, had in itself the power to
give life, then righteousness really would have come by legalistically following such a
Torah. 22 But instead, the *Tanakh* shuts up everything under sin; so that what had been

promised might be given, on the basis of *Yeshua* the Messiah's trusting faithfulness, to
those who continue to be trustingly faithful.

[23] "Now before the time for this trusting faithfulness came, we were imprisoned in
subjection to the system which results from perverting the *Torah* into legalism, kept
under guard until this yet-to-come trusting faithfulness would be revealed. [24]
Accordingly, the *Torah* functioned as a custodian until the Messiah came, so that we
might be declared righteous on the ground of trusting and being faithful. [25] But now that
the time for this trusting faithfulness has come, we are no longer under a custodian.

[26] "For in union with the Messiah, you are all children of God through this trusting
faithfulness; [27] because as many of you as were immersed into the Messiah have clothed
yourselves with the Messiah, in whom [28] there is neither Jew nor Gentile, neither slave
nor freeman, neither male nor female; for in union with the Messiah *Yeshua*, you are all
one. [29] Also, if you belong to the Messiah, you are the seed of *Avraham* and heirs
according to the promise." [a] Genesis 12.7, 13.15; 17:7; 24:7. [3 (page 1673)]

Let's look at some of the references for the above scriptures. First a look at *Galatians* 3:17. "'The legal part of the *Torah* does not nullify an oath sworn by God.' Even if the *Torah* had required legalistic obedience without trust, it could not nullify an oath sworn or a covenant established so as to abolish the promise to *Avraham*, which says that Gentiles will be blessed through him (vv.8:9) without having to become Jews." [3 (page 1673)]

Next, we look at a reference for *Galatians* 3:19. "'So then, why the legal part of the *Torah*?' In vv. 19-21, *Sha'ul* continues using Jewish methods of interpretation. The *Abrahamic Covenant* gives a promise to all who believe in the Messiah. The *Mosaic Covenant* gives another promise, added later, to a specific people, *Isra'el*. So, the *Galatians* are included in the larger promise of *Avraham* and do not need to become circumcised, putting themselves under the later covenant, which is for Jews. Jew and Gentile are included in the larger promise through *Avraham* already, which is fulfilled in Messiah. [3 (page 1673)]

In *Galatians* 3:21-22, we learn that "faith is best translated as *trusting faithfulness*. *Trusting faithfulness* to those who continue to be *trustingly faithful* to him (*Yeshua*) and to the Father." [3 (page 1673)]

Trusting faithfulness is the concept of faith *Sha'ul* brings to all his letters. As for *Torah*, *Sha'ul* says, "Bear one another's burdens – in this way you will be fulfilling the *Torah's* true meaning, which the Messiah upholds." *Galatians* 6:2 [3 (page 1677)]

"*Yeshua* did not negate or institute a different *Torah* (Law) of *Moshe*. The *Law of Messiah* and the *Law of Moshe* are one in the same. *Yeshua* did not come to abolish the *Torah*. (*Matthew* 5:17; Rydelnik 1841)." [3 (page 1677)]

If the *Torah* actually had the power to give life, "the *Torah* could automatically impart the *Ruach HaKodesh* to legalists, transforming them into people who trust God and are faithful to him, 'then righteousness really would have come by legalistically following such a *Torah*. But instead, the *Tanakh* shuts up everything under sin,' imprisoning all of humankind (v. 23, cf. *Romans* 11:30-32), 'so that what had been promised might be given, on the basis of *Yeshua* the Messiah's trusting faithfulness, to those who continue to be trustingly faithful' to him and to the Father. Faith is there best translated as 'trusting faithfulness.''' [3 (page 1673)]

Galatians 3:24 says, "'the *Torah* functioned as a custodian until the Messiah came.' Whenever the *Torah* was perverted into legalism, it served in the role of harsh disciplinarian for the Jewish people, providing some protection but generally making the Jewish people aware of their many transgressions. (v.19) [3 (page 1673)]

Once again, we see the issue is not the *Torah*, but the legalism that perverted *Torah* and the added traditions of men that made it hard for people to focus on a loving God. Instead, they were under the pressure of performance to be certain of being observant! Pressure our Heavenly Father never intended.

Next, let's look at the book of *Corinthians*, written in 56AD before the Passover of 57AD. [4] There are three main scriptures we will look at while in *Corinthians*. The first is *1 Corinthians* 6:12-20, where we will see if everything is permitted!

1 Corinthians 6:12 "You say, 'For me, everything is permitted'? Maybe, but not everything is helpful. 'For me, everything is permitted'? Maybe, but as far as I am concerned, I am not going to let anything gain control over me. 13 'Food is meant for the stomach and the stomach for food'? Maybe, but God will put an end to both of them. Anyhow, the body is not meant for sexual immorality, but for the Lord, and the Lord is for the body. 14 God raised up the Lord, and he will raise us up too by his power.

1 Corinthians 6:15 "Don't you know that your bodies are parts of the Messiah? So, am I to take parts of the Messiah and make them parts of a prostitute? Heaven forbid! 16 Don't you know that a man who joins himself to a prostitute becomes physically one with her? For the *Tanakh* says '**The two will become one flesh**,' [a] 17, but the person who is joined to the Lord is one spirit. 18 Run from sexual immorality! Every other sin a person commits is outside the body, but the fornicator sins against his own body. 19 Or don't you know that your body is a temple for the *Ruach HaKodesh* who lives inside you, whom you received from God? The fact is, you don't belong to yourselves; 20 for you were bought at a price. So, use your bodies to glorify God." [a Genesis 2:24; 3 (page 1638)]

Two notes are given for this section of *Sha'ul's* letter to the *Corinthian* church. The first is regarding *1 Corinthians* 6:12 – "You say, 'For me, everything is permitted'? *Sha'ul* does not deny the principle but cautions against its misuse by pointing out that not everything is helpful. His point is expressed saying, 'I am not going to let anything gain control over me.''' [3 (page 1638)]

A second note for this section in *1 Corinthians* 6:13 regards the issue of foods. "'Food is meant for the stomach and the stomach for food.' This is not said in order to oppose the Jewish dietary laws. Rather, the libertines offered it as a euphemistic argument against self-restraint." [3 (page 1638)]

Next, we go to *1 Corinthians* chapter 8, where *Sha'ul* speaks regarding the issue of eating food that has previously been sacrificed to idols. "The questions raised in this chapter is whether a believer is free to eat meat that he knows, or suspects may have been part of an offering in a pagan Temple."

1 Corinthians [8:4] "So, as for eating food sacrificed to idols, we 'know' that, as you say, 'An idol has no real existence in the world, and there is only one God' [5] For even if there are so called 'gods,' either in heaven or on earth – as in fact there are 'gods' and 'lords' galore – [6] yet for us there is one God, the Father, from whom we exist; and one Lord, *Yeshua* the Messiah, through whom were created all things and through whom we have our being. [7] But not everyone has this knowledge. Moreover, some people are still so accustomed to idols that when they eat food which has been sacrificed to them, they think of it as really affected by the idols; and their conscience being weak are thus defiled. [8] Now food will not improve our relationship with God – we will be neither poorer if we abstain nor richer if we eat. [9] However, watch out that your mastery of the situation does not become a stumbling block to the weak. [10] You have this 'knowledge'; but suppose someone with a weak conscience sees you sitting, eating a meal in the temple of an idol. Won't he be built up wrongly to eat this food which has been sacrificed to idols? [11] Thus by your 'knowledge' this weak person was destroyed, this brother for whom the Messiah died; [12] and so, when you sin against the brothers by wounding their conscience when it is weak, you are sinning against the Messiah! [13] To sum up, if food will be a snare for my brother, I will never eat meat again, lest I cause my brother to sin." [3 (page 1641)]

As we can see, the identity of the food was not in question. Instead, the issue was about avoiding the possibility of tempting someone weaker in faith by our questionable actions.

Our last scripture in *Corinthians* is *1 Corinthians* 10:25-33, and is about asking your host about the food being served if you aren't sure you should eat it.

1 Corinthians [10:25] "Eat whatever is sold in the meat market without raising questions of conscience, [26] **for the earth and everything in it belong to the Lord**. [a; 27] If some unbeliever invites you to a meal, and you want to go, eat whatever is put in front of you without raising questions of conscience. [28] But if someone says to you, 'This meat was offered as a sacrifice,' then don't eat it, out of consideration for the person who pointed it out and also for conscience's sake – [29] however, I don't mean your conscience but that of the other person. You say, 'Why should my freedom be determined by someone else's conscience? [30] If I participate with thankfulness, why am I criticized over something for which I myself bless God?' [31] Well, whatever you do, whether it's eating or drinking or anything else, do it all so as to bring glory to God. [32] Do not be an obstacle to anyone – not Jews, not to Gentiles, and not to God's Messianic Community. [33] Just as I try to please everyone in everything I do, not looking out for my own interest but for those of the many, so that they may be saved; [11:1] Try to imitate me, even as I myself try to imitate the Messiah." [3 (page 1644)]

Daniel Leonard Harris, in his book *God Cares What You Eat*, asks, "Did the Apostle Paul say that we should eat whatever food an unbeliever gives us at his house without asking any questions? Answer: No… the Apostle Paul says that you should not ask your host whether or not the meat he is giving you was first offered to idols. Of course, you can ask what kind of food it is. And you are certainly free to politely refuse to eat any forbidden foods." [11 (page 20)]

The important thing, once again, is to avoid being an obstacle to anyone needing salvation. "Though it is true that Jews and Gentiles are equally in need of salvation, and in this regard, there is no difference between them, it is nevertheless true that salvation does not eradicate one's identity as either a Jew or as a Gentile. Yet *Sha'ul* continues to refer to believing Gentiles as 'Gentiles' (*Romans* 11:12; *Ephesians* 2:11) and to Messianic Jews as 'Jews'. (*Galatians* 2:13)." [3 (page 1644)]

The second letter was thought to be to the *Corinthian* church in late summer of 57AD. [4] The verses pointed out in the discussion of *Torah's* relevance in the area of dietary laws are found in *2 Corinthians* 6:14-7:1.

2 Corinthians [6:14] "Do not yoke yourselves together in a team with unbelievers. For how can righteousness and lawlessness be partners? What fellowship does light have with darkness? [15] What harmony can there be between the Messiah and *B'liya'al*? What does a believer have in common with an unbeliever? [16] What agreement can there be between the temple of God and idols? For we are the temple of the living God – as God said,

'I will house myself in them, ...and I walk among you, I will be their God, and they will be my people.' [b]

[17] Therefore *ADONAI* says,

'Go out from their midst; separate yourselves; don't even touch what is unclean. [c] **Then I myself will receive you.** [d] [18] In fact, **I will be** your **Father, and you will be my son's** and daughter's.' says *ADONAI-Tzva'ot*.' [e] b *Leviticus* 26:12; *Exodus* 6:7; *Jeremiah* 31:32 (33), 32:38; *Ezekiel* 37:27. c *Isaiah* 52:11. d *Ezekiel* 20:34, 41. e 2 *Samuel* 7:14; *Isaiah* 43:6. 3 (page 1660)

2 Corinthians [7:1] "Therefore, my dear friends, since we have these promises, let us purify ourselves from everything that can defile either body or spirit, and strive to be completely holy, out of reverence for God." [3 (page 1661)]

Everything we do needs to be with conscious thoughts of having reverence for God.

Several places in the letters to the Corinthian fellowship, *Sha'ul* instructs that humankind is designed to be the temple of God's Holy Spirit (*Ruach HaKodesh*). We were all designed to be followers of the One True Father and individual temples of worship to the Father. [11]

In *1 Corinthians* 6:19, we learn that our bodies are the temple of God. Therefore, as temples, we should nourish ourselves with the clean foods and drinks instructed by *Yehovah* God. In *1 Corinthians* 10:31, we are told that no matter what we eat and drink, it should be presented as to the glory of *Yehovah*. *2 Corinthian* 6:17, is a follow up letter. The people are told not to touch the unclean thing, and if they follow this instruction, they would be received and treated with favor by *Yehovah*. [11]

In the winter of 57AD, *Sha'ul* penned his letter to the church in Rome. [4] There were conflicts "between Gentile disciples and the Jewish community. *Sha'ul*'s focus in the book of *Romans* is on how God's promises to the people of *Israel* relate to Gentiles who have come to faith in Messiah." It is "intended to help them understand the unbelief of many Jews, God's continuing work with *Israel*, the Jewish roots of the gospel, the full inclusion of Gentiles as children of *Avraham* (Abraham), and the necessity of serving the Jewish people." [3 (page 1604)]

Three sections of the letter come into question periodically regarding the issue of dietary laws. Let's take a look at each area. The first is *Romans* 6:14-15. Let's back up a bit and start at *Romans* 6:1.

Romans 6:1 "So then, are we to say, 'Let's keep on sinning, so that there can be more grace'? 2 Heaven forbid! How can we, who have died to sin, still live in it? 3 Don't you know that those of us who have been immersed into the Messiah *Yeshua* have been immersed into his death? 4 Through immersion into his death, we were buried with him; so that just as, through the glory of the Father, the Messiah was raised from the dead, likewise we too might live a new life. 5 For if we have been united with him in a death like his, we will also be united with him in a resurrection like his. 6 We know that our old self was put to death on the execution-stake with him, so that the entire body of our sinful propensities might be destroyed, and we might no longer be enslaved to sin. 7 For someone who has died has been cleared from sin. 8 Now since we died with the Messiah, we trust that we will also live with him. 9 We know that the Messiah has been raised from the dead, never to die again, death has no authority over him. 10 For his death was a unique event that need not be repeated; but his life, he keeps on living for God. 11 In the same way, consider yourselves to be dead to sin but alive for God, by your union with the Messiah *Yeshua*." [3 (page 1613-1614)]

12 "Therefore, do not let sin rule in your mortal bodies, so that it makes you obey its desires; 13 and do not offer any part of yourselves to sin as an instrument for wickedness. On the contrary, offer yourselves to God as people alive from the dead, and your various parts to God as instruments for righteousness. 14 For sin will not have authority over you, because you are not under legalism but under grace.

15 "Therefore, what conclusion should we reach? 'Let's go on sinning because we're not under legalism but under grace'? Heaven forbid! 16 Don't you know that if you present yourselves to someone as obedient slaves, then, of the one whom you are obeying, you are slaves – whether of sin, which leads to death, or obedience, which leads to being made righteous? 17 By God's grace, you, who were once slaves to sin, obeyed from your heart the pattern of teaching to which you were exposed; 18 and after you had been set free from sin, you became enslaved to righteousness. 19 (I am using popular language because your human nature is so weak.) For just as you used to offer your various parts as slaves to impurity and lawlessness, which led to more lawlessness; so now offer your various parts as slaves to righteousness, which leads to being made holy, set apart for God. 20 For when you were slaves of sin, you were free in relationship to righteousness; 21 but what benefit did you derive from the things of which you are now ashamed? The end result of those things was death. 22 However, now, freed from sin and enslaved to God, you do get benefit – it consists of being made holy, set apart for God, and its end result is eternal life. 23 For what one earns from sin is death; but eternal life is what one receives as a free gift from God, in union with the Messiah *Yeshua*, our Lord." [3 (page 1614)]

Once again, we note that the "Greek word *nomos* literally 'law' and often translated *Torah* (*Matthew* 5:17), must be rendered here as 'legalism,' and defined as skewing and diminishing the *Torah* into a system of rules for earning God's praise without trusting, loving, or communing with him, the 'Giver of the *Torah*.'" (Note *Romans* 6:14) [3 (page 1614)]

When we consider the terms 'law' and 'grace', we might think they are opposite each other. But actually, the opposite of 'law' is 'lawlessness.' And the opposite of 'grace' is what is termed 'works.' *Romans* 6:14 speaks against legalism, not against the *Torah* itself. Being free of legalism, one can be blessed by the blessings of Grace. *Yeshua's* death, through His crucifixion, already paid for the death of our sin nature. And His *Holy Spirit* within us, His believers, now make us His delight. And, leaving legalism behind, we follow *Torah* out of love and gratefulness, not legalism. Just as *Sha'ul* says in *Romans* 7:22. "For in my inner self I completely agree with God's *Torah*." [11 (page 24)]

"What is 'God's Law?" It is His revealed word, unchanging throughout history." The author, *Daniel Leonard Harris*, says, "It was partially fulfilled in Christ's first coming to earth. (*Matthew* 5:17-20). And the purpose of the Law is being finally completed by the Holy Spirit's work of sanctification of the church until Christ's second coming to earth. This sanctification of believers includes their increasing obedience and holiness, not so much to earn salvation (which was purchased by Christ) but have already been saved to grow in grace. This must include observance of God's dietary laws as well as the Ten Commandments, and the rest of His law. 'Wherefore the law is holy, and the commandments holy, just, and good.'" (*Romans* 7:12) [11 (page 24)]

Is *Romans* 6 an anti-*Torah* section of the letter to the Romans? "Faith in Messiah pertains to every sphere of life (cf. *James* 2:12-26). Yet despite the truth – and the fact that the love of God is linked to obedience (1 *John* 5:3) – many of the body of the Messiah in recent years have been influenced by the false teaching of antinomianism (anti-*Torah*). Some hold that believers are no longer obligated to follow even the moral laws of *Torah* in light of *Yeshua's* work of grace." [3 (page 1613)]

"In *Romans* 6:1-2, *John* 14:15, and 1 *John* 5:3, *Sha'ul* answers his critics – Jews who felt that his message of grace abolished the need to observe *Torah*. This misconception by his critics assumes that *Sha'ul* was advocating an antinomian worldview: that *Torah* was now a relic of the past. *Sha'ul* retorts with the *Hebraic* idiom, 'Heaven Forbid,' or *Chalilah* ('A curse be upon it!'). *Sha'ul* reminds his followers that by virtue of being united with the Messiah (*Romans* 6:3-6), the believer has actually died to sin. Although the penalty was paid on Messiah's execution stake (v. 6), this is not a license to violate the *Torah*, to sin. From such a strong defense, it is impossible to conclude that *Torah* observance has been revoked. What *Sha'ul* disparages is a legalistic observance of *Torah* commands, something God never intended for *Isra'el* in the first place." [3 (page 1613)]

Next, we turn our attention to *Romans* 10:4. "For the goal at which the *Torah* aims is the Messiah, who offers righteousness to everyone who trusts." [3 (page 1620)]

The note regarding this scripture again states, "an error made here by all major English New Testament translations of this text is rendering of the Greek word as 'end' not 'goal!' This implies 'termination' of the *Torah*, which is often understood to mean that the law has been abolished." [3 (page 1620)]

"The coming of Christ did not cancel God's law, as some incorrectly interpret this verse. In His own words, Jesus specifically said that he did not come to abolish the law, but to fulfill and complete it. (*Matthew* 5:17-20). And He did not complete it so as to discard it, because that would contradict His clear statements otherwise." [11 (page 21)]

Christ's death and resurrection did make some changes. "The system of animal sacrifices has been permanently ended by Christ's death as the Lamb of God. Jesus is the perpetual and eternal sacrifice, the 'Lamb slain from the foundation of the world.' (*Revelation* 13:8)." … "But the principle of justification by sacrificial death for sins still remains. A believer is saved by the sacrificial death of Christ for his sins. But the unbeliever must pay for his own sins by his own eternal death and damnation in Hell. In one sense, the sacrificial system has been 'upgraded,' but no principles have changed. And this certainly includes dietary laws." [11 (page 21)]

The *Curtain* separating the *Holy of Holies* was torn from top to bottom. What a sign! Therefore, from that time to the present, animal sacrifices could no longer be offered. *Yeshua* was the final *Passover Lamb*. None other was necessary. His crucifixion was the final sacrifice needed. He paid the penalty for our sinful nature. For "…those whose names are written in the Book of Life belonging to the Lamb slaughtered before the world was founded." [Revelation 13:8 3 (page 1797)]

Yeshua's sacrifice was for the entire world of humans no matter when they enter this realm we call earth. Those who trust *Yeshua* and *His Word* and follow *Him* will be freed from the slavery of sin and live eternally with *Yehovah*. The unbeliever, who refuses *Yeshua's* free gift, will not spend their eternal life with *Yehovah*, but will be in separation from Him for eternity. Salvation atones for our sin nature but does not remove the responsibility of obedience to *Torah*. If anything, in gratitude, we serve *Yehovah* and *Yeshua* by showing honor to *Their Word* and obedience to the *Torah*.

The last verse we will look at in *Romans* is 14:10. It says, "You, then, why do you pass judgment on your brother? Or why do you look down on your brother? For all of us will stand before God's judgment seat; [11] since it is written in the *Tanakh*

'As I live, says *ADONAI*, every knee will bend before me,

And every tongue will publicly acknowledge God.' [a]

[12] "So then, every one of us will have to give an account of himself to God. [13] Therefore, let's stop passing judgment on each other! Instead, make this one judgment – not to put a stumbling block or a snare in a brother's way. [14] I know – that is, I have been persuaded by the Lord *Yeshua* the Messiah – that nothing is unclean in itself. But if a person considers something unclean, then for him it is unclean, [15] and if your brother is being upset by the food you eat, your life is no longer one of love. Do not, by your eating habits, destroy someone for whom the Messiah died! [16] Do not let what you know to be good, be spoken of as bad; [17] for the Kingdom of God is not eating and drinking, but righteousness, *shalom*, and joy in the *Ruach HaKodesh*. [18] Anyone who serves the Messiah in this fashion both pleases God and wins the approval of other people." [a Isaiah 45:23; 3 (page 1627)]

The note regarding *Romans* 14:14 states, "'Nothing is unclean in itself.' *Sha'ul* is certainly not espousing moral relativism. His remark has to do not with human behavior but with ritual uncleanliness. It is not surprising that *Sha'ul*, having alluded in the previous verse to *Leviticus* 19 (a chapter full of commandments about uncleanness) continues with a dictum on that subject. The Bible does not always explain why some things are pure and others not." [3 (page 1627)]

The circumstances of *Romans* 14:14 is the key to interpreting the passage correctly. *Sha'ul* is teaching the stronger believers to be an encouragement rather than a confusion to the person weaker in faith. He cautions them not to be an obstacle to their new faith. The issue is a religious one and not about the food served. [11]

The parallel chapter is *1 Corinthians* 10, where *Sha'ul* is addressing the issue of eating meat offered to pagan idols.

The person *Sha'ul* is writing to sounds like a Messianic believer. He would have been confident in his faith and aware that idols are not gods, so he has no problem eating the 'clean' meat that had been offered to idols. However, a new Gentile believer may not understand yet that eating those meats would be okay. The new believer had just left behind a past that most likely included regularly offering meat to pagan idols before eating it. He might not yet understand, and the more confident believer may be unwittingly tempting the new believer to continue that practice. [11 (page 19)]

Sha'ul is not addressing anything about eating something God has called unclean. The audience he was addressing were Jewish believers, and they only ate 'clean' meats. He is correcting the believers to avoid eating meat previously offered to idols if there are new believers in the group who might be confused. It was to avoid tempting the new convert who had recently been a Gentile idol worshiper.

The next scripture we will look at is *Colossians* 2:16-23. The book of *Colossians* was written in 62AD. It is now 32 years after the crucifixion of *Yeshua* and 29 years since *Sha'ul's*
Damascus experience. [4] Still, *Sha'ul* was clarifying, answering questions, and teaching the Gospel to the various churches. This letter was to the *Colossian* congregation.

Colossians 2:16 "So don't let anyone pass judgment on you in connection with eating and drinking, or in regard to a Jewish festival or *Rosh-Hodesh* or *Shabbat*. 17 These are a shadow of things that are coming, but the body is of the Messiah. 18 Don't let anyone deny you the prize by insisting that you engage in self-mortification or angel worship. Such people are always going on about some vision they have had, and they vainly puff themselves up by their worldly outlook. *19* They fail to hold to the Head, from whom the whole Body, receiving supply and being held together by its joints and ligaments, grows as God makes it grow. *20* If along with the Messiah, you died to the elemental spirits of the world, then why, as if you still belonged to the world, are you letting yourselves be bothered by its rules? – *21* 'Don't touch this!' 'Don't eat that!' 'Don't handle the other!' *22* Such prohibitions are concerned with things meant to perish by being used [not by being avoided], and they are based on **man-made rules and teachings**. [a] 23 They do indeed have the outward appearance of wisdom, with their self-imposed religious observances, false humility, and asceticism, but they have no value at all in restraining people from indulging their old nature." [a Isaiah 29:13; 3 (page 1697)]

"Many people zero in on the phrase in verse 16 (the King James Version), 'Let no man therefore judge you in meat,' and claim that this spells the end of the dietary laws. But verse 22 explains that the rules we are free from are the religious 'commandments and doctrines of men.' It is not God's Law that is being rejected here, but men's ascetic restrictions on the legitimate enjoyment of life. Verse 23 says that although these man-made guidelines can appear to have some value, they do not restrain the inner depravity of man. However, we know that God's dietary laws promise and deliver great benefits, including freedom from many terrible diseases (*Exodus* 15:26; *Deuteronomy* 7:15). And God's laws are perpetual commandments (*Leviticus* 3:17) given by a good God (*Mark* 10:18) Who does not lie (*Romans* 3:4) nor change (*Malachi* 3:6)." [11 (page 27)]

The last scripture we will address in this section is *1 Timothy* 4:1-5. This letter to Timothy was written in 63AD. [4]

"Historically speaking, *1* and *2 Timothy* show a typical first-century relationship between a rabbi and his chief student, perhaps his *talmid hakam* ('most learned student'). Literally speaking, these letters are examples of rabbinic *responsa*, written decisions and rulings given by legal scholars in response to questions. The closeness of the relationship between rabbi and student is supported by history. Timothy accompanied *Sha'ul* on some of the latter's journeys, and *Sha'ul* wrote about Timothy in a number of his letters (e.g., *1 Corinthians* 4:17; 16:10; *Philippians* 2:19, 22; *1 Thessalonians* 3:6)." [3 (Page 1709)]

"In this letter, *Sha'ul* consults with Timothy about challenges Timothy has encountered. All of *Sha'ul's* advice is presented with the goal of helping Timothy lead the community of mostly Gentile believers to which he had been appointed, as well as, to walk in his own personal destiny and fulfill his calling." [3 (page 1709)]

1 Timothy [4:1] "The Spirit expressly states that in the *acharit-hayamim* some people will apostatize from the faith by paying attention to deceiving spirits and things taught by demons. [2] Such teachings come from the hypocrisy of liars whose own consciences have been burned, as if with a red-hot branding iron. [3] They forbid marriage and require abstinence from foods which God created to be eaten with thanksgiving by those who have come to trust and to know the truth. [4] For everything created by God is good, and nothing received with thanksgiving needs to be rejected, [5] because the word of God and prayer make it holy." [3 (page 1712-1713)]

Was *Sha'ul* giving permission to eat anything they wanted? The answer to that question is No! Let's look at what the circumstances were. In verses 1 and 2, *Sha'ul* warns against deceiving spirits and things taught by demons. Seducing spirits and demons contradict *Yehovah's Scriptures* and place wrong restrictions on people. God gave humankind freedom to marry and gave them an abundance of foods that are nourishing. Our hearts should be filled with thanksgiving as we receive our *good gifts* from the Father. [11 (page 20)]

The main point is that *Yehovah* did not give all meat to be eaten. Only His Word sanctifies what meats, or foods, are specified 'clean.' Although we pray prayers of thanksgiving at our meals, no amount of our words can sanctify anything. If everything was acceptable to be ingested, no one would suffer with indigestion and other gastrointestinal problems. [11 (page 20)]

Once again, neither the dietary laws nor the *Torah* are discounted or removed. Each time, in each instance the *Torah* is upheld and valued. It is only the man-made rules and traditions that are negated. I believe we can conclude that the *Torah* is embraced, upheld, and lived out in the lives of *Yeshua*, *Kefa*, *Ya'akov*, and *Sha'ul*.

With that conclusion, we move to the next section and look at the portion of *Torah* called the *Dietary Laws.*

CHAPTER FOUR

WHY "UNCLEAN"? PIGS AND PEOPLE

As a reminder, we will look at the scriptures detailing thc living things God provided for our nutritional health and those that are not designed for eating. Then, in this section, we will focus on those items in the "Do Not Eat" group and additional scriptures cautioning against the eating of fat and blood.

"The temptation for Adam and Eve in the *Garden of Eden* is the same one that we face today. Will we live our lives by the standard of God's Word as revealed in the *Bible*, or will we decide for ourselves, apart from God, what is good or evil (*Genesis* 3:5)? As regards our topic, will we let God choose our menu for us, and believe that as a God of love He wants only the best for us? Or will we decide that we know better and go our own self-destructive way? The results of this choice for many people can be life or death."[2 (page 1)]

Once again, let's take a look at what God, *Yehovah*, said.

Vayikra (*Leviticus*) 11:1 "*ADONAI* said to *Moshe* and *Aharon*, 2 "Tell the people of *Isra'el*, 'These are the living creatures which you may eat among all the land animals: 3 any that has a separate hoof which is completely divided and chews the cud — these animals you may eat. 4-6 But you are not to eat those that only chew the cud or only have a separate hoof. For example, the camel, the coney and the hare are unclean for you, because they chew the cud but don't have a separate hoof; 7 while the pig is unclean for you, because although it has a separate and completely divided hoof, it doesn't chew the cud.

8 "'You are not to eat meat from these or touch their carcasses; they are unclean for you.

9 "'Of all the things that live in the water, you may eat these: anything in the water that has fins and scales, whether in seas or rivers – these you may eat. 10 But everything in the seas and rivers without both fins and scales, of all the small water-creatures and of all the living creatures in the water, is a detestable thing for you. 11 Yes, these will be detestable for you – you are not to eat their meat, and you are to detest their carcasses. 12 Whatever lacks fins and scales in the water is a detestable thing for you.

13 "'The following creatures of the air are to be detestable for you – they are not to be eaten, they are a detestable thing: the eagle, the vulture, the osprey, 14 the kite, the various kinds of buzzards, 15 the various kinds of ravens, 16 the ostrich, the screech-owl, the

seagull, the various kinds of hawks, 17 the little owl, the cormorant, the great owl, 18 the
horned owl, the pelican, the barn owl, 19 the stork, the various kinds of herons, the hoopoe
and the bat.

20 “‘All winged, swarming creatures that go on all fours are a detestable thing for you; 21
except that of all winged swarming creatures that go on all fours, you may eat those that
have jointed legs above their feet, enabling them to jump off the ground. 22 Specifically,
of these you may eat the various kinds of locusts, grasshoppers, katydids, and crickets. 23
But other than that, all winged swarming creatures having four feet are a detestable thing
to you.

24 “‘The following will make you unclean; whoever touches the carcass of them will be
unclean until evening, 25 and whoever picks up any part of their carcass is to wash his
clothes and be unclean until evening: 26 every animal that has a separate but incompletely
divided hoof or that doesn’t chew the cud is unclean for you; anyone who touches them
will be unclean. 27 Whatever goes on its paws, among all animals that go on all fours, is
unclean for you; whoever touches its carcass will be unclean until evening; and whoever
picks up its carcass is to wash his clothes and be unclean until evening — these are
unclean for you.’”

29 “‘The following are unclean for you among the small creatures that swarm on the
ground: the weasel, the mouse, the various kinds of lizards, 30 the gecko, the land
crocodile, the skink, the sand-lizard, and the chameleon. 31 They are unclean, crawling
creatures; whoever touches them when they are dead will be unclean until evening. 32
Anything on which one of them falls when dead will become unclean – wooden utensils,
articles of clothing, leather, sacking – any utensil used for work; it must be put in water,
and it will be unclean until evening; then it will be clean. *(vii)* 33 If one of them falls into
a clay pot, whatever is in it will become unclean, and you are to break the pot. 34 Any
food permitted to be eaten that water from such a vessel gets on will become unclean, and
any permitted liquid in such a vessel will become unclean. 35 Everything on which any
carcass-part of theirs falls will become unclean, whether oven or stove; it is to be broken
in pieces – they are unclean and will be unclean for you; 36 although a spring or cistern
for collecting water remains clean. But anyone who touches one of their carcasses will
become unclean. 37 If any carcass-part of theirs falls on any kind of seed to be sown, it is
clean; 38 but if water is put on the seed and a carcass-part of theirs falls on it, it is unclean
for you.’”

39 “‘If an animal of a kind that you are permitted to eat dies, whoever touches its carcass
will be unclean until evening. 40 A person who eats meat from its carcass or carries its
carcass is to wash his clothes; he will be unclean until evening.’”

41 “‘Any creature that swarms on the ground is a detestable thing; it is not to be eaten – 42
whatever moves on its stomach, goes on all fours, or has many legs – all creatures that
swarm on the ground; you are not to eat them, because they are a detestable thing. 43 You
are not to make yourselves detestable with any of these swarming, crawling creatures; do
not make yourselves unclean with them, do not defile yourselves with them. 44 For I am
ADONAI your God; therefore, consecrate yourselves and be holy, for I am holy; and do not
defile yourselves with any kind of swarming creature that moves along the ground. 45 For

I am *Adonai*, who brought you up out of the land of Egypt to be your God. Therefore, you are to be holy because I am holy.'"

46 "'Such, then, is the law concerning animals, flying creatures, all living creatures that move about in the water, and all creatures that swarm on the ground. 47 Its purpose is to distinguish between the unclean and the clean, and between the creatures that may be eaten and those that may not be eaten.'"[1 (Page 141-143)]

Yehovah is such a wonderful God of grace, and he provided easy-to-understand ways to show us what we should avoid and what things are safe. It is in the design and function of the animal itself! This is not complicated at all! As from the beginning, deception from the Adversary made something complicated out of something simple.

"Every living organism eats from a different 'menu.' While most of us would not order a rat from our menu, it would make a wonderful meal for a vulture or boa constrictor." [2 (page 2)]

"Many people in Southeast Asia consider dog meat a delicacy, while most Americans would balk at the idea of eating 'filet of Rover.' On the other hand, the Western standard of a hamburger is repulsive to millions of Hindus who consider the cow to be sacred, and possibly even a reincarnated relative. Many cultural eating habits have been eventually shown by scientific discoveries to be harmful or even deadly." [2 (page 3)]

There seem to be four factors that determine choices of food:

- Personal Preference
- Cultural Customs
- Religious Guidelines
- Scientific Recommendation" [2 (page 3)]

All over the world, we find people consuming meat from sources God calls unclean. For instance, in America, people eat catfish, pork, lobster, shrimp, scallops, and more. Some even eat opossum, raccoon, and squirrel. In Asia and Africa, people eat elephants, hippopotamus, and a variety of animals not on the "clean" list.

"Certain parts of Creation were designed by God to be food for Man, and certain parts were not. That divine design is revealed in the Bible, it is totally trustworthy because God cannot lie, and it is totally authoritative because God is the Creator. Scientific standards, cultural customs, and personal preferences are inadequate, apart from the standard of the Bible's dietary laws." [2 (page 5)]

As we notice in the scripture, the words 'unclean' and 'detestable' are used throughout when specifying the animals we are not to use for food, or touch in many cases. That is a strong message! Keep in mind that "the dietary laws cannot save us – Christ alone does that. They do, however, keep us healthier and holier in God's service." [2 (page 52)]

With that in mind, let's take a look at a few of these unclean and detestable choices. Maybe we can see why these labels are placed on these particular creations. Maybe these restrictions are for our good!

While people in the West eat lobster and crab, camels are on the list, too! We are all probably happy about avoiding camel meat. However, Camels are excellent beasts of burden but not entrees!

What then about swine? It is advertised as the ‘other white meat’, but should we be consuming it at all? Pigs will eat just about anything. They are not restricted to vegetation. As scavengers, they are the garbage disposal of the planet! They clean the land as they root the land. This is a great thing! They turn over the soil and add organic matter, which stimulates microbes.

Even with modern science and today’s technologies, pork is still dangerous to eat. No amount of clean eating will change a swine from “unclean” to “clean”. Their “cleanness” isn’t about their environment. Rather, it is about how their body’s design is structured to process what they eat.

As I began my personal journey of regenerating health in my body, I struggled with colitis as well as anemia. Eating Biblically was a very new idea, and I was haphazard in implementing the idea. I continued to struggle with the symptoms of intestinal distress until one day I met people who not only taught biblical eating, but helped me add some safe supplements to my routine. The first food I decided to give up was pork in all its many forms. Within a very short time, my symptoms began to reduce until one day they were gone! I don’t exactly know the timeframe, but I have been one happy pork-free lady for over forty-five years!

“Jesus, as one who was ‘born under [the] law’ (*Galatians* 4:4), did not eat pork. One time, He used pigs as a dumping ground for demons, evicting the demons and destroying the swine (see *Matthew* 8:28-32). This event occurred after weeks of healing various diseases.” [5 (page 147)]

“One reason for God’s rule forbidding pork is that the digestive system of a pig is completely different from that of a cow. It is similar to ours in that the stomach is very acidic. Pigs are gluttonous, never knowing when to stop eating. Their stomach acids become diluted because of the volume of food, allowing all kinds of vermin to pass through this protective barrier. Parasites, bacteria, viruses, and toxins can pass into the pig’s flesh because of overeating. There, the toxins and infectious agents can be passed on to humans when they eat a pig’s flesh.” [5 (page 147)]

“In the *Biblical Archeological Review*, *Jane Cahill* examined the toilets of a Jewish household in Jerusalem, finding no parasites nor infectious agents, but only pollen from the many fruits, vegetables, and herbs they had eaten. A similar study about Egyptians revealed eggs from Schistosoma, Trichinella, Wire Worm, and tapeworms, all found in pork. All of these organisms cause significant chronic diseases.” [5 (page 148)]

Trichinosis is just one of the ‘perils of pork.’ “The primary symptoms of this infection include muscle pain, headaches, fever, and swelling in the extremities.” “These are all nonspecific symptoms that do not necessarily indicate any one disease.” [5 (page 148)]

“In the United States, three of the six most common food-borne parasitic diseases of humans are associated with pork consumption. These include toxoplasmosis, taeniasis or cysticercosis (caused by the pork tapeworm Taenia Solium) and trichinellosis.” [5 (page 148)]

“In Japan, the source of these infections was traced to the flesh of pigs, bears, horses, raccoons, and foxes. All of these animals are listed in scripture as putrid or unclean.” [5 (page 148)]

“Swine are also good incubators of toxic parasites and viruses – although the animal doesn’t usually appear to be ill while carrying these diseases. A scientist at the *University of Giessen Institute for Virology* in Germany showed in a study of worldwide influenza epidemics that pigs are the one animal that can serve as a mixing vessel for new influenza viruses that may seriously threaten world health.” [5 (page 148)]

“If a pig is exposed to a human’s DNA virus and then a bird’s virus, the pig mixes the two viruses – developing a new DNA virus that is often extremely lethal for humans. These viruses have already caused worldwide epidemics and destruction. Virologists have concluded that if we do not find a way to separate humans from pigs, the whole earth’s population may be at risk.” [5 (page 149)]

“Often when a virus moves from one species in which it is harmless to another species, the new species can be devastated by the new variant of virus. The green monkey – another unclean animal – has been shown to do this in connection with the HIV virus. (The swine flu epidemics from Hong Kong, now have been documented to develop by this mechanism.)” [5 (page 152)]

“Other unclean animals can possibly change benign viruses into toxic viruses.” [5 (page 152)]

“The *1942 Yearbook of Agriculture* reported that 50 diseases were found in pigs, and many of these diseases were passed on to humans by eating the pig’s flesh.” “Little wonder that God would inspire His prophet to include eating pork among the disobedient acts of stubborn people who, in addition to idolatry and conjuring up spirits of the dead, ‘continually provoke me to my very face…who eat the flesh of pigs, and whose pots hold broth of unclean meat.’” (*Isaiah* 65:3-4) [5 (page 149)]

“Doesn’t cooking make it safe?” Some think that because we can thoroughly cook food today that it no longer is viable to follow the rules of clean and unclean. But is that true? I would say no. [5 (page 152)]

“Sophisticated ovens and cooking devices have been found in the most ancient archeological ruins, including most of the *Israelites’* ruins.” “They understand that cooking meat is certainly important. Can we safely assume that diseases caused by unclean animals have disappeared because we now cook things better?” [5 (page 153)]

Job 14:4, KJV “Who can bring a clean thing out of an unclean? Not one.” [5 (page 153)]

“Even the microwave oven heats meat unevenly, allowing bacteria and parasites (such as trichinosis) to survive in meat. Many outbreaks of various infections have developed in so-called cooked food. If the food is unclean, don’t count on cooking it to protect you. Some of the most toxic poisons are not destroyed by heat.” [5 (page 153)]

“A sobering report from Scotland revealed that food poisoning by toxins, virus, or bacteria occurred in spite of thorough inspection at every stage of food preparation, including handling and cooking.” [5 (page 153)]

According to the *'No-No'* list used with *Reams Biological Theory of Ionization*, compiled by *Betty Reams Hernandez*, the following are the various pork products to avoid:

"Ham, bacon, sausage, pork ribs, pork chops, jowls, crackling, crisp pork skins, chitterlings, any other part of swine, or anything that contains pork fat or lard. Do not eat hot dogs or bologna, which contain pork." [RBTI No-No List]

When we avoid eating those things called unclean, our bodies can begin to heal. I can attest to this. For many years, pork was included in my lifestyle in the form of ham, bacon, and pork chops. Once I learned that there was a list of foods mentioned in the Bible that I should avoid, I decided to see if following these instructions might help me. I had suffered from digestive issues for years. As I began eliminating the unclean foods and adding more of those foods designed for us to use for fuel, my stomach and intestines thanked me! My story includes more than just the elimination of pork, but it was a great start!

"Shellfish are another group of the deadly 'unclean'. Most of the fancy appetizers and specialties offered in restaurants tend to be shellfish – shrimp cocktail, oysters Rockefeller, stuffed or cracked crab, lobster thermidor, clam chowder, etc. Many Cajun and oriental food recipes include pork and/or shellfish. If more people knew what disease those fancy animals carried, they would pale at the thought of eating such poison. Most shellfish carry one or more parasites in their body which are usually not killed by cooking. In addition, it is unfortunate that many shellfish are eaten raw, which further increases the risk of catching disease from them. One such common and deadly parasite is the tapeworm Diphyllobothrium Latus, which can grow up to seventy-five feet in length inside a person's intestines. Another micro-organism, Bilharziasis, causes urinary schistosomiasis, a painful and debilitating disease of the spleen, liver, intestines, and urinary tract." [2 (page 40)]

"One of the worst of all dangers carried by shellfish is the disease Cholera. This is one of the worst killer diseases of history, with epidemics having wiped out literally millions of people in short periods of time. For instance, two million people died of Cholera in the Middle East and Russia in the early 1800's. And this is not a disease limited to third-world countries. Cholera outbreaks occurred repeatedly in America, as recently as 1981 in Texas and Louisiana." [2 (page 40)]

"Hepatitis is another disease often carried by shellfish. It is an infectious viral disease that attacks a person's liver and may remain in a person for years. There are an estimated 200 million people worldwide with hepatitis, with about 200,000 of them being Americans. There are numerous epidemic outbreaks of this disease every year around the world, and several have been directly linked to shellfish. This is not to say that all shellfish carry hepatitis, but again, there is a serious risk. In general, it is important to remember that shellfish live off scum, and that none of them are disease-free or 'clean.'" [2 (page 40)]

Mattityahu (*Matthew*) [13:47] "Once more, the Kingdom of Heaven is like a net, thrown into the lake, that catches all kinds of fish. [48] When it was full, the fishermen brought the net up onto the shore, sat down and collected the good fish in the baskets, but *threw the bad fish away*." [1 (page 1411)]

In the category of fish, those on the "unclean" list include shellfish, catfish, crab, shrimp, and others. Again, we see they are designed for the clean-up crew, rather than an appetizer. They are the scavengers of the water system's waters. As scavengers, they are very important to the health of lakes, rivers, and seas. However, their high toxicity makes them unfit for human consumption.

We know we can eat fish with fins and scales, but what about fish without scales? The *US Navy Manual for Survival on Land and Sea* lists that "all the important fish with poisonous flesh…lack ordinary scales. Instead, these poisonous fish are covered with bristles or spiny scales, strong, sharp thorns, or spines, or are encased in a bony box-like covering. Some have naked skin, that is, no spines or scales." (*Survival on Land and Sea*, 1944)

Many of these unclean sea creatures like eels, sharks, and catfish, are predatory scavengers. Due to the toxic substance in the blood, eel's blood can be dangerous if it comes in contact with the eyes or another mucus membrane in the human body.

A 1991 study, shared by FDA Consumer, disclosed that raw oysters, clams, and mussels accounted for 85% of all illnesses caused by eating seafood.

When preparing and cooking clean fish, it is important to use proper methods of cleaning, processing, and cooking. Raw or poorly cooked fish can transmit several kinds of parasites, like tapeworms or flukes, as a result of the environment they live in.

Our God cares so much for us that He gives us guidelines to help us avoid the mistakes of consuming things dangerous to our health. God is definitely concerned about our health.

Beyond swine and lobster, there are additional animals and insects created for purposes other than for our food. Even in the category we call fowls, there are specific fowl we can eat and others that are not to be on the menu. Birds specified as scavengers are designed to help in the cleanup and removal of dead animals and garbage. Vultures and seagulls are considered unclean, and as birds of prey or scavengers, they are carnivorous and control the populations of other animals.

Predatory birds usually accumulate high levels of toxic chemicals in their bodies due to dietary habits of eating both the flesh and blood of their prey. This, in turn, makes them not a good food source for humans. [3]

Fortunately, for me, reptiles are on the unclean list. I personally can't imagine eating reptiles, but many people do. They are scavengers and carnivorous, reasons enough to leave them off the menu.

Although I am not a fan of eating grasshoppers and locusts, they are on the clean list and okay for consumption. As a matter of fact, *Yochanon the Immerser* (John the Baptist) enjoyed locust with wild honey!

Mattityahu (Matthew) [3:4] "*Yochanon* wore clothes of camel's hair with a leather belt around his waist, and his food was locusts and wild honey." [1 (page 1387)]

Chargol is a Hebrew word mistranslated sometimes as 'beetle". It is actually a kind of grasshopper. The grasshopper, which eats a clean diet, can be a good substitute for shrimp if needed. Other insects, like ants, worms, bees, caterpillars, cockroaches, and others, are unclean according to scripture. I imagine everyone will agree that cockroaches are not something we even want to eat!

Bees are mentioned above as "unclean", but their honey is clean and healthy too! Proverbs 16:24 likens pleasant words to a honeycomb, "sweet to the taste and healing for the body." [1(page 1089)] Proverb 24:13 says to eat honey for it is good and sweet like God's wisdom. Last is Proverbs 25:16, which gives a warning to eat only as much as you need. Eating too much honey may distress the stomach. [1 (pages 1103 and 1105)]

In addition to *Leviticus* chapter 11, there are other teachings in the *Torah* regarding laws affecting health and relationship with the Creator. We have touched on the laws regarding eating blood previously, but let's visit this topic again in this section.

Vayikra (*Leviticus*) [3:17] "It is to be a permanent regulation through all your generations wherever you live that you will eat neither fat nor blood." [1 (page 132)]

Vayikra (*Leviticus*) [7:26] "You are not to eat any kind of blood, whether from birds or animals, in any of your homes. [27] Whoever eats any blood will be cut off from his people." [1 (page 137)]

Vayikra (*Leviticus*) [17:13] "When someone from the community of *Isra'el* or one of the foreigners living with you hunts and catches game, whether animal or bird that may be eaten, he is to pour out its blood and cover it with earth. [14] For the life of every creature – its blood is its life. Therefore, I said to the people of *Isra'el*, 'You are not to eat the blood of any creature, because the life of every creature is its blood. Whoever eats it will be cut off.'" [1 (page 153)]

Vayikra (Leviticus) [19:26] "Do not eat anything with blood. Do not practice divination or fortune-telling." [1 (page 155)]

Vayikra (*Leviticus*) [22:8] "But he is not to eat anything that dies naturally or is torn to death by wild animals and thereby make himself unclean; I am *ADONAI*." [1 (page 158)]

D'Varim (*Deuteronomy*) [12:23] "Just take care not to eat the blood, for the blood is the life, and you are not to eat the life with the meat. [24] Don't eat it, but pour it out on the ground like water. [25] Do not eat it, so that things will go well with you and with your children after you, as you do what *ADONAI* sees as right." [1 (page 244-245)]

Throughout scripture, *Yehovah* instructs us not to eat blood. This is an important restriction we should respect. Our bloodstreams are our waste disposal systems. The bloodstream carries toxins and waste away from the muscles and organs, and also removes viruses and more. Knowing this, we can agree that blood is not hygienic, nor clean!

What about products made of blood? I didn't know that there were "foods" made of blood, but there are! Products such as blood pudding, canned meats with blood by-products, and blood sausage would definitely not be acceptable or condoned by our Heavenly Father! This is true even when the animal slaughtered is considered clean.

We have a guideline in Exodus 12:46 of the procedure in place for slaughtering a lamb. This scripture is regarding the Passover Lamb, but is the best way to allow an animal's body to be free of as much blood as possible and have no bones broken. The goal of the butcher is to slit the animal's throat quickly, bringing a quick, clean, and humane death to the animal. The animal is then hung to let the blood drain efficiently.

Today, some people prefer to eat meats that have gone through a process that we know as *Kosher*. This is a very humane slaughter, but goes a bit further. The meat is put through extensive washing, and then salt is used to remove any additional blood. Spices and herbs are added to flavor the meat and make it tender. Kosher rules go beyond slaughter, having guidelines for foods, dairy, household products, supplements, and even the facility where they are prepared. Although not specifically found in the Bible, they are good processes for purity and cleanness.

Blood does contain minerals and nutrients as well as waste products. When the blood is poured on the ground, it is not wasted, but helps mineralize the soil. It follows the path it was intended to and nourishes the ground.

Scriptures also teach that we are not to eat meat from animals that die in manners other than proper slaughter. If the animal was killed by another animal, died of old age, or through an accident, it was considered unclean and was not for consumption. If properly slaughtered, the animal would have the least amount of stress, and therefore the meat would not be tainted by stress hormones pulsing through the body, making it less nutritious and perhaps harmful. We see the care *Yehovah* has is not just for the animals, but concern for us too!

Also, what did *ADONAI,* God, say about fat? A difficult topic to tackle for sure.

Vayikra (*Leviticus*) 3:12 "If his offering is a goat, then he is to present it before *ADONAI*. 13
He is to lay his hand on its head and slaughter it in front of the tent of meeting, and the
sons of *Aharon* are to splash its blood against all sides of the altar. 14 He is to present
from it his offering, an offering made by fire to *ADONAI*; it is to consist of the fat covering
the inner organs, all the fat above the inner organs, 15 the two kidneys, the fat on them
near the flanks, and the covering of the liver, which he will remove with the kidneys. 16
The *cohen* will make them go up in smoke on the altar; it is food, an offering made by
fire to be a fragrant aroma; all the fat belongs to *ADONAI*. 17 It is to be a permanent
regulation through all your generations wherever you live that you will eat neither fat nor
blood." [1 (page 132)]

Vayikra (*Leviticus*) 7:22 "*ADONAI* said to *Moshe*, 23 'Say to the people of *Isra'el*, 'You are
not to eat the fat of bulls, sheep, or goats. 24 The fat of animals that die of themselves or
are killed by wild animals may be used for any other purpose, but under no circumstances
are you to eat it. 25 For whoever eats the fat of animals of the kind used in presenting an
offering made by fire to *ADONAI* will be cut off from his people.''' [1 (page 137)]

"From medical research, we now understand that fat is a tissue in which the body stores energy. When a meal is missed, the body breaks down fat and uses the fat as fuel for energy. Unfortunately, animal fat is also a storage place for toxins and parasites. These toxins are found in the fat of all animals we eat. Examples include DDT, insecticides, herbicides, antibiotics, hormones, and various other chemicals the animals have ingested, breathed, or touched." [5 (page 30)]

"In 1979, a hormone called DES (diethylstilbestrol) was removed from the market because researchers learned that this substance caused cancer in the vagina and cervix in daughters of women who had received the drug to prevent miscarriage. They found that the stockyards throughout the United States injected beef cattle with large amounts of DES because it enabled the animals to gain weight rapidly. And sure enough, the hormone was stored in the animal's fat tissue." [5 (page 31)]

"Scientists have also discovered other hormones added to food that produce cancer, and many of these hormones are found in higher concentrations in the fat that covers meats." [5 (page 31)]

"Hard fat (i.e., fat that is firmest at room temperature and is most saturated) is the most toxic fat for the human body. The increased consumption of hard fats in our day has been accompanied by increased vascular disease, cancers of the breast, colon, and prostate, along with many other chronic diseases." [5 (page 31)]

"The hardest fats are found in cows (oxen), sheep, and goats." We see "God's protective hand and divine design in *Leviticus* 7:23, where He exclusively lists these three animals." [5 (page 31)] There are different types of fats - visceral and muscular fat. The visceral fat, mentioned in Leviticus, protects internal organs. It serves as an energy reserve for the animal and a cushion for the organs. This is the fat used in burnt offerings sacrificed along with the entrails and internal organs of the animals. It was an offering completely burnt, symbolizing dedication and purification.

The other type of fat is muscular fat. This is generally marbled throughout the muscle meat. It is not possible to remove this fat completely, but much will be removed through broiling, baking, grilling, and other ways of cooking. Intramuscular fat develops later and can be seen as a determinant of meat quality, flavor, and tenderness.

In the manufacture of hot dogs and hamburgers, many times fat is injected to the mix to reach 30% fat content in the product. No wonder people are dying from clogged arteries, heart disease, and strokes. Animal fats contain small amounts of naturally occurring trans fats produced in the digestive system of the animal. Vegetable oils become chemical trans fats when they are hydrogenated. Hydrogenated fats in any form are not natural, and these fats are breaking the ordinance of avoiding fats. According to the law of reaping and sowing, we will reap ill health if we sow bad foods in our lives. When we are preparing meats or other fatty foods, we need to remember to remove as much of the blood and fat as possible.

Let's take a look at three curious scriptures. These are noted three times in scripture, and it makes them sound like they are part of the Dietary Laws. But are they? Let's take a look and see if we can determine the true meaning.

Sh'mot (*Exodus*) [23:19b] "You are not to boil a young animal in its mother's milk." [1 (page 103)]

Sh'mot (*Exodus*) [34:26] "You are not to boil a young goat in its mother's milk." [1 (page 119)]

D'varim (*Deuteronomy*) [14:21b] "You are not to boil a young animal in its mother's milk." [1 (page 246)]

What do these scriptures mean? In my mind, I was pretty sure this was a command that we should never have a cheeseburger or some kind of dish that would combine dairy with meat! I had never heard this one, but actually, it makes much more sense once we dig deeper. It is definitely a fact that a cheeseburger or spaghetti with meat and cheese are both meals that probably have too much fat and can lead to heart disease, excess weight, and more. But did the Hebrew people see it that way? Was that what God meant?

The preincarnate *Yeshua* Jesus enjoyed a meal with *Avraham* and Sarah before promising them a child. One big difference was the calf, already born, was prepared separately from the curds and milk.

B'resheet (*Genesis*) [18:1] "*ADONAI* appeared to *Avraham* by the oaks of *Mamre* as he sat at the entrance to the tent during the heat of the day. [2] He raised his eyes and looked, and there in front of him stood three men. On seeing them, he ran from the tent door to meet them, prostrated himself on the ground, [3] and said, 'My lord, if I have found favor in your sight, please don't leave your servant. [4] Please let me send for some water, so that you can wash your feet; then rest under the tree, [5] and I will bring a piece of bread. Now that you have come to your servant, refresh yourselves before going on.' 'Very well, they replied, 'do what you have said.' [6] *Avraham* hurried into the tent to Sarah and said, 'Quickly, three measures of the best flour! Knead it and make cakes.' [7] *Avraham* ran to the herd, took a good, tender calf, and gave it to the servant, who hurried to prepare it. [8] Then he took curds, milk, and the calf which he had prepared, and set it all before the men; and he stood by them under the tree as they ate." [1 (page 24)]

With that, I think that dairy and meat at the same meal is not against dietary rules. I still caution you to be careful about the fat and consume it in moderation.

So what do the scriptures mean? One day, I was listening to a talk by *Nehemia Gordon*, who mentioned these very scriptures. He stated that no one really knew what they meant for sure, but one theory is that the rule was more about avoiding the practice of pagan rituals than avoiding cheeseburgers. [(*The Hebrew Yeshua vs The Greek Jesus*, 2005)]

Evidently, pagan worshippers of that timeframe participated in fertility rites in which a baby goat was cooked in the milk of the mother. They would then sprinkle the broth on their gardens and fields in hope of pleasing their gods and maybe increasing the crop yield. *Yehovah* was not pleased with this pagan magic and specified three times that this was unacceptable.

This ritual was not a dietary rule, but a rule to avoid idolatry and pagan ways.

The pagan theory seems to fit, but could there be even more to this scripture?

"The secret to solving the puzzle is context. We simply have to look at these verses in context. In all three places where this sentence is mentioned in the Bible, it seems to be very disjointed, just coming at us abruptly and seemingly out of nowhere. That is because to us it has no context related to it. However, if we look at the verse from a different light, we see something different." [6 (Seeking Scripture)]

Let's look at each of these verses in context with the verses previously noted and the complete verse itself.

Sh'mot (*Exodus*) 23:14 "'Three times a year, you are to observe a festival for me. 15 Keep the festival of *matzah*: for seven days, as I ordered you, you are to eat *matzah* at the time determined in the month of *Aviv*; for it was in the month that you left Egypt. No one is to appear before me empty-handed. 16 Next, the festival of harvest, the first fruits of your efforts sowing in the field; and last, the festival of ingathering, at the end of the year, when you gather in from the fields the results of your efforts. 17 Three times a year all your men are to appear before the Lord, *Adonai*. 18 You are not to offer the blood of sacrifice with leavened bread, nor is the fat of my festival to remain all night until morning. 19 You are to bring the best first fruits of your land into the house of *Adonai* your God. You are not to boil a young animal in its mother's milk.'" [1 (page 103)]

Sh'mot (*Exodus*) 34:22 "'Observe the festival of *Shavu'ot* with the first-gathered produce of the wheat harvest, and the festival of ingathering at the turn of the year. 23 Three times a year all your men are to appear before the Lord, *Adonai*, the God of *Isra'el*. 24 For I am going to expel nations ahead of you and expand your territory, and no one will ever even covet your land when you go up to appear before *Adonai* your God three times a year. 25 You are not to offer the blood of my sacrifice with leavened bread, and the sacrifice of the feast of *Pesach* is not to be left until morning. 26 You are to bring the best first fruits of your land into the house of *Adonai* your God. You are not to boil a young goat in its mother's milk.'" 27 "*Adonai* said to *Moshe*, 'Write these words down, because they are the terms of the covenant, I have made with you and with *Isra'el*.'" [1 (page 119)]

D'varim (*Deuteronomy*) 14:21 "'You are not to eat any animal that dies naturally; although you may let a stranger staying with you eat it, or sell it to a foreigner, because you are a holy people for *Adonai* your God. You are not to boil a young animal in its mother's milk. 22 Every year you must take one tenth of everything your seed produces in the field, 23 and eat it in the presence of *Adonai* your God. In the place where he chooses to have his name live you will eat the tenth of your grain, new wine and olive oil, and the firstborn of your cattle and sheep, so that you will learn to fear *Adonai* your God always.'" [1 (page 246)]

"Now, we can see that the first two times it appears is **directly following a mention of first fruit offerings**, the best of the best. The third time we see mention of offerings is after the statement, but in reference to year-by-year offerings, this is key.

"You see, the *Israelites* were accustomed to being mistreated by their landlords and overseers and so when it came to sustaining themselves, things were understandably difficult and made more so by their 'superior's.' As slaves in this land (Egypt), they would have been forced into making offerings to these false gods which their rulers worshipped. Now with their own resources scarce and them likely not even worshipping these gods actually, it is highly probable to assume they had the practice of trying to shortchange on the offerings in order to keep some for themselves.

"So, if you bring the first fruits of your wheat, you could take some of last year's wheat from the bottom of the barrel and mix it with the latest, better wheat, and thereby present a lower quality offering while keeping more of the better quality to feed your family with.

"So, the premise is that ***this could be a Hebrew idiom***. The mother's milk represents a previous generation, and the young goat is the latest, newest, best of a new generation. This figure of speech could mean, according to speculation, not to combine the old with the new or one generation of produce with the next.

I think we can see that "the primary support for the theory that is the most plausible at this point lies in the context of the scriptures. Let's look at those verses, *Exodus* 23:19 and *Exodus* 34:26, again with this in mind… The context is offering your first fruits. Not your leftovers. Not food from last year, but your first fruits." [6 (Seeking Scripture)]

Now let's look at the *Deuteronomy* appearance and see what we learn.

"In this example, the phrase leads to a commentary about first fruits, particularly, making your offerings from the seed year by year, not last year's seed mixed with this year's, but each year you are to make an offering **from that year's seed**.

"If it is a *Hebrew idiom* which means do not combine the old with the new or one generation of produce with the next, we finally have the sentence that agrees in context within the verses it appears in. However, this is merely speculation, and it is surely not a salvation issue." "Bring the first fruits of your time to the Father, not leftovers and don't boil a young goat in its mother's milk!" [6 (Seeking Scripture)]

The scripture, *Deuteronomy* 14:21, does fall in the chapter reminding the people of the various Dietary Laws and other teachings in the *Torah*. It certainly may have the hidden message for first fruit offerings but may be a caution against pagan worship as well. These are scriptures that have caused confusion for years.

Agriculturally, I understand that actually cooking the kid in its mother's milk would pose a problem for the mother. I'm told that female animals self-ween their young when the animal is old enough and mature enough to survive on its own. By that point, the mother has typically healed and recovered enough to get pregnant again. Killing the baby or removing it from its mother before weaning puts the mother in an odd cycle for reproduction. From an agricultural point of view, it makes sense that *ADONAI* has concern for the animals' life, growth, and reproduction cycle.

With these various theories, we can see that they don't fall under Dietary Laws, and it may need to be left as a mystery in scripture for now.

In the next section we look at how swine, monkeys, bats, and other 'unclean' creatures not only cause disease, but they have been used in research, pharmaceuticals, and foods.

CHAPTER FIVE

DISEASE, PHARMACEUTICALS AND MEDICINE. CLEAN OR UNCLEAN?

To Keep *Torah* or Not to Keep *Torah*?

As we look at the diseases we experience as a result of disregarding *Yehovah's Torah*, let's start with a look at the promise He gave in *Exodus* 15:22-27.

Sh'mot (*Exodus*)[15:22] "*Moshe* led *Isra'el* onward from the *Sea of Suf*. They went out into the *Shur Desert*; but after traveling three days in the desert, they had found no water. [23] They arrived at *Marah* but couldn't drink the water there, because it was bitter. This is why they called it *Marah* ('bitterness'). [24] The people grumbled against *Moshe* and asked, 'What are we to drink?' [25] *Moshe* cried to *ADONAI*; and *ADONAI* showed him a certain piece of wood, which, when he threw it into the water, made the water taste good. There *ADONAI* made laws and rules of life for them, and there he tested them. [26] He said, 'If you will listen intently to the voice of *ADONAI* your God, do what he considered right, pay attention to his *mitzvot* and observe his laws, I will not afflict you with any of the diseases I brought on the Egyptians; because I am *ADONAI* your healer.'" [1 (page 92)]

The Israelites had just made an escape from the Egyptians and *ADONAI* had provided not only safe passage in a miraculous way but had 'healed' the water so they could be nourished in the desert. Truly He was their Way Maker, Provider and Healer! He is ours as well! As with any relationship or covenant, there must be observance to something or someone, and obedience to the same. In this case, *ADONAI* provided his *Torah*, the rules and guidance he provides for our good. Our part is to know His *Torah* and grow in obedience.

Mikhah (*Micah*) [6:8] "*ADONAI* says, 'Human being, you have already been told what is good, what *ADONAI* demands of you – no more than to act justly, love grace and walk in purity with your God.'" [1 (page 846)]

Mattityahu (*Matthew*) [11:25] "It was at that time that *Yeshua* said, 'I thank you, Father, Lord of heaven and earth, that you concealed these things from the sophisticated and educated and revealed them to ordinary folks. [26] Yes, Father, I thank you that it pleased you to do this. [27] My Father has handed over everything to me. Indeed, no one fully knows the Son except the Father, and no one fully knows the Father except the Son and those to whom

the Son wishes to reveal him. 28 Come to me, all of you who are struggling and
burdened, and I will give you rest. 29 Take my yoke upon you and learn from me, because
I am gentle and humble in heart, and you will find rest for your souls. [b] 30 For my yoke is
easy, and my burden is light.'" b Jeremiah 6:16; 1 (page 1405)

What is this yoke he speaks of? What does it mean? Most of us know that a yoke is used with oxen or other animals. I once purchased a goat yoke! I had no goats, but I understood that for proper use, two goats would be required. The older goat is more experienced and the other younger one needs to learn. The older one helps the young one learn how things work properly. Using this term from *Yeshua*, He is the wiser teacher, and we need to be yoked to him to understand the will of the Father.

A note regarding *Jeremiah* 6:16 has the answer! "'Ask about the ancient paths.' Both Christian and Jewish commentators see the 'ancient paths' as *Torah* observance and the spiritual paths of the patriarchs, as well as those who experienced redemption from slavery in Egypt. The 'ancient paths' are demonstrated by a life of faithfulness to *ADONAI* and his instruction." [1 (page 622)]

The term *yoke* that *Yeshua*, Jesus, uses in *Matthew* speaks of the *Torah* and *ADONAI'S* instruction. He and the Father are One. Therefore, if we focus on the consequences of disobedience to his Word, we won't experience the provisions offered by the Father in the covenant. We will be distracted by disobedience and will have been deceived. The Adversary once again will have thrown out stumbling blocks and we possibly will fall for the trap!

Sadly, we are a disobedient people. We have chosen disobedience, and we have been deceived. As we know, the Adversary seeks to kill, steal, and destroy.

Yochanon (*John*) 10:10 *Yeshua* says, "'The thief comes to steal, kill, and destroy; I have come so that they may have life, life in its fullest measure.'" [1 (page 1537)]

Knowing this, we must be on our guard always and seek the Truth for our own good.

"Despite the fact that the United States has the world's best medical facilities, the average life span has only recently increased to 74 years!!!" [7 (page 29)]

In *Psalm* 90:7 we see what has happened because of disobedience.

Tehillim (*Psalm*) 90:7 "For we are destroyed by your anger, overwhelmed by your wrath. 8
You have placed our faults before you, our secret sins in the full light of your presence. 9
All our days ebb away under your wrath; our years die away like a sigh. 10 The span of
our life is seventy years, or if we are strong, eighty; yet at best it is toil and sorrow, over
in a moment, and then we are gone." [1 (page 997)]

From the time of Adam, who lived 930 years, we have certainly slipped to an all-time low.

"Scripture and medical research agree that modern lifestyles lived without reference to God's laws and design shorten life and hasten death." [7 (page 30)]

"The Bible is bold in promising us health according to His design. God's reputation is dependent on His promises to us for health." [7 (page 40)] But the ball is in our court, and we need to follow Him.

Mishlei (*Proverbs*) [4:20] "My son, pay attention to what I am saying; incline your ear to my words. [21] Don't let them out of your sight; keep them deep in your heart; [22] for they are life to those who find them; and health to their whole being." [1 (page 1068)]

Diseases Ancient and Modern - Egypt and the U.S.

Again, *Yehovah's* Word says, "If you will listen intently to the voice of *ADONAI* your God, do what He considered right, pay attention to His *mitzvot* and observe His laws, I will not afflict you with any of the diseases I brought on the Egyptians; because I am *ADONAI* your healer." *Sh'mot* (*Exodus*) 15:26. [1 (page 92)]

"What were the diseases God brought upon the Egyptians? Do they exist today?" [7 (page 40)]

"We have a clear idea of the Egyptian diseases from radiographs and autopsies performed on mummies by paleopathologist, *Marc A. Ruffer* and others. These studies show that many Egyptians had the same diseases that still cause illness today." [7 (page 40)]

"The most common affliction of the Egyptians appears to be vascular diseases that resulted in severely calcified arteries. Other common maladies included arthritis, tooth decay, infections, cancer, emphysema, tuberculosis, parasites, pneumonia, and obesity. Childbirth, deaths and infections after birth are fairly common. "[7 (page 40)]

"Mummified pharaohs often show the most advanced degenerative diseases. Historically, "pharaohs and other royalty (see 1 *Kings* 4:22; *Amos* 6:4) were the only ones whose diets included large quantities of meat and other delicacies." [7 (page 40)]

"Modern research is showing that following the same ordinances God gave His people to protect them from the diseases of the Egyptians would help protect us from disease today." [7 (page 41)]

"LEADING CAUSES OF DEATH IN THE U.S. – 1990

1. Heart Disease
2. Cancer
3. Cerebrovascular Disease
4. Chronic Lung Disease
5. Accidents
6. Pneumonia
7. Diabetes Mellitus
8. Atherosclerosis
9. Suicide
10. HIV
11. Hepatitis and cirrhosis" [7 (page 41)]

"These modern diseases show the consequences of disobedience to God's ordinances." [7] (page 41)

"Hardening of the arteries is also known as arteriosclerosis and is implicated in heart disease, cerebrovascular disease, and atherosclerosis. The first case of myocardial infarction was reported in the medical literature in 1906. Now the disease is so common that the smallest hospitals have special units for such patients. Hard animal fat has a fatty acid that is sticky and causes platelets to clump together. Most of the things we are warned to avoid in Scripture contribute to this disease." [7 (page 43)]

Let's take a look at the history of many diseases and plagues that have been destructive to humankind throughout history. *Michael Rood*, in his DVD series called "*These Things Are Unclean To You*" gives us an overview.

Here we go:

Bubonic Plague, aka as the *Black Plague*: It is said it was caused by fleas from rodents. The fleas were carrying a bacteria called *Bacterium Yersinia Pestis.* Interestingly, the European Jewish people did not suffer with the plague and were therefore blamed for the deaths and illness. However, it was not by their actions that the plague spread. It was the guidelines in *Torah* that provided a foundation of health that kept the Jewish community safe from the plague. Christians who didn't follow *Torah*, did not survive the plague. [6]

Hygiene in the Word?

"Many passages in the *Word of God* instruct in hygiene, including cleansing the body inside and out, cleaning houses, clothing, cooking utensils, stoves, the proper handling of human waste, and more. Part of the cleansing when one was healed of the plague of leprosy sounds like this." [2]

Leviticus 14:8 "And he that is to be cleansed shall wash his clothes, and shave off all his hair, and wash himself in water, that he may be clean: and after that he shall come into the camp and shall tarry abroad out of his tent seven days. 9 But it shall be on the seventh day, that he shall shave all his hair off his head and his beard and his eyebrows, even all his hair he shall shave off: and he shall wash his clothes, also he shall wash his flesh in water, and he shall be clean." [2]

"The hygiene of the community was also addressed. The Scriptures direct the obedient to bury the waste that comes from the body." [2]

D'varim (*Deuteronomy*) 23:13 (12) "Also you are to have an area outside the camp to use as a latrine. 14 (13) You must include a trowel with your equipment, and when you relieve yourself, you are to dig a hole first and afterwards cover your excrement. 15 (14) For *Adonai* your God moves about in your camp to rescue you and to hand over your enemies to you. Therefore, your camp must be a holy place. [*Adonai*] should not see anything indecent among you, or he will turn away from you." [1 (page 256)]

Disobedience to Torah and Disease

Disease, plagues, and leprosy are a result of disobedience to and ignoring the *Torah's* help. Other diseases, as a result of disobedience and cultural habits. [6]

Measles, which has killed about 200 million people, and Smallpox are both a result of mishandling and misuse of sheep. [6]

Nikah Virus (*NIV*) is a zoonotic virus, which means it can spread between animals and people. It comes from mishandling and misuse of pigs and can come from Fruit bats as well. [6]

Whooping cough, or pertussis, can also come through the mishandling and misuse of pigs. [6]

H1N1, also called the bird flu, is from mismanagement of birds. [6]

Coronavirus can come from the blood of bats and bush meats. It too is a result of misuse and manipulation. [6]

SARS can come from an *Indonesian Palm Civet Cat*. They are fed coffee beans which do not digest but result in a coffee bean called Fox Dung coffee. [6]

Monkey pox, or *West Nile* virus develops from jungle pets. [6]

Leprosy in *Egyptians* came from misuse and manipulation of water buffalo. [6]

HIV is a result of misuse and manipulation of chimpanzees and the great apes. [6]

As the viruses go through various communities, immunity is built up. However, for those in other areas, their immunity will not properly have the defensive reaction. We will look more at viruses in a bit. [6]

The one thing all these diseases have in common is they are a result of in some way coming in contact with animals that are considered by our Creator as unclean. Sadly, an entire industry has formed around concocting solutions from not only the animals, but the viruses themselves. We were warned about ingesting or touching the unclean, but now the unclean is injected in us under the name of vaccines and given to us in the form of pills. What good can possibly come from this?

Pharmekia - What Is This?

Sadly, *pharmakeia*, also known as sorcery and the occult, is nothing new. The Bible is full of warnings against the occult, drugs, and idol worship.

"*Strong's* G5331 describes *pharmakeia* as:

1. The use or the administering of drugs
2. Poisoning
3. Sorcery, magical arts, often found in connection with idolatry and fostered by it.
4. *Metaph,* the deceptions and seductions of idolatry.

Strong's G5332 gives the pronunciation of *pharmakeia* as 'far-mak-i-ah'. It means medication (pharmacy). i.e. (by extension) magic (literally or figuratively): sorcery, witchcraft." 3 Article: Revelation Scriptures – Discover Babylon's Deception by Pharmakeia / Sorcery. Revelation 18:23

The history of pharmacology shows several meanings for the word *pharmakon*. *Pharmakon* is where we get the name of the pharmacology industry and pharmacology itself. The meanings are *remedy*, *charm* and *poison*. Something to think about.

Over the centuries, natural healers have used herbs, minerals, herbs, vegetables and sometimes animal parts in the quest for healing. They weren't concerned about research and science so much. Results were what they were seeking. Results to restore well-being and balance.

Sometimes the power of suggestion and a placebo is all that is needed. My dad was a drug salesman many years ago. He would talk about the many sugar pills that were dispensed. Many times the sugar pills did the trick. Beliefs can be a strong motivator and our bodies react to our thoughts and words!

The study of drugs and their interactions with living organisms is the study of pharmacology. It seeks to discover how drugs act in the body including looking at possible side effects. Through trial and error the correct dose of medication is determined.

As we look back at the history of the medical industry, pharmacology is one of the oldest branches within the industry. The Egyptians and the Sumerians kept records of how they utilized their drugs as far back as 4000 years ago. Diseases were treated with interesting substances like lizard's blood and frog's bile, and many other strange concoctions. [11]

Moldy bread, an early form of penicillin, was used by the Egyptians. Eber's Papyrus, an Egyptian record dating back to 1500BC was found in the 1800's. The scroll had a record of 800 different herbal mixtures. They also used oils extracted from plants known to help the body heal. We use these same oils today with the essential oils used externally and in aromatherapy. [11]

King Tut's tomb was opened in 1922. 350 alabaster jars of various plant oils were discovered inside. In Mexico it is known that *King Montezuma* had gardens of medicinal plants. Herbs with medicinal characteristics were also grown by the Aztec Indians.

All over the world healers have been using the garden gifts provided us by *Yehovah*. They have gone by many names over time - traditional healers, herbalists, holistic healers, medicine men and many more. Many times the various traditions in healing were passed down through families. Passed down through generations as there might not be a healer in the community.

Let's look at some examples of medicines created from animals considered *unclean*.

Some Thyroid supplements are made of animal thyroid gland tissues. It is called Desiccated Thyroid Extract (DTE) and is hard to regulate. Many times, the thyroid medicine is made from the thyroid gland of pigs. And, as we know, we are not to touch swine, much less eat one hoping for better health. [11]

Another commonly prescribed medication is Premarin™ (conjugated estrogens). This medication is sometimes suggested to relieve symptoms of menopause. It is made from the urine of pregnant mares! The name Permarin™ stands for 'pregnant mare.' As we have discussed, horses were not created as food and are not considered clean. It is possible the side effects from these products might be because the source is not something designed to be in our bodies. [11]

Originally many drugs were created from natural plants, herbs, and oils. Many now are modified with chemicals and molecularly restructured to make new and stronger drugs. It used to be that the pharmacist would actually prepare the medications and provide information to educate the patient. Now pharmacists primarily dispense synthetic medications made by drug companies. The combinations may have tissues from animals or fetuses with added elements like mercury. With the average person over sixty on 19 medications, how can they keep up with all the side effects and dangerous interactions?

The pharmaceutical industry changed their education program during the Vietnam War years. Prior to the war, students had to identify herbs and plants by their leaves, roots and flowers. I understand that those pharmacists trained after the war, have none of that education. Those requirements were removed. Pharmacists were no longer educated in herbal based medicine.

The process in creating many drugs and vitamins supplements come from by-products and chemical compounds of the petroleum industry. Antihistamines, cough syrups, antibacterials, analgesics, creams, gels and ointments, aspirin and other over the counter drugs have petrochemicals in their mixture.

The raw materials used as starting points to the manufacture of medicines are called pharmaceutical feedstocks. These materials can be chemicals or biological. They are from petrochemicals like natural gas or can be animal derived ingredients like cartilage, pancreases etc. Time-release drugs slowly dissolve as a result of the tartaric acid-based polymers. Capsules and coatings are frequently polymer based too.

These manufacturing processes are used for most vitamin supplements too! Once I did an experiment using two well known supplement brands and one natural food based supplement. I don't recommend doing this at home, but I slowly baked the supplements at a very low temperature in the oven. The natural supplement was baked and just sort of looked toasted. The other two were made from these chemical petroleum products. Oh my, did my kitchen smell with the fragrance of burned rubber. They also turned black. Again, do not do that experiment in your home! It took forever to get the smell out of the house.

There are two ways to discover new drugs.

1. Researching soil samples and other parts of the environment may lead to discoveries of new chemical substances.
2. Utilizing existing drugs, manipulation of the molecules, may give way to a new chemical that has different or additional properties benefiting in a new way. These can be synthetic or partly synthetic depending on the source.

Advancements in drug development such as gene splicing, a form of genetic engineering, is called Recombinant DNA technology. Through this process researchers use enzymes to remove.

DNA - Miraculous Language

DNA from one type of organism and transfer it to a different organism. Through this procedure the organism that received the DNA is now directed by the new DNA to produce a different substance. Common bacterium are normally used as they multiply rapidly. These chemicals are created in large vats allowing the production of unlimited amounts of drugs. [11]

What could possibly go wrong? Mixing concoctions and brewing up mixtures in order to get some kind of result! And all with substances that were never intended for use in the body in any way, shape, or form! Our very image is being compromised. What is this DNA the sorcerers are meddling with?

"DNA has been called the most mysterious molecule in the universe. The information that it contains cannot be explained by any natural process. The sequence of chemicals on the DNA molecule is used to construct every other molecule in the human body. Yet, neither the structure nor the information contained therein can be reproduced in a laboratory by mixing the four chemical components from which DNA is constructed. All attempts to do so have been as fruitless as trying to develop any of the 22 million books in the *Library of Congress* by having a monkey randomly doodle symbols on a piece of paper. [12 (Page April 22)]

"One gram (0.0022 lb.) of DNA can hold as much information as one trillion CD's. Stated another way, this information storage system is so efficient that a microscopic speck smaller that a dust particle could hold a copy of every high-resolution movie ever produced – with room to spare for every movie made for the next hundred years. As advanced as modern technology has become, mankind's greatest achievements and mighty technological advances are child's play when compared with that which God has produced." [12 (Page April 22)]

"DNA is a language:

- A language is a series of non-repeating symbols that carry a meaning. DNA is a series of non-repeating chemicals that carry information.
- A language causes a response by those receiving the message. DNA causes responses to happen throughout the cells within our bodies.
- Language has structure provided by spaces, punctuation, and divisions in the text. DNA is structured in this way.
- A language transfers information. DNA is the most compact information transporting system in the universe.
- Most importantly, a language has an author. No information can exist without an intelligent source.

"Who authored DNA? Who put the unbelievably complex design and unfathomable quantity of information upon the DNA code of every human being? The Bible gives us the answer. One of the many names of Jesus Christ is the 'author of life'. He is the ultimate author for he wrote the very language found upon the DNA molecule – the language of life." [12 (page February 27)]

"There are approximately 200,000 different proteins that make up the majority of the structures within the human body. As far as we know, every one of these proteins has some useful, functional purpose. Why are our bodies not full of useless leftover chemicals from our evolutionary past? The proteins vary from the crystal-clear protein solution within our eyeballs to the enamel on our teeth. Starting out as a single cell (dividing and doubling in size approximately every 30 minutes) and forming increasingly complex structures, our bodies know how, where, when, and how much of each of these proteins form. Too much and we die. Too little and we die. Tissue produced in the wrong location, and we die.

"Most amazing is how each protein is produced. They are formed from coded information upon the DNA molecule. But to form each protein, a little protein machine must attach to the DNA at just the right point to start the process. **Then a different protein machine must start the unzipping process**. Next, a third protein machine must line up a special molecule (RNA) of exactly the right length, and a fourth protein must know when to stop the copying process. The RNA passes through a fifth protein machine that allows an exact copy of the information to be made.

"Here is the trillion-dollar conundrum. Biologically useful proteins NEVER exist in nature unless DNA makes them, and DNA cannot be made, or unzipped, without these proteins. So, where did either one come from? Just as you can't have a chicken without an egg, you can't have an egg without the chicken (chickens were formed with eggs already inside the female chicken). The obvious answer is that the entire system was created simultaneously – yet this is the one answer not to be allowed to be considered by students." [12 (page March 9)]

As scripture says in *Psalm* 139, "We are wonderfully made!"

Modern Medical Industry - A Bit of History

Several scriptures come to mind when considering what has happened in the medical industry. Let's take a look at a few. Nothing is a surprise to *Yehovah*!

Romans [1:18] "What is revealed is God's anger from heaven against all the godlessness and wickedness of people who in their wickedness keep suppressing the truth: [19] because what is known about God is plain to them, since God has made it plain to them. [20] For ever since the creation of the universe his invisible qualities – both his eternal power and his divine nature – have been clearly seen, because they can be understood from what he has made. Therefore, they have no excuse; [21] because, although they know who God is, they do not glorify him as God or thank him. On the contrary, they have become futile in their thinking; and their undiscerning hearts become darkened. [22] Claiming to be wise, they have become fools! [23] In fact, they have exchanged the glory of the immortal God for mere images, like a mortal human being, or like birds, animals, or reptiles!" [1 (page 1601)]

Revelation [18:23] "the light of a lamp will never again shine in you; the voice of bridegroom and bride will never again be heard in you. 'For your businessmen were the most powerful on earth, all the nations were deceived by your magic spell.'" [1 (page 1804)]

Galatians [5:19] "And it is perfectly evident what the old nature does. It expresses itself in sexual immorality, impurity and indecency; [20] involvement with the occult and with drugs; in feuding, fighting, becoming jealous and getting angry; in selfish ambition, factionalism, intrigue [21] and envy; in drunkenness, orgies, and things like these, I warn you now as I have warned you before; those who do such things will have no share in the Kingdom of God!" [1 (page 1676)]

"Sickness is a natural consequence of living surrounded by adversaries that attack us from within and from without. Not to worry, our lives are safe because of unprecedented advances in medical science, new knowledge and amazing technology is at our service to counteract the ravages of our world. But how safe are we really?" [10 (page 129, 130)]

There are two types of techniques or focuses on medicine – Patient-centered conservative focus or Disease-centered criteria. [10 (page 131)]

"Disease-centered criteria, set by the all-powerful medical institutions of America prevails in most parts of the world." [10 (page 131)]

"To ignore the medical 'new order' mandated by American institutions is to commit professional suicide. The United States is the leader in the modernization and mechanization of medicine. No one has invested more time, effort, and money in the development of awesome technology such as computerized Tomography Scans, Magnetic Resonance Imaging, lasers, video surgery components, etc. These costly 'toys' fascinate doctors everywhere the way Super Nintendo has captured the attention of our children. Though the rest of the world loves to criticize the Americans for the automation of medicine, they are desperately trying to emulate them. Even the *University of Austria* is giving in to the temptation because medical technology has a spell-casting attraction so powerful that we, the doctors, are as dependent on it as addicts are to their drugs." [10 (page 132)]

"The second half of this century has seen the greatest technological explosion in the history of medicine – chemical syntheses of pharmaceuticals, genetic engineering, computerization of microbiology, nuclear medicine, gamma knife, transplants, endoscopic surgery, surgical training simulators, and hundreds of other scientific advances. In the clinical field, new devices facilitate the work of physicians. Computer programs exist which diagnose and recommend a treatment. It is now possible to examine organs using a tiny probe that functions as a video camera. New technology permits accident victims to be attended to rapidly by teams of highly trained doctors, nurses, and technicians that often bring patients 'back' to life." [10 (page 134)]

"Yes, medicine has come a long way. But we are in awe and can't take our eyes and minds off the glitter of the machinery, while losing sight of the patient." [10 (page 135)]

"These technological creations undeniably represent a huge advance in the diagnosis and treatment of diseases, but no apparatus or computer program can replace the human touch of a doctor. The abuse of technology has undermined the ability of the physician to listen to and observe the patient. The lure of technology has alienated physicians from their mission." [10 (page 135)]

Francisco Contreras, M.D., states "My father, *Ernesto Contreras Sr.*, M.D., a doctor from the old school of medicine, instilled in me a philosophy that is not opposed to progress but disagrees with anything that places the patient as a secondary concern." [10 (page 135)]

"The original mission of medicine was established some 500 years before Christ. It was shaped into the following oath: a pact physicians make with society." [10 (page 136)]

According to the *Encyclopedia Britannica* on-line (under *Hippocratic oath, Philosophy & Religion, then Ethics*), originally, the oath was used swearing to the Greek gods *Apollo*, called the physician, and to *Aesculapius*, the god of medicine, as well as many other pagan gods. The oath has been revised over time and approved by the *American Medical Association* as follows:

"You do solemnly swear, each by whatever he or she holds most sacred,

That you will be loyal to the *Profession of Medicine* and just and generous to its members

That you will lead your lives and practice your art in uprightness and honor

That into whatsoever house you shall enter, it shall be for the good of the sick to the utmost of your power, holding yourselves far aloof from wrong, from corruption, from the tempting of others to vice

That you will exercise your art solely for the cure of your patients and will give no drug, perform no operation, for criminal purpose, even if solicited, far less suggest it

That whatsoever you shall see or hear of the lives of men or women which is not fitting to be spoken, you will keep inviolably secret.

These things do you swear. Let each bow the head in sign of acquiescence." [10 (page 136)]

Sadly, even with good intentions, this oath came from a belief in pagan gods and is not connected with the Creator God, *Yehovah.* The doctors of old may have had at their core a desire to help people, but over time, as this oath states, loyalty is not to the people, but to the Profession of Medicine. I think that explains a lot!

Let's look at an area of interest that *Dr. Contreras* calls "*Epidemics and the Birth of the Medical Industry.*"

"Epidemics have killed a vast number of people. *Jean Hamburger*, a French researcher, in his book *Honey and Hemlock*, exposes the tragedy of these deaths. The impression left in those that experienced the raging fury of death during that period can easily be perceived reading his words:

'I have seen the wounded stare of too many men, women, young people and children even who foresaw themselves as damned because they could not understand that whole races of people had made the diseases a sign of the wrath of the gods.'" [10 (page 137-138)]

"The *Black Plague* killed 25 million Europeans in the 1300's, cholera claimed the lives of 100,000 Frenchmen in 1832, typhus claimed 3 million Poles and Russians in 1914, and again in Europe, the flu epidemic killed 25 million people in 1918." [10 (page 138)]

"In the Middle Ages, the common epidemics were malaria, leprosy, typhus, influenza, and *St. Anthony's Fire*. Perhaps the pestilence that desolated Europe the most was *The Black Death*, a bubonic plague of the pulmonary type. The *Black Death* began around 1333 in the central region of Asia, later extending itself to the *Mediterranean Sea*, *Russia*, and *Ireland*, reaching its climax in 1348. It is said that one-fourth of the population died in places stricken by it. Physicians considered isolation as the only recourse. So it was that the 'quarantine' was born near the end of the 15th century." [10 (page 138)]

"At the end of the 15th century, syphilis took on epidemic characteristics, not respecting social class, rank, or sex. The name of the disease follows a legend about a young shepherd called *Syphilo* who had this disease imposed on him for insulting the Sun. It spread rapidly among his companions. It is said that the Renaissance was lashed by two plagues, syphilis, and witch hunts. The latter was converted into a true collective psychosis. The witches were nothing more than women with mental dysfunction who, since not recognized as ill, fell under the jurisdiction of the theologians and lawyers instead of the care of a physician. They are also known from the *Salem* (*Massachusetts*) trials of the 17th century when a series of women were executed for witchcraft. We know now that these actions and behavior were caused by foods containing spores of hallucinogenic mushrooms with alkaloids similar to LSD. Thanks to 20 years of research, *Dr. Johannes Weyer* in his book *Diabolical Frauds* along with contemporary scientific discoveries, the hereditary stain has been removed from many families who believed they had witches in their ancestry." [10 (page 139)]

"In the 17th century, some new diseases were identified: rickets, tuberculosis, and beriberi. Smallpox attacked Europe in the 18th century, but an important medical event contributed to the fight against it – immunization, a method based on the principle that people who survive a forced attack are protected from future attacks. Therefore, if a person was exposed to a light attack, he was protected from the epidemic. In that century, *Edward Jenner* appeared on the scene. He was a rural British doctor who found out about this folk belief that people who contracted 'cowpox' would not contract smallpox. *Jenner* made the belief the subject of experimentation for two years and in 1796 injected into a child a purulent secretion of cowpox. Six weeks later, he injected the subject with the pus of smallpox. So it was that a new therapy was born. Since it was obtained from cattle (*vacca* in Latin) it was called vaccination." [10 (page 139, 140)]

"Before the advent of these scientific advances, the authorities used desperate methods to try and control epidemics. They buried corpses together with all their belongings and burned them, in some cases even entire cities. They petitioned the heavens and offered all sorts of sacrifices. Some placed the blame on Jews and in desperation and hatred, massacred 600 in *Brussels* and 2000 in *Strasbourg*." [10 (page 140)]

"With the enemy in sight, the fear of God was extrapolated to the fear of germs. So, doctors, immunologists, microbiologists, physiologists, and many other specialists began to wage war against an infinitely smaller but tremendously resourceful foe. Their scientific drive, restricted for so many centuries, emerged with a passionate force that could not be stopped. There was excitement and hope for the physician; hope of achieving the victory over infectious diseases caused by these insolent, minuscule microbes." [10 (page 140, 141)]

"In this scientific environment of the mid-19th century, two opposing schools of thought were born, headed by two gigantic figures, *Bernard* and *Pasteur*. In the matter of the development of disease, what was black for one was white for the other." [10 (page 141)]

"*Claude Bernard* (1813-1878), French physician and physiologist, was the first to consider that the body's ability to mend depends on its general condition, that is to say, how nourished it is. If our body can depend on an adequate internal environment, *Bernard* asserted that it would know how to make the necessary adjustments to maintain the proper state of balance. He concluded that germs are only responsible for the development of disease if our body offers conditions favorable to the germ. If our body maintains an adequate '*milieu interieur'* or internal environment, it will be able to fight off the germ and there will be no disease. It seemed like an irrefutable argument. How else could one explain the fact that, though we all come in contact with the same germs, only a few of us fall ill? This is the fundamental theory of the ***humorist*** school of thought. Of course, *Bernard* was a man with a sense of humor, but the purpose of calling the movement 'humorist' was to give honor to *Hippocrates* who 500 years before Christ, without the help of microscopes, knew that there were 'forces within us that truly heal.' The ancient Greeks believed that the body was formed by four 'humors' (Latin for liquids). Any alteration in their perfect balance caused pain, disease, even emotional changes; hence the modern application of saying 'good or bad humor'" [10 (page 142)]

"*Louis Pasteur* (1822-1895), on the other hand, disagreed with *Bernard*, affirming that germs are the true villains in the history of disease and that by neutralizing them, we not only could prevent infections, but we could also cure them. His hypothesis was confirmed by his vaccines and treatments. This is the fundamental theory of the ***causalist*** school of thought, so named because if the cause of a disease can be determined, the saving antidote can be developed!" [10 (page 142)]

"*Pasteur's* prestige is founded on his accomplishments in microbiology. The research and experiments he conducted led to the confirmation of his hypothesis in 1877. *Pasteur* demonstrated that germs reproduce themselves like any other organism. These advances formed the guiding principles of disease control research. Today many owe their life to the achievements of *Pasteur*, but the methods employed in his research were reckless." [10 (page 142)]

One of *Pasteur's* achievements is the vaccine against rabies, but with no more clinical data then that of *Jenner*, he prepared the vaccine, gave it to a healthy volunteer (fool) and then infected him with the disease! Pasteur and his colleagues must have had many anxious hours and days waiting for the deadly outcome, but the 'guinea pig' survived and was declared successfully inoculated. This experiment got everybody's attention and gave him even more notoriety than before, in the eyes of scientists and the public.

Soberly and humbly the genius he was said, 'Luck favors the prepared minds.' *Pasteur* frequently departed from scientific method established in his day and carried out experiments that were neither very ethical nor humane." [10 (page 143)]

"One of the great misfortunes of being human is the fact that we spend so much time waiting. What we want is action and quick results. Because of this, when *Pasteur* opened the door to the search for the illusive germ and provided the weaponry for the fight, the world, scientific and not, was ready to take the initiative. Almost everyone followed *Pasteur* and the *causalist* school of thought, of course! The *French* government responded and funded a research institute for *Pasteur* to continue with the exploration of microorganisms, so *Pasteur Institute* opened its door in 1886. To date this research institute is at the forefront of scientific discovery; the last one attributed to them was the *Human Immunodeficiency Virus* (*HIV*)." [10 (page 143, 144)]

"*Elie Metchnikoff* (1845-1916), Russian biologist and pathologist, discovered phagocytes and situated himself in Paris to be able to work with *Pasteur* and his institute. With the passing of the years, he was able to absorb the 'advances' in the struggle against infection but his observations and research obliged him to question the theory of *Pasteur*. Soon, he switched to *Claude Bernard's humorist* school of thought. *Metchinikoff* wanted to show the importance of the humorist's perspective, but few paid attention to his work because *Pasteur* wasn't in agreement. In order to make his point clear, *Metchinkoff* and several co-workers stood before an assembly of physicians and drank liquid contaminated with millions of *cholera bacilli*. They did this to demonstrate their conviction that if the immune system is strong, it has the power to resist germs. *Metchinkoff* demonstrated his hypothesis in an overwhelming way. Not a single one of the participants in the experiment fell ill with cholera. Although the course of history was not changed, *Metchinkoff* gained respect, so much so that *Pasteur* named him as his successor in 1904. He continued with his studies in immunology and physiology and won the *Nobel Prize for Medicine* in 1908." [10 (page 144,145)]

"In the second half of the 19th century and the first two decades of the 20th, the two most feared germs of all time were discovered. *Robert Koch* (1843-1910) discovered these germs which cause tuberculosis and cholera and received the *Nobel Prize* for his work in 1905. Other germs were discovered that cause typhoid fever, gonorrhea, malaria, diphtheria, amoebiasis, tetanus, meningitis, syphilis, and rubella. These accomplishments pushed scientists toward a search for treatments that would specifically seek out germs without causing any damage to normal cells. This concept was called 'magic bullet' and continues to be the guiding principle of the modern-day pharmaceutical industry. The truth is that any medication that enters the body is exposed to thousands of barriers, both physical and chemical, and its success depends on the reaction of each particular person. Some medications can have beneficial effects, but they can also be converted into morbid substances and be lethal as we shall observe later." [10 (page 145)]

"*Paul Ehrlich* is considered the father of the pharmaceutical industry. He was the first to produce pharmaceuticals in an organized way. Another highly important event was the accidental discovery of *Penicillin* in 1928 by *Alexander Fleming* (1881-1955). *Fleming* had been engaged in the search for causative agents in the influenza epidemic of 1918 which did away with 25 million people. On a holiday he left his bacterial cultures on the worktable in his London laboratory. They became contaminated with green fungus which destroyed the microorganisms of the culture. There is no doubt that 'luck favors the prepared'. This 'luck' earned him the *Nobel Prize* in 1945. [10 (page 145,146)]

"As a direct result, the massive production of antibiotics began and since then, doctors and researchers have not looked back; they devoted themselves to the mission of conquering the infectious insolent bugs that cause diseases. The success of antibiotics guaranteed the *causalist's* school of thought to flourish. It has become an immovable and incontrovertible institution. Those who oppose it today are disregarded without a backward glance because the statutes of the establishment are medical dogma. To belong to it is a privilege, to oppose it is heresy. Its principles and laws are even protected by a myriad of governmental agencies and societies like the *National Health Institutes* and the *American Cancer Society*." [10 (page 146)]

"The improvement in worldwide health is attributed by the medical industry to the development of drugs that destroy causal agents. The truth is that the control of plagues and disease has been achieved because of sociological changes like hygiene, better distribution of food and, however unrelated to health it may seem, city planning. I (*Francisco Contreras, MD*) would almost dare to affirm that public health problems diminished in great measure because of these factors long before a vaccination was injected, and first 'magic bullet' administered. For example, the appropriate management of sewage in the 18th century and the practice of quarantine yielded impressive results, but the deplorable living conditions of those far away times are for us now inconceivable. Some time ago I (*Francisco Contreras, MD*) read a book by *Patrick Sueskind*, *The Perfume* that, even though it's a novel, describes with exquisite precision the environment of Paris in the 18th century." [10 (page 147)]

The description given in *The Perfume* of the stench and horrible conditions of Paris in the 18th century is enough to turn the stomach. No concern was given of the healing hygiene guidance of God's Word. Did they know the hygiene laws? Certainly, people in the Jewish communities would live differently, but unfortunately the information was not encouraged among the peoples.

"If the inhabitants of the most progressive city of Europe lived under such nauseating conditions, the circumstances of the rest of the old world belong to the unthinkable. Obviously in these miserable conditions, diseases spread like wildfire, but to science this was not so obvious, especially to medical science. In 1847 *Dr. Ignas Semmelweis* was ousted from the medical profession for the 'quackery' of promulgating that doctors should wash their hands before exploring their patients. At that time, they would do an autopsy and, without washing their hands, explore a patient! And these are the guys that supposedly have a better than average I.Q., scary!" [10 (page 147, 148)]

"Let history speak instead. Thanks to improvements in sewage and general sanitation, smallpox epidemics began a dizzying descent before *Edward Jenner* discovered inoculation. Smallpox might actually have disappeared without any treatment at all. But doctors had to intervene, and the general use of vaccination was popularized. Curiously, the incidence of this disease began to ascend at the end of the 19th century. By 1892, the number of people infected with smallpox had ascended to 165,774 more cases than in the years preceding vaccination. In 1865, an alarming increase in death by smallpox was reported in England. More than 22,000 died after vaccination became obligatory there. By 1872, over 44,000 deaths were reported, and the number of fatalities continued to climb each year in spite of vaccination. It took officials 76 years to wake up to the fact that the vaccine was the real cause of the deaths." [10 (page 148, 149)]

"In 1939, *Germany* instituted obligatory vaccination against diphtheria and the incidence of this disease rose astronomically to 150,000. *Norway*, on the other hand, decided not to vaccinate. Only 50 cases were reported there in the same period. Another greatly feared epidemic in the 19th century was tuberculosis. In 1812, the death rate from tuberculosis in *New York* was 700 lives for every 100,000 inhabitants. By 1892, the rate had diminished to 370 and further to 180 in 1910. By 1950, the rate stood at 50 lives per 100,000. The need for treatment has to be seriously questioned since downward trends would probably have continued without treatment. Statistics demonstrate that infant mortality from scarlet fever, diphtheria, whooping cough, and mumps diminished 90% between 1869 and 1896, before the introduction of antibiotics and immunization. It shouldn't be surprising that *Pasteur*, on his deathbed, was quoted as confessing to *Metchinkoff*, 'the pathogen (germ) is nothing, terrain is everything' referring to the internal environment that *Bernard* had postulated." [10 (page 149, 150)]

"Yet, medical science did not change its trajectory. The search for 'magic bullets' that will destroy germs continues. I guess it's the profitable thing to do. In our time, *Native Americans* have the highest infant mortality, suffer infectious diseases in epidemic proportions and are cursed with the shortest longevity in the nation. Philanthropists decided to resolve the *Navajos'* health problems by making generous donations to back a program designed by the *University of Cornell's Medical School*. The program was implemented in 1960." [10 (page 150)]

"A full-fledged clinic, with all the technological advances of the time, was constructed for the project and highly trained *Cornell* physicians were sent to attend the *Navajo* full time. After five years of dedicated and arduous work by all involved, the *Cornell-Navajo* project was terminated. Medical knowledge, technology and drugs had no impact on infant mortality which continued at 300% higher than the nation's average. Infectious diseases were not put under control and longevity of *Native Americans* did not improve. On average, they die 11 years before most Americans. The rate of death by tuberculosis diminished insignificantly and continues to be 11 times higher than the rest of the country." [10 (page 150, 151)]

"The power of the medical industry's propaganda is truly omnipotent; it not only has obscured the eyes of doctors and scientists, but also the rest of the world. Our hearts tell us that we have the power to listen to our body and know what is happening to it. Sadly, scientific criteria have clouded our instincts, convincing us that we were foolish. How else do we explain that it has taken 100 years to realize the *causalist* school offers only a mirage. How can 'the establishment' keep offering us a myth and call it truth?" [10 (page 151)]

Romans [1:22] "Claiming to be wise, they have become fools! [23] In fact, they have exchanged the glory of the immortal God for mere images, like a model human being, or like birds, animals, or reptiles! ...[25] They have exchanged the truth of God for falsehood, by worshipping and serving created things, rather than the Creator – praised be he forever, Amen." [1 (page 1606)]

"I realize that *Paul* (*Sha'ul*) was not referring to physicians or scientists but, although uncomfortable, it applies well." [10 (page 151)]

"Throughout the world, governmental authorities 'look out' for our interests and our health. The need to control pharmaceuticals from the very start of the manufacturing process is important because they are dangerous. But the ruling powers that determine when and how they will be delivered to the ill are not always aimed toward the well-being of the patient. Ahead of the patients come investors who keep a watchful eye on the security of their money and astutely measure the probability of success (economics of course). Next come the producers with their scientific equipment who also worry about their share of the profits, and way down the list the 'well-being' of the patient." [10 (page 152)]

"The pharmaceutical industry, indecently profitable, deals with diseases not as afflictions, but as market opportunities. For instance, *AIDS*, the newest market (at the time of this writing 1997), has had the advantage of rapid growth and less resistance from the *FDA* to try treatments with some 'shortcuts' because of the enormous pressure patients and activists are putting on the U.S. government to find a cure. In 1985, the *National Institute of Health* (*NIH*) invited *Burrows-Welcome*, an English company with experience in antivirals (owners of the patent for the popular anti-flu *Sudafed*) to develop and manufacture a treatment against the devastating plague." [10 (page 153)]

"Researchers of the laboratory immersed themselves in the archives of the pharmaceutical junk yard and came up with an anti-cancer drug (chemotherapy) known for its antiviral activity, *AZT*, rejected by the *FDA* 23 years earlier as being primitive and extremely toxic. But the *NIH* gave in to the 'pressure' of the epidemic and began its clinical application. The risk is acceptable since the patients were sentenced to die." [10 (page 154)]

"Without losing time, *Burrows-Welcome* requested a patent which was granted in 1978. The first study concluded that *AZT* did not prolong the life of *AIDS* victims but did improve their quality of life, an interesting conclusion, given the fact that it had been discontinued in the 70's precisely because of severe side effects. *Harvard University* also carried out clinical testing with *AZT* on patients in advanced stages of *AIDS* in which it was noted that this 'improvement in their quality of life' consisted of retarding the onset of typical symptoms. The results were counterproductive since the patient suffered more from the side effects of *AZT* therapy (nausea, vomiting, fatigue etc.). By 1992, the sales of *AZT* had topped 100 million dollars, thanks to the sales pitch based on its ephemeral benefits." [10 (page 154)]

"As is to be expected, pharmaceutical laboratories – small and large – wanted a 'piece of the market' but instead of cooperating and sharing scientific experience, greed divided them. As in all wars, disunity weakened them and none has been able to defeat this minuscule, but powerful virus. In the 80's everyone was in a race against time to find a treatment or a vaccine. After barely ten years of arduous research, *Merck* announced that they would stop participating in the race, owing to enormous mutation capacity of the virus, its resistance to antivirals, a very doubtful market and very poor perspective for finding an effective treatment they were suspending their anti-*AIDS* program. The pharmaceutical industry, its investors, and scientists forgot about the global consequences that this epidemic could cause and almost all of them abandoned *AIDS* 'research'. In other words, they no longer had any interest in this 'market.'" [10 (page 154, 155)]

"The financial future of many products, especially pharmaceuticals, depends on the outcome of the researchers. This encourages scientific fraud. Incentives for scientists at important universities like *Harvard*, *MIT*, and *Yale* include prestigious publications, international recognition, travel, scholarships, and patent rights which ensure them riches, power, and the ultimate possibility – a *Nobel Prize*. To attain all this, universities provide them with super laboratories and the most promising students, who act as slaves." [10 (Page 160)]

"How can government agencies protect us from dangerous medications if they depend on research conducted by an industry that has sold out? How can they depend on fraudulent scientists who fall prey to the lure of fame and fortune? The description of this phenomenon is masterfully done by *Dr. Herbert M. Shelton* in his book *Hygienic Review* in which he states, 'Science is the ever-subservient handmaiden of commercialism; and we should not be surprised by the fact that the scientists can find and have found justification, even if only fictional, for all the practices that are fostered by the commercial world for profit.'" [10 (page 161)]

"The majority of the world's population uses medications that have probably been evaluated by dishonest scientists and approved by government officials who dance to the music of money. The words of *Linnaeus* in his *Diaeta Naturalis* (*Natural Diet*, 18th century) ring true when he says, 'to live dependent on medicine is to live hideously.' Such words have never before taken on such depth of meaning as now, when the majority of human beings suffer from one disease or another, and when so many people depend on medication to keep them going each day. The most prescribed drugs are tranquilizers, sleeping pills, high blood pressure drugs, arthritic pain killers and antibiotics, all of which are consumed in industrial quantities. Billions of these pills —are sold annually by drug stores." [10 (page 161)]

There have been many consequences of the pharmaceutical system. To name a few:

Thalidomide incident – taken to combat nausea during pregnancy produced severe deformities. [10 (page 162)]

DES (*diethylstilbestrol*) – a synthetic female hormone – caused cancer in rats. "Thirty years later, the daughters of those who took *DES* showed an extraordinarily high incidence of vaginal, cervical and breast cancer as well as liver damage, and their children suffered congenital deformities." [10 (page 162)]

Flagyl – "an antibiotic frequently prescribed." "Although definitive and clinical evidence of its carcinogenic quality are irrefutable, there is no indication that authorities plan to withdraw it from the market." [10 (page 163)]

Among the drugs most prescribed are the ones used to combat high blood pressure. "It may be that the anti-hypertension drugs contribute to bringing down your blood pressure, but they do not reduce the mortality from heart attacks or embolism (blood clots). What does this mean? Patients who have the same mortality index as those who don't take them. Besides being an unnecessary cost, they produce headaches, nausea, and impotence." [10 (page 164)]

Sorcery at work! Concoctions, of who knows what, created to hopefully stop one problem, but in turn create many more. None of this is truly benefiting the body nor returning the person to excellent health. Symptoms treated and more symptoms come about! The roller coaster of the medical health industry.

Viruses - From Whence Do They Come?

Even as I write this treatise, our world is dealing with the horrors of the result of a mandate to be inoculated for a *Sars corona* virus called *COVID-19.* The statistics seem to show that more vaccinated people have died or suffered severe side effects than those who had the disease itself. That seems to be the result each time these germs get out of hand!

The *Sars-Corona*, *COVID-19*, is still somewhat a mystery at the time of this writing, but we do know some things. Could we be outside *Yehovah's* will once again? What about the bats!

D'varim (*Deuteronomy*) 14:11 "You may eat any clean bird; 12 but these you are not to eat:
eagles, vultures, ospreys, 13 kites, any kind of buzzard, 14 any kind of raven, 15 ostriches,
screech-owls, seagulls, any kind of hawk, 16 little owls, great owls, horned owls, 17
pelicans, barn owls, cormorants, 18 storks any kind of heron, hoopoes and **bats**." [1 (page 246)]

Vayikra (*Leviticus*) 11:13 "The following creatures of the air are to be detestable for you – you are not to eat their meat, and you are to detest their carcasses…19 the stork, the various kinds of herons, the hoopoes and the **bat**." [1 (page 141)]

Galatians 6:7 "Don't delude yourselves: no one makes a fool of God! A person reaps what he sows." [1 (page 1677)]

An article from *God Said Man Said* titled '*Diet, Hygiene, Quarantine, and Hell to Pay*', provides the following information. The headlines of "*Nature*, February 3, 2020: '*A Pneumonia Outbreak Associated with a New Coronavirus of Probable Bat Origin.'*" and "*Science Daily*. February 10, 2020: '*Coronavirus Outbreak Raises Question: Why are Bat Viruses so Deadly?*' The subhead states: 'Bats' fierce immune systems drive viruses to higher virulence, making them deadlier in humans.' A paragraph from the article follows:

"'This makes bats a unique reservoir of rapidly reproducing and highly transmittable viruses. While the bats can tolerate viruses like these, when these bat viruses then move into animals that lack a fast-response immune system, the viruses quickly overwhelm their new hosts, leading to high fatality rates.'" [2]

"The sub-headline in the February 12, 2020, feature on *Vox* states: 'Horseshoe bats are known to carry coronavirus which can infect humans.' A few excerpts follow from an interview *Vox* feature writer *Brian Resnick* did with *Johnathan Epstein*:

'To better understand why health officials want to know which animals were involved in the new outbreak, I called up *Jonathan Epstein*. He's a veterinarian and an epidemiologist with the *Eco-Health Alliance* who was involved in tracking down the animal source for the *SARS* outbreak.'

'**Question**: What do we know right now about where this novel coronavirus came from?

'***Epstein***: I think we have very strong evidence that supports the idea that this virus ultimately comes from bats. But we don't know what other animals may have been involved.

'**Question**: What do you mean by 'what other animals may have been involved? Is it possible that this didn't come directly from bats?

'***Epstein***: A good example here is the story of *SARS*. When *SARS* emerged in 2003, it was also in a live market in Southern China, in *Guangdong*. It turned out people that were handling and trading civet [small, mostly nocturnal mammal native to tropical Asia and Africa] had a higher instance of exposure and infection to this virus. Then they tested animals within the markets, and civets were found to be infected with the same virus that was infecting people.

'So, the assumption was made that people were getting it from civets, and civets were very promptly and publicly removed from markets and stamped out.

'But a very important study came out a few months after the epidemic looking at civets on farms that supplied the live animal markets, and it turned out that none of the civets that were being farmed had any evidence of exposure or infection to *SARS coronavirus*.

'That was important because this was not, in fact, a civet virus that was getting into the markets. Civets were getting infected in the markets themselves, just like people.

'***Renick*** asks: So, what was giving the civets *SARS*? Was it the bats?

'***Epstein***: So, this is where I come in, and my colleagues. We started working on *SARS* back in 2003, trying to understand what the wildlife reservoir was.

Epstein continues: 'And we found it to be bats, horseshoe bats specifically. We now know that there's a whole group – a whole diversity – of viruses related to *SARS* that are circulating in horseshoe bats.

'One of the viruses we identified with our partners at the *Wuhan Institute of Virology* back in 2013 is 96% similar to this novel coronavirus. That gives us confidence that this new coronavirus also is a bat virus originally.

'These bats are hunted and eaten in China, and in fact were brought into the markets in the case of *SARS*, and that is how other animals, including people, were infected.'" [End of quotes]. [2]

"You'll find the following paragraph in the February 15, 2020, issue of *Science News* under the heading, '*New Coronavirus Fuels Outbreak*.' [2]

‘Bats are considered a source of coronaviruses but don’t usually pass the viruses directly to humans. *SARS* probably jumped from bats into raccoons, dogs, or palm civets before leaping to humans. *MERS* went from bats to camels then to humans. A paper published January 22 in the *Journal of Medical Virology* suggests that the new virus has components from bat coronaviruses. Some evidence suggests the virus crossed into humans only once, in mid-November, and has since spread from person-to-person. [End of quote]’ [2]

‘Here we go again. Another new, global field study is in, and the discovery is that every commandment and precept in God’s Word has inherent within it a blessing or a curse. Because the Word of God is the supernatural, inerrant truth, obeying it yields the blessing of doing the right thing. Because the Word of God is the supernatural, inerrant truth, disobeying it yields the curse of doing the wrong thing. God is not mocked. [End of quotes]’” [2]

Once again, men manipulating viruses cause catastrophic results. What are these viruses, these germs, the medical industry has been chasing all these years? *Dr. Richard Brouse*, in his book, *Build a Better You*, describes viral infections this way – “Examples of common diseases caused by viruses include the common cold, warts, corns, the flu, *cytomegalovirus* (*CMV*), chickenpox and cold sores. Serious diseases, such as *Ebola*, *AIDS*, *Avian flu*, and *SARS* are all also caused by viruses, as are most colorectal and some cervical cancers. The relative ability of viruses to cause disease is described in terms of virulence. Survivors of the most virulent viruses usually have life-long resistance. Other diseases are under investigation as to whether they have a virus as the causative agent, such as the possible connection between *Human Herpesvirus Six* (*HHV6*) and neurological diseases such as multiple sclerosis and chronic fatigue syndrome.” [13 (page 330)]

“Viruses have many different mechanisms by which they produce disease. Mechanisms at the cellular level primarily include cell lysis, the breaking open and subsequent death of the cell. If enough cells die, the people start to suffer the effects. Although many viruses cause the disruption of healthy processes, resulting in disease, they may also exist relatively harmlessly within us. An example would include the ability of the herpes simplex virus, which causes cold sores, to remain in a dormant state within the human body for many years, then erupt during episodes of heavy stress or nutritional inadequacy. Small children are vectors for viruses, especially warts, as their immune system is immature and fails to react when a virus is present.” [13 (page 330)]

“A virus is a small infectious organism – much smaller than a fungus or bacterium – that needs a living cell in order to reproduce. The virus attaches to a cell, the virus releases its DNA or RNA (which contains the information needed to create new virus particles) and takes control of some aspects of the cell’s metabolism. The components of the virus are then manufactured inside the cell and must be properly assembled for the virus to be released and remain infectious.” [14 (page 912)]

“What happens to the cell depends on the type of virus. Some viruses kill the cells they infect. Others alter the cell function so that the cell loses control over normal cell division and becomes cancerous. Some viruses incorporate a part or all of their genetic information into the host cell DNA, but they remain silent (or latent) until the cell is disturbed in a way that permits the virus to emerge again.” [14(page 912)]

"Most viruses have a preferred host. Some, such as the influenza virus, can infect humans and a variety of other animals. However, some strains of influenza have adapted in a way that allows them to infect one species of animal more efficiently than others. Most viruses commonly found in people are transmitted from person to person. Some viruses, such as the rabies virus or encephalitis viruses, infect animals primarily and humans only occasionally." [14 (page 912)]

"The body has a number of specific and nonspecific defenses against viruses. Physical barriers, such as the skin and mucous membranes, discourage easy entry. Infected cells also make interferon(s), a family of glycoproteins that can make noninfected cells more resistant to infection by many viruses." [14 (page 912)]

"If a virus does enter the body, various types of white blood cells, such as lymphocytes, are able to attack and destroy infected cells. The two main types of lymphocytes are B lymphocytes and T lymphocytes. When exposed to a viral attack, T lymphocytes increase in number and mature into either helper cells, which aid antibody producing B lymphocytes, or cytotoxic (killer) cells, which can attack cells infected by a specific virus. T lymphocytes also produce chemicals (called cytokines) that speed this maturation process. The cytokines from helper cells can help B lymphocytes and their derivatives, the plasma cells, to produce antibodies that target specific viruses and make them noninfectious before they can infect another cell." [14 (page 912)]

"Probably the most common viral infections are those of the lungs and airways. These illnesses include the common cold, influenza, throat infections (pharyngitis or laryngitis), croup in small children, and inflammation of the windpipe (tracheitis) or other airways (bronchiolitis, bronchitis)." [14 (page 913)]

"What is a retrovirus? Viruses are tiny microbes that can infect cells. Once in a cell, they use cellular components to replicate. They can be classified according to several factors, including:

- The type of genetic material they use (DNA or RNA)
- The method they use to replicate within the cell.
- Their shape or structural features

"Retroviruses are a type of virus in the viral family called *Retroviridae*. They use RNA as their genetic material and are named for a special enzyme that's a vital part of their life cycle – reverse transcriptase. [4]

"There are many technical differences between viruses and retroviruses. But generally, the main difference between the two is how they replicate within a host cell. Here's a look at the steps of the life cycle of human immunodeficiency virus (HIV) to help illustrate how retroviruses replicate:

1. Attachment. The virus binds to a receptor on the surface of the host cell. In the case of HIV, this receptor is found on the surface of immune cells called CD4 T cells.
2. Entry. The envelope surrounding the HIV particle fuses with the membrane of the host cell, allowing the virus to enter the cell.

3. Reverse transcription. HIV uses its reverse transcriptase enzyme to turn its RNA genetic material into DNA. This makes it compatible with the host cell's genetic material, which is vital for the next step of the life cycle.
4. Genome integration. The newly synthesized viral DNA travels to the cell's control center, the nucleus. Here a special viral enzyme called integrase is used to insert the viral DNA into the host cell's DNA.
5. Replication. Once its DNA has been inserted to the host cell's genome, the virus uses the host cell's machinery to produce new viral components, such as viral RNA and viral proteins.
6. Assembly. The newly made viral components combine close to the cell surface and begin to form new HIV particles.
7. Release. The new HIV particles push out from the surface of the host cell, forming a mature HIV particle with the help of another viral enzyme called protease. Once outside the host cell, these new HIV particles can go on to infect other CD4 T cells. [4]

"The key steps that differentiate retroviruses from viruses are reverse transcription and genome integration." There are three retroviruses that can affect humans. They are HIV and Human T-cell lymphotropic virus (HTLV) types 1 and 2. [4]

"A retrovirus is a 'stealth virus' that, like HIV, enters the host without alerting the immune system. [8 (Forward by *R.F. Kennedy, Jr.*)]

"Retrovirus may lie dormant for years without causing harm. Before killing a person, a retrovirus will usually destroy their immune system. As a result, many retroviruses cause cancer." [8 (page x)]

There is a strong association between a previously unknown retrovirus and *Myologic encephalomyelitis*, commonly known as *chronic fatigue syndrome*. (ME/CFS). They are also linked to certain blood cancers – *Xenotropic Murine Leukemia Related Virus* (XMRV). [8 (page x)]

The retrovirus was found in mice and had somehow jumped into humans via contaminated vaccines. [8 (page xi)]

"Even more troubling to the medical establishment, *Dr. Mikovits'* research revealed that many of the female patients afflicted with XMRV had children with autism. Suspecting XMRV might be passed from mother to child, as with HIV, *Mikovits* tested seventeen of the children. Fourteen showed evidence of the virus. Those findings dovetailed with parental reports of autistic regression following vaccination. Subsequent studies linked XMRV to epidemics in leukemia, prostate cancer, autoimmune disease, and the explosion of Alzheimer's disease!" "Worse yet, research also found widespread XMRV contamination in the blood supply and blood products. Based on her research and findings of others, it seems that anywhere from 3 to 8 percent of the population now carry the virus – XMRV has become part of human ecology, passed from mother to child in vitro or through breast milk." [8 (page xi)]

"In January of 2011, HIV-AIDS expert *Ben Berkhout* published these explosive revelations in the journal *Frontiers in Microbiology*. He included *Mikovits'* evidence that mouse tissue used in vaccine production was the likely vector for human contamination.

Unbeknownst to *Judy* (*Mikovits*), her co-author on this book, *Kent Heckenlively*, had already independently discovered published medical research showing that the first recorded outbreak of *ME/CFS* was among 198 doctors and nurses at the *Los Angeles County Hospital* in 1934-1935, following their injection with an experimental polio vaccine grown in mouse brain tissue…*Mikovits'* evidence threatened financial catastrophe for the world's pharmaceutical companies because of their negligent use of animal cell cultures to produce vaccines and other pharmaceutical products." [8 (page xi)]

"Pharmaceutical companies and their captive regulators unleashed a furious broadside against *Mikovits* and *Ruscetti*, besieging them from every stronghold." … "The *Semmelweis* reflex is the term describing the knee-jerk revulsion with which the press, the medical and scientific community, and allied financial interests greet new scientific evidence that contradicts an established scientific paradigm. The reflex can be particularly fierce in cases where new scientific information suggests that established medical practices are actually harming public health." [8 (page xii)]

"*Dr. Bernice Eddy* was an award-winning virologist, and one of the highest-ranking female scientists in NIH history. She and her research partner, *Elizabeth Stewart*, were the first researchers to isolate the *Polyomavirus* – the first virus proven to cause cancer. In 1954, NIH asked *Eddy* to direct testing of the *Salk* polio vaccine. She discovered, while testing eighteen macaques, that *Salk's* vaccine contained residual live polio virus that was paralyzing the monkeys. *Dr. Eddy* warned her NIH bosses that the vaccine was virulent, but they dismissed her concerns. The distributors of that vaccine by *Cutter Labs* in California caused the worst polio outbreak in history. Health officials infected 200,000 people with live polio; 70,000 became sick leaving 200 children paralyzed and ten dead." [8 (page xv)]

"In 1969, *Eddy* discovered that a cancer-causing monkey virus, SV40, had contaminated ninety-eight million *Salk* polio vaccines. When she injected the SV40 virus into newborn hamsters, the rodents sprouted tumors. *Eddy's* discovery proved an embarrassment to many scientists working on the vaccine. Instead of rewarding her for her visionary work, NIH officials banned her from polio research and assigned her to other duties. The NIH buried the alarming information and continued using the vaccines." [8 (page xv)]

SV40 is the viral agent in monkey kidney cells. [8 (page xvi)]

"In total, ninety-eight million Americans received shots potentially containing the cancer producing virus, which is now part of the human genome. In 1996, government researchers identified SV40 in 23 percent of the blood specimens and 45 percent of the sperm specimens collected from healthy adults. Six percent of the children born between 1980 and 1995 are infected. Public health officials gave millions of people the vaccine for years after they knew it was infected. They contaminated humanity with a monkey virus and refused to admit what they'd done." [8 (page xvi)]

"Today, SV40 is used in research laboratories throughout the world because it is so reliably carcinogenic. Researchers use it to produce a wide variety of bone and soft tissue cancers including mesothelioma and brain tumors in animals. The cancers have exploded in the baby boom generation, which received the *Salk* and *Sabin* polio vaccines between 1955 and 1963. Skin cancers are up by 70 percent, lymphoma and prostate by

66 percent, brain cancer by 34 percent. Prior to 1950, mesothelioma was rare in humans. Today, doctors diagnose nearly 3,000 Americans with mesothelioma every year; 60 percent of the tumors that were tested contained SV40. Today, scientists find SV40 in a wide range of deadly tumors, including between 33 percent and 90 percent of brain tumors, eight of eight ependymomas, and nearly half of the bone tumors tested." [8 (page xvi)]

Judy Mikovits stated, "My greatest concern was that well-meaning efforts to create weakened viruses for vaccines had created new problems. Had science properly considered the question of whether any mixing of human and animal tissue brought with it the inevitable risk of transferring animal viruses to humans? Or that these animal viruses would combine with human viruses to create new pathogens?" [8 (page 12)]

"Ultimately who is responsible for the pain, the sickness, the death, and yes, even the pandemics? It will at first seem too simplistic, but it seems that way because it is. Sin and death entered a perfect world through the vehicle of unbelief and disobedience." [2]

This battle of good and evil continues today. It continues in many realms including the industry of medicine. This is certainly not an exhaustive look at this topic but does make the point that *Yehovah's* Word is Truth and there are consequences for not following *Torah.*

"The natural mind is at war with the mind of Christ. It will choose error naturally. Carnal man instinctively mocks God." [5]

"One quite dominant example of the flaunting disobedience and mocking of the *Word of God* is 'carnaldom's disregard for the *Creator's* dietary laws. The *Maker* of the totality of your person is God, and one should think this *Maker* would have an understanding of what one should consume in foods and words." (This includes what should go into our bodies through eating, touching, or injecting.) "The dietary laws also extend to the handling of waste that comes from the body after the nutrients in eaten foods are extracted. [*Deuteronomy* 23:13 (12)] Keep in mind that neither the biology of the human nor of the animal has changed from the Old Testament to the New." [5]

As long as people continue to ingest animals God calls unclean and the chemical concoctions of the medical industry, humankind and creation will continue to suffer. At the time of this writing, changes are happening in the government oversight organizations as assessments are being evaluated about the industry as a whole. This may be good news for the health of humankind. I certainly hope so!

CHAPTER SIX

AWESOMELY AND WONDERFULLY MADE

Tehillim (*Psalm*) [139:13] "For you fashioned my inmost being, you knit me together in my mother's womb. [14] I thank you because I am awesomely made, wonderfully; your works are wonders – I know this very well. [15] My bones were not hidden from you when I was being made in secret, intricately woven in the depths of the earth. [16] Your eyes could see me as an embryo, but in your book all my days were already written; my days had been shaped before any of them existed." [1 (page 1051)]

Science Says…Solids, Fields or Something Else

Newtonian Thought

How are we made? Why does it matter about our lifestyles or the foods we eat? Is the order specified in the Creation story important to our overall health? Who are we? What are we?

"Until recently…much of our self-definition was based on the physics of a few hundred years ago. What *Barbara Ann Brennan*, author of *Hands of Light – A Guide to Healing*, refers to is "our insistence on seeing ourselves as solid objects. This definition of the universe, as made up of solid objects, was held largely by *Issac Newton* and his colleagues in the late 17th and early 18th centuries. *Newtonian* physics was extended in the 19th century to describe a universe composed of fundamental building blocks called atoms. These *Newtonian* atoms were thought of as composed of solid objects – a nucleus of protons and neutrons, with electrons revolving around the nucleus much like the earth traveling around the sun." [2 (page 21-22)]

Newtonian laws "were seen as the basic laws of nature, and *Newtonian* mechanics was considered to be the ultimate theory of natural phenomena. These laws held from the ideas of absolute time and space and of physical phenomena as strictly casual in nature. Everything could be described objectively. All physical reactions were seen to have a physical cause, like balls colliding on a pool table. Energy-matter interactions, such as a radio playing music in response to invisible radio waves, were not yet known. Nor did it occur to anyone that the experimenter himself affects the experimental results not only in psychological experiments but also in physical ones as well, as physicists have now proven." [2 (page 22)]

"This view was very comforting and still is to those of us who prefer to see the world as solid and largely unchanging, with very clear, definite sets of rules that govern its functioning. Much of our daily lives still run on *Newtonian* mechanics. Except for the electrical systems, our homes are largely *Newtonian.* We experience our bodies in a mechanical way. We define most of our experience in terms of absolute, three-dimensional space and linear time. We all have clocks. We need them to continue our lives as we have structured them – mostly linearly." [2 (page 22)]

This may be why changing clocks twice a year from Standard Time to Daylight Savings Time is so disruptive. Our basic foundation of time seems confusing! In reality all of Creation remains the same. It is the false man-made change that affects only human beings. You will notice that all around us animals, fish, birds, the sun, moon and stars make no change! Only human beings seek absolute time from an artificial time change. Moving the hands on the clock is a false application with many negative results. Our life's very structure is altered.

"In the early 19th century, new physical phenomena were discovered that could not be described by *Newtonian* physics. The discovery and investigation of electromagnetic phenomena led to the concept of a field. A field was defined as a condition in space which has the potential of producing a force." [2 (page 22)]

Faraday and Maxwell

"*Michael Faraday* and *James Clerk Maxwell* found it more appropriate to use a field concept and say that each charge creates a 'disturbance' or 'condition' in the space around it, so that the other charge, when it is present, feels a force. Thus, the concept of a universe filled with fields that create forces that interact with each other was born." [2 (page 22)]

"In the last 15 to 20 years" (now 50 to 70 years) "(100 years behind the physicists), most of us have just been beginning to use such concepts in describing our personal interactions. We are just beginning to admit that we ourselves are composed of fields. We sense another presence in the room without seeing or hearing them (field interaction); we speak of good or bad vibes or sending energy to others or reading each other's thoughts. We immediately know whether or not we like someone, whether we will get along with him or clash. This 'knowing' can be explained by the harmony or disharmony in our field interactions." [2 (page 22)]

Could this be the reason animals have varying reactions to different human beings? One person can enter a room and the dog's tail wags with friendly approval! However, the opposite reaction can take place too! Animals seem to sense the true intent of the person. These responses may be explained by harmony or disharmony in the experienced field.

Einstein - Mass and Matter

"In 1905, *Albert Einstein* published his *Special Theory of Relativity* and shattered all the principal concepts of the *Newtonian* world view. According to relativity theory, space is not three dimensional, and time is not a separate entity. Both are intimately connected and form a four-dimensional continuum, 'space-time.' Thus, we can never talk about space without time, and vice versa. Furthermore, there is no universal flow of time, i.e., time is not linear, nor is it absolute. That is, two observers will order events differently in time if they move with different velocities relative to the observed events. Therefore, all measurements involving space and time lose their absolute significance. Both time and space become merely elements to describe phenomena." [2 (page 23)]

"The *Native American* culture, which didn't have clocks to create linear time, divided time into two aspects: the now and all other time. The *Australian* aborigines also have two kinds of time: the passing time and the Great Time. What occurs in the Great Time has a sequence, but it cannot be dated." [2 (page 23)]

"*Einstein's* space-time continuum states that apparent linearity of events depends on the observer. Another important consequence of *Einstein's* relativity is the realization that matter and energy are interchangeable. Mass is nothing but a form of energy. Matter is simply slowed down or crystalized energy. Our bodies are energy." [2 (page 24)]

Crystalized Energy - Vibration

Crystalized energy - what a concept! Have you ever considered yourself a crystal? I had not! I had considered the beautiful gemstones, like amethyst, as pretty, but nothing beyond. Now, having worked in a "rock shop", I have observed over time the impact and benefit the gemstones have on plants and people! For thousands of years, these beautiful gems and minerals have been used for various applications as jewelry, lighting, goblets, home decor and healing!

The Bible mentions sixty-two gemstones and minerals! I had no idea of that and I grew up in "the church.". Just take a look at the *Ephod* worn by the high priest. The first one to wear the *Ephod* was Aaron, Mose's brother. Also called the Breastplate, this piece of spiritual armour was designed by *Yehovah* Himself! Twelve gemstones adorned the *ephod* representing the twelve tribes of Israel and the stones were inlaid in gold! Did you know gold is an excellent conductor of electricity? It allows currents to flow freely and reliably. This might be the reason the Arc of the Covenant needed to be carried with poles and not touched. The electric current was probably so strong that completing a circuit would cause electrocution!

The breastplate covered the high-priest's heart and vital organs. It was part of the amour *Shaul* spoke about in Ephesians 6. Instead of a Roman soldier, Ephesians 6 describes the spiritual armour of the high priest. It brought physical as well as spiritual power from *Yehovah*. At some point, this use of stones representing the tribes became the tradition we call "birthstones." Birthstones, used as necklaces, are still providing energy over the heart area. Scriptures throughout the Bible speak of minerals that are used for commerce, and extraordinary gemstones that bring brilliance to the throne room of our Creator

Elohim! Lapis Lazuli is the oldest known gemstone used for commerce even at the time of Abraham. Lapis may have been on the breastplate also but called sapphire in the Bible. The names may have changed, but the beauty and frequency still remain. Two stones of onyx were the part of the ephod that supported the breastplate. On these onyx stones were written the names of the twelve tribes. He carries us all on His shoulders! The other parts of the ephod were the Urim and Thummin. These are unknown stones to us today but were used to communicate with God for answers that were either 'yes' or 'no'. Urim means Lights and Thummin means perfection or truth. They were the determinants of innocence or fault, blessings or curses. It is possible these vibrations gave the direction or answer when needed. There is more description in Exodus 28-30.

Crystals, gemstones, minerals and all of creation vibrates with energy forces we call frequency and electro-magnetism. The crystals are composed of various elements of the periodic table and guess what? We are a combination of various elements of the periodic table too! As such, we all vibrate with energy and seek balance in our dance with Creation. Our Creator is the Source of all mathematics, physics, quantum physics, chemistry and everything designed. Everything created and designed uses energy and has frequency! Music, gemstones, minerals, plants and all of nature vibrate at various levels sharing life with human beings and the planet. Even the earth has a low-frequency microseismic signal every 26 seconds. The Earth's pulse!

As human crystals, we need balance in our bodies. The major minerals we require include calcium, phosphorus, magnesium, sodium, potassium, chloride and sulfur. There are other minerals required too and together they keep our hydration levels balanced, bones strong, and provide proteins for building structure, nerves and muscles. All these vibrate at different rates providing the basis for a healthy life. Our bodies are full of energy! We are spirits and souls living in a vibrating physical form.

Dr. Mayo, of Mayo Clinic, humorously once said that to make a human body we would need "enough potassium for one shot from a toy cannon,

Enough fat for seven bars of soap,

Enough iron to make a medium-sized nail,

Enough sulphur to delouse a dog,

Enough lime to whitewash a chicken coop,

Enough magnesium for one dose of medicine,

Enough phosphorus for a few boxes of matches.

The total purchase would fill not more than a couple of grocery bags. So, there you have it: our do-it-yourself kit for making the human body - a little dust and a lot of water!" [12]
(page June 23rd)

Now let me introduce you to Dr. Carey Reams. He was a gifted researcher that was willingly used by God to open the world to the idea of balance agriculturally and for our human bodies. He understood these nutrients (elements) were necessary for life. Let's look at a bit of his story.

Dr. Carey Reams - RBTI

"As a young researcher, *Carey Reams* had a voracious appetite to understand how biological life worked, as well as a pronounced ability to think outside the box. Along with his unique inquisitiveness, he found he had a natural bent for math. This was one of the reasons he was attracted to the general and special theories of relativity of *Dr. Albert Einstein*." [3 (page 5)]

"In 1905, *Albert Einstein* produced four scientific papers that forever revolutionized how scientists would understand the Universe and the matter within it. The first described how to measure the size of molecules in a liquid; a second put forward how to determine their movement, and a third demonstrated how light comes in packets called photons – the foundation of **quantum physics** and the idea that eventually won him the Nobel Prize. A fourth article introduced special relativity, leading physicists to reconsider notions of space and time that had sufficed since the dawn of civilization. Then, a few short months after the first four papers, appearing almost as an afterthought, *Einstein* published a fifth paper pointing out that matter and energy can be interchangeable at the atomic level – specifically that $\mathbf{E=MC^2}$ – the scientific basis of nuclear energy and the most famous mathematical equation in history." [3 (page 6)]

"As a young scientist in the 1930's, *Reams* thought a lot about *Einstein's* special mass-energy equation; however, he was pioneering on his own without a teacher. The more he contemplated its possible meanings and applications, the more he began to question how the equation might demonstrate that **mass (M)** of biological life may be built out of **energy (E).** In his first encounters with the now famous $\mathbf{E=MC^2}$ equation, *Reams* did not understand what was happening to the energy as it moved from A to B. He felt that if he understood what was happening to energy moving from A to B, he could begin to understand what was happening if energy was moved from B to A. '*Dr. Einstein*,' *Ream's* asked, 'Since you have shown science how energy moves from A to B, would you explain what it means to move energy back from B to A?' "*Einstein's* response was brief and to the point. 'I'm going to give you that assignment,' he stated.' [3 (page 6)]

"*Reams* took Einstein's challenge and realized that *Einstein's* equation provided the first relativistic definition of what matter really is. Matter is made up of two types of energy: $\mathbf{E_1}$ (heat) and $\mathbf{E_2}$ (electrical); therefore $\mathbf{E_1=MC^2-E_2}$. In other words, Einstein's formula says that $\mathbf{E_2}$ (electrical) energy equals the difference between $\mathbf{MC^2}$ (matter) – $\mathbf{E_1}$ (heat) energy. That is, electricity is the energy that holds things together. Electricity is what makes chelation. Electricity is the substance between heat and matter, while matter is heat plus electrical energy. Up until this time, *Ream's* realized that electricity had really never been defined or understood. Now *Einstein's* equation demonstrated that electrical energy is the substance between heat and matter." [3 (page 6)]

"Few realize that *Einstein's Theory of Relativity* and his famous equation $\mathbf{E=MC^2}$ helped solidify the mathematical thoughts of *Carey Reams* on how life is put together or taken apart by energy in ionic form. *Einstein* revealed how to take atomic structure apart and release the energy within it, whereas *Ream's* revealed how to take the energy within atomic structure and build healthy, high-energy biological life out of it." [3 (page 6)]

"To the physicist the study of nature is mathematical numbers, and to God, who is a God of mathematics, He says even the hairs of our head are numbered. Well, if *Jesus* had said, 'When your atoms and amino acid molecules are numbered' the people would not know what He was talking about. He knows not only what your atoms are, the numbers of your atoms that you are made of, but He also knows the number of your anions and cations. Every tree, every drop of water in the ocean (no two drops are alike), every snowflake (no two are alike), every blade of grass (no two are alike) reveals God in His greatness. When we understand the mathematical and chemical structure of matter, we see how truly great God is, and how little we are. How insignificant we are, and how helpless we are, and how much we need Him to help us understand these mysteries. The study of nature is so beautiful, so fantastic that only God can call it into existence." [4 (page 32)]

"In the Book of *Amos*, in the Old Testament, Chapter 3:7 we read: 'Surely the Lord God will do nothing, but he revealeth his secret unto his servants the prophets.' And in *Jeremiah* 33:2-3 it says, 'Thus saith the Lord, the Maker thereof (the Lord is the Messiah) 'the Lord that formed it, to establish it; the Lord is the name. Call unto me and I will answer thee, and show thee great and mighty things, which thou knowest not.' God has kept His Word." [4 (page 32)]

Dr. Carey Reams developed an assessment tool called *Reams Biological Theory of Ionization*. It is a mathematical equation that gives the status of the body's processes at that point in time. It is the theory of ionization." [4 (page 32)]

"This theory of ionization, of the story of creation, is becoming a reality because God is the God of math, a God of science, and He made it!" [4 (page 35)]

"Nature makes energy in many compound patterns. And it makes these compound patterns from nine elementary geometric patterns." [4 (page 38)]

"The liver manufactures a substance called bile, which in its purest state is a form of dilute hydrochloric acid. The body stores bile in little sacs in the stomach, gall bladder and capillaries of the liver." [4 (page 38)]

"All foods that we eat are cationic, with the exception of lemons. Lemon juice is anionic. In other words, the electron in lemon juice is traveling clockwise and all the electrons in other foods are traveling counterclockwise. However, some foods are more cationic than others, and some are less cationic. But we can say that lemon juice is nature's own natural dilute hydrochloric acid, and the liver can daily convert it into some 5 to 6 billion different enzymes, or vitamins if one is in good health. Lemon juice has less chemical change than any other natural substance known to man. The only other substance that can be used is man-made hydrochloric acid tablets." [4 (page 38-39)]

"Each food has its frequency number, according to its kind, the same as people have their frequency numbers. Once you know the frequency then you know the proper diet of all plants and animals. A horse can live on grass all of its life after it is weaned. Man's frequency is the highest decimal and as such requires the most complex diet. Frequency is how much time it takes for one electron to make one complete revolution around one molecule. This is measured in micro numbers (e.g., man's frequency log of 24, or .0000024 of a second.)" [4 (page 45)]

"The greater variety of foods that we can eat, the safer it is to maintain good health. Our foods are depleted of minerals today, and by having a great variety we come nearer fulfilling the mineral needs of our deficiencies. We lose *reserve energy* by limiting our choice of food intake." [4 (page 45)]

"In order to understand food chemistry, we must understand that there is a great similarity in amino acids in animals and plants. There is a great similarity in every frequency, and the micronage, milli-micronage, and milli-milli-micronage structure. That is, the biological, physical, and mathematical principles are very much alike in both animals and plants. No amino acids can be formed without **FIRST** having an atom of nitrogen. It is the first requirement in the formation of any amino acid cell. Amino acid in its true form may or may not be a complete cell. In its perfected form it could be a complete cell because all biological cells are amino acid cells, but seldom do you find one that is complete. The **SECOND** requirement after the first atom of nitrogen (protein) to form the amino acid cell is calcium, or one or more of the groups of calcium. The **THIRD** requirement to form the amino acid cell is oxygen. The **FOURTH** requirement is phosphate, and the **FIFTH** is potassium." [4 (page 45-46)]

"In this manner all biological structure is made, plants using carbon dioxide and animals oxygen." [4 (page 46)]

"The magnetism of the union of these and many other elements on any given frequency determines the organ structure, regardless of the various frequencies. Phosphates in plants have a different chemical action from what phosphates do in people. In plants the colloidal particles make cellulose, and in animals they are the bone structure. The greater the amount of cellulose in the plant the more tree-like the plant. The less cellulose it contains the more vine-like the plant. [4 (page 46-47)]

"The amino acids in plants are formed by ionization exactly as in animals. Plants do not have blood like we have, they have what we call sap. The sap rises because the amino acid is in anionic form. The sap goes up into the branches and the leaves through the process of photosynthesis. It uses the phosphate to join carbon, hydrogen, and oxygen. The plants breathe in the carbon form from the air and breathe out oxygen. Carbohydrates ($C_6H_{22}O_{11}$) in plants are formed in very simple terms as follows:

Carbon + Water (Phosphates is the catalyst) = sugar in plant

6 Carbons + 11 (H_2O) = $C_6H_{22}O_{11}$"

"The water is used to form the carbohydrates that are in the plant, using calciums as a catalytic base for the plant carbohydrates. There is a rule that the higher the carbohydrate content of the plant or the fruit, the higher the mineral content, and the heavier the fruit, the greater the specific gravity." [4 (page 46-47)]

"These are factors in determining the mineral content of foods. The higher the carbohydrate content the more energy it is possible for the person to get from the food they eat." [4 (page 47-48)]

Dr. Carey Reams recommends a wide variety of fruits and vegetables to provide the most energy for our bodies. "His RBTI test is the measure of excessive loss of ENERGY." "A loss of ENERGY is the result of a mineral deficiency." … "The loss of energy from one organ affects other organs. All of our organs are more or less dependent upon another." [4 (page 9-10)]

"God is the author of mathematics and chemistry. He made the laws of life, solids, liquids, gases, minerals, and vegetables. Chemistry could not exist without mathematics. There would be no need for mathematics were it not for chemistry." [4 (page 10)]

"The joining together of chemistry and mathematics is called PHYSICS. God is God of PHYSICS. All things that are made by the laws of physics are (and there is nothing made that is made without) adherence to the laws." [4 (page 10)]

"*IONIZATION* is God's laws putting things together and taking them apart ion by ion. An ion in its singular anionic form is the smallest amount of ENERGY in existence, in fact the smallest thing that God ever created. All things that are made are formed from IONS." [4 (page 10)]

God's plan of the use of energy for more perfect health is recorded in the Bible. The RBTI theory is a valuable tool to assess the body's situation and begin the process of bringing the body into the healing zone so the body can begin to heal. [4 (page 10)]

"By definition, frequency refers to the periodic or cyclic motion of electrons about atoms and molecules. This periodic motion is measurable in terms of time per each cycle of motion to be completed. What we want to look at is how this frequency relates to the biologic life of the human body and, more particularly, what it has to do with feeding and wellness of the human organism." [6 (page 9)]

"It is a recognized fact that all atomic structures have vibratory motion. This vibratory motion is a product of the energy of the sub-atomic particles known to most as 'electrons' and 'positrons.' As we shall see, each pure element has its own vibratory pattern called frequency; however, Reams Biological Theory of Ionization refers to these particles as **anions** (electrons) and **cations** (positrons or protons). As these sub-atomic particles combine, new charge ratios develop, which result in new frequencies." [6 (page 9)]

First, understand that "the atom is an electromagnetic structure. Yet (previously) only the electrical relations were being addressed, while the magnetic aspect was ignored. Anywhere there are electrical relations, there are magnetic relations also. In reality, what has been considered an attraction of opposite charges in electricity is actually the alignment of current flow causing magnetism." [6 (page 10)]

"Biological Ionization Principles recognize and deal with the electrical and magnetic charge force interrelationship. For example, it is recognized in Ionization principles, that **each element has a measurable resistance level, and it is unique for that element only**. **That resistance level is directly related to the ratio of the anions (electrons) and cations (positrons or protons) within the internal structure of the atom.** To put it another way, nature has a law of electrical flow that says electricity will always follow **the line of least resistance**. Electricity will flow easier where there is less impairment or interference to its movement." [6 (page 10)]

"**The process of digestion involves both energy release and frequency adjustment**. Digestion is a resistance process. The organized molecular and atomic structure of incoming food encounters the digestive enzymes. These, in turn, exert what some would call an 'Electron Press,' or high amount of energy pressure to disrupt the present molecular and atomic structure. The 'press' effect actually forces the electrons of the molecules and their atoms into a lower orbit. When this happens, many of the existing molecular and atomic bonds of the food material are broken. This renders the bound-up energy into a free state, which can be shunted to the liver for the beginning process of recombining into the higher frequency amino acids unique to the human. When the digestive enzymes are too 'dilute,' they do not exert enough 'Electron Press' or resistance upon the molecular and atomic structure of the incoming food. Thus, the bound-up energy in the food is not released into a usable state. This is how the loss of energy to the liver begins to take place biochemically." [6 (page 15-16)]

"The basic rule is **The Frequency Tells the Diet**. *This simply means that because frequency tells the combination of elements and their arrangement in the line of least resistance*, then the content of the diet and the way the foods should be provided for best nutrition can be known. In other words, if the frequency is known, then the ratio for the minimum amount of the various mineral elements that can make up that particular frequency is known." [6 (page 17)]

Let's look a little further into food as voltage and energy for our bodies. Energy in and energy out! We hear terms like antioxidants, free radicals, and our pH. What impact do these have on our health? Turns out the fuel for our bodies is our food choices. Let's learn a bit more about function before we are blessed by the cornucopia of foods Our Creator has given us for our fuel. This will help us see why some things are detrimental to our energy levels.

"An antioxidant is a molecule capable of giving away electrons. Thus, when your mother says, 'eat your vegetables,' she is saying that the vegetables contain electrons that are good for you." [5 (page 11)]

"We maintain our health and heal primarily by making new cells. To make a new cell requires a voltage of -50mV." (mV=millivolt) [5 (page 11)]

What could go wrong? What would cause a problem with voltage? Well, there are 'Electron Stealers' out there!

"Electron stealers cause damage, have a pH from 0-6.9, are acidic, are free radicals, are the positive pole, are destructive, and at the atomic level they spin left." We need our cells to spin right! [5 (page 11)]

Voltage - Dr. Jerry Tennant

"You will hear statements like 'all disease occurs when you are acidic.' What this is really saying is that all disease occurs when your voltage is low or in an electronic stealer state." And, then there are free radicals. "A free radical is a molecule that is missing electrons. It is like a mugger looking for someone's purse to steal. When a free radical steals electrons from the cell, it damages the cell." [5 (page 11)]

"We maintain our health and heal primarily by making new cells. To make a new cell requires a voltage of -50mV." [5 (page 11)]

"Salivary and urinary pH are about 0.8 pH units less than cell pH. Salivary pH is a rough indicator of cellular voltage. Urinary pH is a rough indicator of the voltage in the fluids around cells. When normal, both should be 6.5. If you add 0.8 to 6.5, you get a pH (cell) of 7.3. This equates to -20 millivolts." [5 (page 12)]

Dr. Jerry Tennant, the author of a series of books called *Healing is Voltage*, uses a description of his thumb to help explain how all this works. "My thumb is running at a voltage of -25mV. It is pink, feels fine and works well. Now, I hit it with a hammer. The thumb is red, swollen, hot, and has a pulsing pain. It has automatically gone to -50mV. This is necessary to make new cells needed to replace the ones I damaged with a hammer. At -50mV, blood vessels dilate and dump raw materials such as proteins, carbohydrates, fats, vitamins, minerals, etc. into the neighborhood. I need these raw materials to build new cells. I also need -50mV to have the energy to turn these raw materials into new cells." [5 (page 12-13)]

"As soon as I finish making enough cells to replace those I damaged with the hammer, my thumb goes back to -25mV. It is normal and I am happy." [5 (page 13)]

"Now let's assume that I ran out of voltage before I was able to make enough new cells to replace those I injured with a hammer. My voltage dropped to -10 millivolts. Now I am stuck in chronic disease. I cannot heal unless I can make new cells. I cannot make new cells unless I have -50mV and all the raw materials I need to make new cells. In chronic disease, my thumb hurts all the time, it is white and doesn't work very well." [5 (page 13)]

"Thus, we see that chronic disease is always defined by having low voltage. One cannot cure chronic disease without inserting enough electrons to achieve -50mV. One must also have the raw materials necessary to make new cells and to eliminate the toxins or infections present that will damage the new cells. One can take all of the medications you like and do as much surgery as you like but you will not heal unless you have -50mV, raw materials, and lack of toxins." [5 (page 14)]

"Without the ability to achieve -50mV and the necessary raw materials to make new cells, you cannot maintain your health and you suffer aging and chronic disease. You also are unable to repair injuries so they can also lead to chronic disease. You don't need drugs to heal. You need to make new cells that work to heal. To make good cells, you need voltage and a good diet. You also need to remove toxins from your body that damage cells and make you obese." [5 (page 14)]

"The earth is a large electromagnet…" "An area of high voltage always causes electrons to flow to an area of low voltage. If your body has lower voltage than the earth, walking barefoot on the dirt or grass will cause electrons to flow from the earth into your body, recharging you. However, if you walk with shoes, this cannot occur." [5 (page 19)]

"Water from the ground contains electrons. We call this 'alkaline water.' However, when we place chlorine and fluoride into the water it turns it into an electron stealer. Thus, every time we drink such water, it steals electrons from us. The water we should be drinking should contain electrons and be clean and free from toxins." [5 (page 20)]

"If you stick a voltmeter into a raw potato, you will measure voltage. However, if you bake a potato or freeze the potato and then insert the voltmeter, most of the voltage will be gone. Unprocessed food contains voltage. Once we process food, most of the voltage disappears. We are designed to eat unprocessed food so that it brings its own electrons with it. When you eat food that has been processed, your body must provide electrons from other sources to digest it. You can actually tell the quality of food such as vegetables by simply using a voltmeter to compare the voltage in one product versus another. [5 (page 21)]

"Moving water is always an electron donor. Still water is an electron stealer. Thus, taking a shower will energize me whereas taking a bath will make me tired. Swimming in the ocean will give you electrons, but swimming in a chlorinated pool will steal voltage from you." [5 (page 22)]

"Moving air is an electron stealer. Thus, people often feel tired if they sleep under a fan. Riding in a convertible is great fun, but you are always tired when you get to your destination." [5 (page 22)]

"If you take a voltmeter that measures in millivolts and hold it in the air inside your home, you will measure a small amount of voltage. Now take it outside. You will find there is much more voltage out in the sun." [5 (page 22)]

"If you take a quartz crystal and squeeze it with a pair of pliers, it will emit electrons. This is called the piezoelectric effect. Our muscles are piezoelectric crystals. Thus, when we exercise, our muscles create electrons. The muscles are also rechargeable batteries. Thus, the movement of our muscles recharges our muscle batteries. Exercise is a major way the body acquires electrons." [5 (page 22)]

"Thus, you can see that humans are designed to get voltage primarily the way our grandparents got it. They worked out in the sun, drank water from a well, ate unprocessed foods, weren't afraid to touch the earth with their hands or feet, hugged their family, leaned against a tree, or stood in moving water while they were fishing, and weren't afraid to stand in the rain." [5 (page 23)]

There are things that hinder healing and stop the proper intake of electrons in our bodies. Let's take a look at what those might be.

"Common Ways Electrons are Taken <u>from</u> the Human Body:

1. Acidic Water (tap water, chlorinated water, fluoride, most bottled water.)
2. Carbonated Beverages
3. Caffeinated Beverages (pop, coffee, tea)
4. Alcoholic Beverages
5. Cooked Food
6. Processed Food

7. Healers/Doctors who touch their patients lose their electrons to the patient.
8. Hugs: transfer electrons from one person to another.
9. Holding a sick child gets the child well quicker, but the parent is left tired.
10. Moving air: wind, air conditioning, fans, convertibles, and hair dryers." [5 (page 23)]

"Cell membranes are primarily capacitors to store electrons for use by the cells. This voltage is used primarily to control the electronic circuitry of the cell membrane since it functions as a semi-conductor, a diode, a transistor, and a microprocessor." [5 (page 44)]

"Inside the cell, we have another electron storage system known as ATP/ADP. This rechargeable battery system is used to make many of the cell's chemical functions work." [5 (page 45)]

"When oxygen is available, we make 38 molecules of ATP from one unit of fatty acids, but when oxygen is unavailable, we only make two! This inability to provide electrons for critical chemical pathways of the cell is part of chronic illness." [5 (page 45)]

"The human body has two wiring systems. Both are made of fibrous tissue. One is the fibrous encasement of nerves that *Robert Becker* named '*analog perineural nervous system*.' The other is the acupuncture system." [5 (page 46)]

"*Robert Becker* was an orthopedic surgeon. His classic book, *The Body Electric* is a must-read for everyone interested in healing. He became interested in the fact that in humans, if you lose a piece of bone, you will make more bone. If you lose a piece of any other tissue, it is replaced by scar tissue. In humans, it was believed that only bone is capable of regeneration. We now know that all tissue can regenerate with proper conditions." [5 (page 46)]

Our bodies are such exciting and wonderful creations just as the scripture says. We are marvelously and wonderfully made. We are energy and we need energy provided by all the aspects of Creation. The air, the water, the sun, the fruit, and other plants made just for us, and more! We need exercise, proper rest, and most of all we need Him! Our Creator and King!

Now with some understanding of why our bodies require specific types of fuel to build and keep health and energy, let's take a look at what He provides us!

CHAPTER SEVEN

BOUNTIFUL FOODS FOR HEALTH AND HEALING

Choose Life!

We turn our attention now to the benefits of *Yehovah's* bounty and how we benefit from living according to *His Will*. These are the sources of fuel for our energy! As we are created of energy, we are also created needing an energy supply. There is a reason *Yehovah* chose certain foods. They are frequencies our bodies recognize and can use to build energy and health. As always, He is a good God providing the instructions for our best lives.

D'varim (*Deuteronomy*) 30:15 "'Look! I am presenting you today with, on the one hand, life and good; and on the other, death and evil – 16 in that I am ordering you today to love ADONAI your God, to follow his ways, and to obey his *mitzvot*, regulations and rulings; for if you do, you will live and increase your numbers; and ADONAI your God will bless you in the land you are entering in order to take possession of it. 17 But if your heart turns away, if you refuse to listen, if you are drawn away to prostrate yourselves before other gods and serve them; 18 I am announcing to you today that you will certainly perish; you will not live long in the land you are crossing the *Yarden* to enter and possess. 19 I call on heaven and earth to witness against you today that I have presented you with life and death, blessing and the curse. Therefore, **choose life**, so that you will live, you and your descendants, 20 **loving *ADONAI* your God**, **paying attention to what he says** and **clinging to him – for that is the purpose of your life**! On this depends the length of time you will live in the land ADONAI swore he would give to your ancestors *Avraham*, *Yitz'chak* and *Ya'akov*.'" [1 (page 265)]

We learn quite a lot from these passages. First, we learn that we are in control of our tongue, and it has the power of life or death! Our words are powerful and bring life or death depending on the words we use and the choices we make. That would also apply to foods our tongues are attracted to!

Deuteronomy takes us even further into the relationship to which God is calling us! Following Him and following His ways brings us **Life**! He even answers the question He proposes to us! It is an open book test! Answer: **CHOOSE LIFE**!

Some years ago I was listening to a teaching on healing that referenced this scripture. The teacher was Gloria Copeland. I can still hear her voice today challenging us to Choose Life! A precious memory I will never forget!

We are granted only one lease on life and all of us should wonder how we can best invest in our most precious gift – Ourselves! Investing in ourselves can bring the greatest profit! We are temples of God's Spirit. The question: How can we do the most for His glory and the benefit of mankind? "For life is valuable only as it is used for the attainment of these ends.'" [2 (page 15)]

Let's delve into how the things we eat might bring glory to God! Our tongues, our words and our choices can help us Choose Life!

Pre-Flood vs Post-Flood

A good place to start is to study God's original plan for mankind's diet. Since *Yehovah Elohim* created humankind, and is our Creator, it is He Who best understands our needs and gave instructions to *Adam* regarding food. "Behold, I have given you every herb yielding seed…and every tree in which is the fruit of a tree yielding seed; to you it shall be for food." [2; (Genesis 1:29)]

The foods chosen for mankind are grains, fruits, nuts, and vegetables. These healthful and nourishing foods can be prepared in a simple and natural manner and even be eaten raw. These foods bring us strength, endurance, and allow our minds and intellect to be awake and able to think and respond. A less quality diet does not benefit the body or the mind. [2]

"*Ellen G. White*, in a letter dated 1884 said, 'Again and again I have been shown that God is bringing His people back to His original design, that is not to subsist upon the flesh of dead animals. He would have us teach people a better way." [2 (page 82)]

Ellen G. White was right. If not introduced to a particular taste when young, the taste may not be a driver for food choices in the later years. Introduction to healthy choices when little will hopefully lead to healthier choices throughout life. In an RBTI class I took regarding the frequency of foods and our body's ability to digest various foods properly, I learned that children don't have the maturity of their organs to digest certain foods including flesh meat until after the age of twelve; and nuts and seeds until the age of eight. A plant based eating program is easier on the digestive track and will hopefully lead to a healthier life and more energy.

With a recent change to the food pyramid guidelines, fruits, vegetables and grains hold an important place. However, flesh meat holds a large place on the plates of many Americans. We need to remember that the quality and standards of foods are very important. We would prefer foods that come from regenerative farms and companies that pride themselves in providing excellent products that do not contain additives and poisons. If one is to include flesh meats, the meats need to be raised with as much care as possible and with as few chemicals added to their food and water supplies as possible. Grass-fed and finished on land without chemicals is a blessing to us and to the animals themselves. Father cares for us and the animals too! We should prefer foods that come from regenerative farms and companies that pride themselves in providing excellent products that do not contain additives and poisons.

If children are not introduced to meats, but rather introduced to fruits and grains they will have less of a desire for meats. Young children are not able to properly digest meats, so it is to their benefit that we eliminate meat from their food choices. (I am interested in where the research is that says young children cannot properly digest meat because that is not something I have ever heard and my husband was a chapter leader for The Weston A Price Foundation for many years) I am unfamiliar with the Weston A. Price Foundation. I will look into it. I changed the wording of the statement to clarify where the info came from. Hope that makes more sense.

God added flesh meats to man's foods after the flood of *Noah's* day, but meat was not to completely replace fruits, grains, and vegetables. Meat would sustain them until the earth was replenished with grasses, plants, trees, and herbs. The world before the Flood had deteriorated into a violent, chaotic, evil place. Most likely eating flesh meat had been going on for sometime even though *Yehovah* had not given His permission. The people living then were so out of control that He must have determined that their appetites could not be reigned back in. Moderation was no longer a possibility. They had become a violent, corrupt society even entertaining unhuman acts of idolatry.

By Moses' time, chaos had once again reigned in the earth. There was once again great disobedience and the people had forgotten who they were. They had been in Egypt and Egypt had gotten in them. God was about to take them on a journey to reintroduce His Way to them and begin to bring them back to obedience. Although *Yehovah* still allowed flesh meat, He reiterated which were "clean" and which were not. The browsing animals were included, but the scavengers were left to do the jobs they were designed for.

In *D'Varim* (Deuteronomy) 8:1-10 Moses reminds the Hebrews of all *Yehovah* has done for them and that they cannot live on food alone but "on everything that comes from the mouth of *ADONAI*." Regarding food, Moses describes the promised land as "For *ADONAI* your God is bringing you into a good land, a land with streams, springs, and water welling up from the depths in the valleys and on hillsides. It is a land of wheat and barley, grapevines, fig trees and pomegranates; a land of olive oil and honey; a land where you will eat food in abundance and lack nothing in it; a land where stones contain iron and the hills can be mined for copper. So you will eat and be satisfied, and you will bless *ADONAI* your God for the good land he has given you." [1 (page 237-238)]

Sadly, our soil is not as rich in minerals as in the beginning. But nuts, fruit, grains, etc. can still be our mainstay. Many vegetables, herbs, fruits, and plants were brought from one country to another and added to the menu list of the early *Israelites*. Their mainstay included bread, wine, and olive oil. The countries in the *Middle East* and *Mediterranean* areas still have these three as a big part of their meals. The *Mediterranean* diet today is possibly a close resemblance to meals eaten by the *Hebrew* families, and *Yeshua* Jesus, in His day. We determined that *Yeshua* did NOT do away with *Torah* and He followed the dietary instructions during His earthly walk. Will eating a biblical and, or *Mediterranean* type diet really benefit us? How limiting is this way of eating and food preparation? Let's take a look!

"The medical and scientific facts confirm it. If we eat as *Jesus* ate, we will be healthier. He is our role model for good habits in eating, exercising, and loving a healthy, balanced life." [3 (page x)]

"The foods that *Jesus* ate were based on *Levitical* law that was given to the *Israelites* from God through *Moses*. The foods that Jesus ate in accordance with the law provided Him with the raw materials to produce a healthy body and a healthy mind. He lived and walked in divine health. God is giving us the grace today to learn about His law and to live according to it." [3 (page 7)]

As we saw in Genesis 1:29, God initially planned for humans to be fruitarian or vegetarian. The animals were designed to be herbivores. This plant based eating program is available to us today throughout the world. A variety of fruits, vegetables, grains, nuts, seeds and more are offered seasonly and provide the amazing cornucopia of proteins, carbohydrates, good fats, vitamins, and minerals our bodies need. Eating a variety of fruits, vegetables, grains, and nuts provide great sources for all the vitamins, minerals and even Omega-3 fatty acids! There really isn't a necessary reason to include fish and animals in our eating programs. The Father's Plan has it all!

From Adam to Noah, people lived very long lives. The oldest person was Noah's grandfather, *Methuselah*, who lived to be nine-hundred, sixty-nine years old (969). Others with notably long lives before the Flood included Adam (930 years), his son Seth (912 years), Enos (905 years)and Jared (962 years). Their lineage seems to be the line from the beginning that *Yehovah* called 'righteous." Could that righteousness be a result of obedience to the Father's plan? The lineage of these people are listed in Genesis chapter 5. Noah lived 350 years after the Flood and was 600 at the time of the Flood. One thought on the reduction of length of life is perhaps less oxygen in the atmosphere and a change in the quality of water. The soil now was different too. Every living thing, all of Creation, was affected by the destruction of the Flood. Amazing to think about that when our lives are certainly much shorter now. In comparison, we know that Abraham lived to 175 and Moses to 120. And now the average is about 75 years. A sad decline in lifetime and the vibrancy of all of Creation.

B'resheet (*Genesis*) [6:3] "*Adonai* said, 'My Spirit will not live in human beings forever, for they too are flesh; therefore, their life span is to be 120 years.'" [1(page 10)]

Some look at the scripture *Genesis* 6:3 as a restriction in age God placed on people. Others look at that scripture as the length of time from the day God made the statement to the day of the Flood. Whatever God's meaning, lack of obedience to the Father is certainly playing a part in the length of life.

(Post flood the Father declared people wouldn't live as long because of their corruption. It wasn't food related. It was our sinful nature that caused ordained shorter lifespans. It also talks about in different texts that our sinful nature will continue to cause decrease in age to where babies will have gray hair CS: Wow, I have never heard anything like that!)

However, God's good plan was still in place after the Flood. An interim time was needed for the grasses, herbs, trees, and vegetation to be restored. I believe the allowance of meat to the diet was a result of the length of time it would take for Creation to be somewhat restored. They would not have the benefit of the fresh grains, nuts and fruits, but would have a second-hand nutritional supply from the animals who were raised on the grasses Noah brought on board the Ark.

Yehovah also introduced an animal sacrifice system that allowed both the person bringing the sacrifice and the cohens (priests) to eat the meat of the animal, bird or grain brought to the tabernacle and later the Temple.

In His grace He designed us to eat plant based food, but gave us a digestive system capable of digesting clean, grass-fed and finished meat of the animals He specified as 'clean.' Although capable of living on both plants and animals, our physical body was designed to be better suited for consuming foods made from plants rather than consuming products made from animals, even if they are "clean."

Water, Water Everywhere! Let's be sure to Drink it!

"God said, 'Let there be a dome in the middle of the water; let it divide the water from the water.' God made the dome and divided the water under the dome from the water above the dome; that is how it was." *B'resheet* (Genesis) 1:6-8 [1(page 2)]

Water was there before everything! Have you ever thought of water as a nutrient? Water is so very important, and the water was divided to create a world fit for humans! Think of the various divisions of water we experience daily. Mostly we think of the liquid form, but there are ice cubes and steam too! All are super healing! Take a look!

"Water is the most important nutrient for the human body. Indeed, the human body consists primarily of water – approximately two-thirds of a person's body weight is water. The average person who is conscious and moving can live for approximately forty-days without food, but only about three to five days without water. Water is necessary for nearly every bodily function, including circulation, digestion, absorption, and excretion. Water is vital for carrying nutrients to all cells of the body. Every cell in the body produces metabolic waste products of some form – commonly lactic acid, urea, and uric acid. An adequate water intake is essential to remove these waste products from the body via the bloodstream and excretory organs." [3 (page 123)]

"The major constituent of all the fluids in the body is water: saliva, gastric juice, bile, pancreatic juices, intestinal secretions, and blood. The synovial fluid, which lubricates the joints, is comprised primarily of water. Patients with joint pain and arthritis definitely need an extra intake of water to provide lubrication for their joints." [3 (page123)]

"Many individuals develop degenerative disc disease in their necks and back as they age. This is usually caused by discs simply wearing out owing to inadequate fluid within the disc. The disc is composed of a fibrous material called the annulus fibrosus, and it is filled with a jellylike substance called *nucleus pulposus*. The jellylike material is composed primarily of water. When the discs become dehydrated, they are more prone to degenerate and eventually herniate, and thus many develop degenerative disc disease and arthritis." [3 (page 123)]

"Joints are covered by cartilage, which is approximately five times slicker than ice and composed of 80 percent water. If cartilage becomes dehydrated and the synovial fluid is insufficient, increased friction results, causing damage to the cartilage, and eventually leading to arthritis. Adequate intake of water is also vital for lung function. Lung tissue that is thoroughly moist is capable of greater oxygen intake and also greater excretion of carbon dioxide." [3 (page 124)]

"Adequate water intake is necessary to improve blood pressure in persons with hypertension, high cholesterol levels, obesity, diabetes, asthma, gastrointestinal problems, hiatal hernia, headaches, angina, allergies, and constipation. Adequate water intake also helps prevent kidney stones and can slow the aging process. The latter is accomplished primarily because adequate water keeps the cells nourished by carrying nutrients to the cells and removing cellular waste products. Finally, those who take in adequate amounts of water generally find they have increased energy because they are healthier at the cellular level." [3 (page 124)]

Most health practitioners recommend we drink at least two to three quarts of filtered or distilled water each day. A great suggestion from Original Medicine is to drink three to four ounces of steam distilled water every thirty minutes while awake. If steam distilled water is not available, consume the safest and cleanest water available.

You can figure out your total hydration needs by taking your total body weight and divide it by two. That will get the overall number of ounces you should plan for per day. Then, as your day progresses, remember every half hour or so, take a drink!! Your body will be grateful!

Water is used in healing externally as well as internally. This therapy is called Hydrotherapy which uses various forms of water to bring relief when prepared warm, hot, or iced depending on the situation. Hydrotherapy works in conjunction with the other areas of our Creator's plan: fresh air, sunlight, exercise, rest, diet, cheerful attitude and trust in the divine power provided in each body for healing!

Bread: The Staff of Life!

"Bread played an important role in the life and teachings of Jesus. But a loaf of bread in Jesus' time was not the baker's loaf we find in our grocery stores today. Bread was baked on large flat rocks, the dough stretched and twirled in a circular fashion to make a large, flat circle. The resulting loaf was larger than a pancake, but thin like paper. The pita bread of today is a modern version of these loaves. One to three loaves of bread per person were eaten at each meal." [3 (page 22)]

Sue Becker, in her book *The Essential Home-Ground Flour Book*, shares the following benefits of baking with freshly ground, whole grain flour.

- "Whole grains are a nearly perfect food. They have the ability to sustain life.

- Many of the life-giving nutrients contained in whole grains are lost to oxidation and spoilage shortly after the flour is ground.
- The common diseases that plague the developed world are directly related to our overconsumption of heavily processed foods, particularly bread products.
- Prior to 1900, most bread was made at home. Flour was either ground at home or purchased from the local miller." [4 (page 11)]

"Throughout history bread has been the 'staff of life.' It is only in more recent years, as people began to enjoy a more varied diet, that bread took on more of the accompaniment role at mealtimes. It is time to return whole grains, and their products found in many stores, to their proper role and place on our plates, as a main dish rather than a side dish." [4 (page 13)]

We need to learn "that real whole grains are nearly perfect foods that have the ability to sustain life and promote health. As you embrace baking with home-ground flour and it becomes part of your life, it is our hope that you will find encouragement and health. As 'real bread' returns to its rightful place as the staff of life, may this small investment of time bring you and others lifelong returns in health and happiness." [4 (page 13)]

Challah, meaning 'loaf', is a versatile, braided egg bread offered at meals, especially on Shabbat and some of the other Feasts of *Yehovah.* For *Rosh Hashanah* raisins might be baked in the loaf and the top of the loaf can also be brushed with honey symbolizing a sweet new year. Challah is first mentioned in *B'Midbar* (Numbers) 15:20 as an offering of the first of the dough for an offering to *Yehovah.* It is also mentioned in Leviticus 23:17. For Shabbat, two loaves are served in remembrance of the double portion of manna the Israelites received for Shabbat while in the wilderness. Generally, the challah is torn and dipped in salt as a covenant. Most likely, *Yeshua* tore the challah and dipped it in salt as he shared it with the disciples during the last supper they had together. He said to remember Him when we eat the bread and drink the wine. The blessings, *Kiddush*, given are the same blessings the Israelites had been praying generation after generation.

"Blessed are You, Lord our God, King of the universe, who brings forth bread from the earth."

Matzah is the bread used for Passover and the Feast of Unleavened Bread. It is an unleavened bread baked without yeast or leavening. Yeast puffs or raises up the dough and is representative of sin or pride in our lives. Matzah is a flat bread much like pita bread or crackers. They can replace crackers and be served in many ways such as with humus or butter. Although I haven't tried it yet, you can substitute matzah crackers for lasagna noodles and make matzah lasagna!

The Matzah cracker itself shares a hidden picture of *Yeshua* and His crucifixion. The cracker is pierced, representing the piercing *Yeshua* experienced in His hands and feet. It is also "bruised" and "striped" showing the damage from the scourging He endured. This message in flat bread was designed by The Father years before the Crucifixion itself. For hundreds of years, each Passover the children of Israel celebrated the feast enjoying this hidden message in their flat bread. Now we can join them in remembering the sacrifice of our Savior.

Ezekiel 4:9 is a combination of grains and beans providing a higher nutrient flour when milled or the mixture can be used for creating soups and stews. The sprouting process increases vitamins and creates breads that are more easily assimilated by the body. You can process your own grains for Ezekiel breads and baked goods, or an Ezekiel 4:9 bread is generally available in the feezer section of some grocery and health food stores. We will look at the Ezekiel 4:9 blend again when we look at beans.

"The corn of the *Bible* times was not like the corn, or maize, that we know in the *United States* today. Maize is native to *North America*, where it has been cultivated for more than three thousand years by the *Native American Indians*. Corn in the *Bible*, however, refers to different grains or seeds. Even in ancient *England*, the term corn referred to wheat, and in *Scotland* and *Ireland*, to oats. In the case of *David* taking corn to his brothers, the grain in question was likely dried kernels of wheat that could be munched upon directly." [3 (page 21)]

"The two foremost grains used in the *Old Testament* were barley and wheat." [3 (page 26)]

As we just learned, "Wheat was considered the staff of life and the king of grains. It became used as a measure of wealth. Barley, the cheaper and more plentiful of the two grains, was used by the poorer classes of people." [3 (page 26)]

"*Jesus* and His disciples ate grains in their raw state, as recorded in *Luke* 6:1." … "These grains may still have been green, or they may have ripened after the harvest. Rubbing the grain in their hands removed the outer husk, but the bran and wheat germ remained." [3 (page 26)]

"Worldwide, more than eight thousand different species of plants supply grains. Only a very small number of these grains are consumed routinely by *Americans*. The most commonly consumed grains worldwide are wheat, rice, corn, and oats. Rice, corn, and oats were not consumed in *Israel* during the time of *Jesus*." [3 (page 29)]

"Millet is mentioned only once in the Scriptures (in *Ezekiel* 4:9). As a grain, however, millet is superior to wheat, corn, and rice in protein content; its average protein content is between 10 and 12 percent. It is also high in minerals and is easily digested. Millet is a hardy plant and can grow in rich or poor soil…Millet has no gluten, which is the primary cause of wheat food allergies." [3 (page 29-30)]

"Rye is another grain mentioned in the *Bible*. Rye is a gluten grain, but its gluten content is much lower than that of wheat. It is approximately 20 percent protein and is high in fiber. Rye contains high amounts of the minerals magnesium, iron, and potassium. It also contains B vitamins and other minerals." [3 (page 30)]

"Most rye breads available commercially are made with refined rye flour, and this flour has usually been mixed with processed wheat flour. Pure rye bread is difficult to find. It is nearly black in color and is very nourishing and flavorful." [3 (page 30)]

"The processing of whole grains of wheat to white flour takes approximately twenty steps. The wheat kernel is composed of an outer layer called the *bran*. The bran is rich in B vitamins, minerals, and fiber. The next layer is the wheat germ, which is the starch or food supply for the sprouting seed. The endosperm is approximately 80 to 85 percent of the grain. The germ is about 3 percent, and the bran is about 15 percent." [3 (page 31)]

"Not only have 80 percent of the nutrients been removed, but the milling process involves such high temperatures that the remaining grain is damaged by oxidation. Flour at the end of the refining process actually has a grayish appearance from the oxidation. That color, of course, would be offensive to most consumers, so a chemical agent such as chlorine dioxide, acetone peroxide, or benzoyl peroxide is used to bleach the flour to make it white. The bleaching process destroys even more of the few vitamins that remain. In addition, the bleaches can react with fatty acids to produce peroxides that are toxic and that can cause free-radical reactions. (Just compare these bleach products to the labels on chemical bleach in your home such as *Clorox*!) In all, the milling and bleaching processes used today remove some twenty-two important nutrients from our bread, including fiber, vitamins, and minerals." [3 (pages 31-32)]

"What about 'enriched' bread? To these breads, bakeries usually replace about four nutrients to the flour they use – thiamin, niacin, riboflavin, and iron. However, the vitamins they use are usually 'coal tar derived' vitamins. Unfortunately, the end result is extremely little actual vitamin enrichment." [3 (page 32)]

"Low-fiber bread that has been laced with a great deal of sugar and hydrogenated fat becomes paste-like in the intestines. This, in turn, leads to constipation, which in turn may lead to gastrointestinal disease such as irritable bowel syndrome, diverticulosis, diverticulitis, and hemorrhoids." [3 (page 32)]

This degeneration of grains is not just about bread. It includes "the buns, for your hamburgers and hot dogs!" And more: "crackers, bagels, pretzels, and many pasta and cereal products, which are also made of white flour. Remember, the most commonly eaten foods in *America* are white bread, coffee, and hot dogs." [3 (page 32)]

"The conclusion we can draw is this: Choose whole-grain products! Besides bread, you should be able to find whole-grain pasta, whole-grain muffins and bagels, and whole-grain pretzels. If the label on those products does not read 'whole-wheat' or 'whole grain,' you should assume that the product is made completely or partially with refined flour." [3 (page 33)]

"Jesus ate whole grains by themselves and in the form of whole-grain bread. We can follow His example by choosing to eat whole-grain breads and pastas and to eat whole grains in cooked and salad dishes." [3 (page 34)]

Beans, Peas, and Lentils

Easily cultivated, beans, legumes, and lentils are other sources of nutrients like fiber and provide flavors to your food. Like grains, beans can be dried and stored for use over time. Beans provide proteins, vitamins, minerals and fiber in soups, breads, salads and wherever added. "In Bible times, they were used to make puree's, pottages, or when mixed with millet, a coarse bread." [3 (page 83)]

"Red stew is a very ancient dish in the *Middle East*. It is made of beans and lentils boiled in garlic – a very tasty, aromatic, and nutritious meal." [3 (page 83)]

The Red lentil stew was often a special dish made by the first-born son for his father when the patriarch was grieving. The Bible shares a story about this meal in *Genesis* 25: 29-34 regarding Issac and his sons, Esau and Jacob. You might remember that Esau, the eldest, sold his birthright to Jacob for a bowl of red-lentil stew. It truly must have been delicious!(Not sure if you know this already. This interaction happened after Esau had been out hunting for a long time. While he was hunting he came across Nimrod with two guards. He killed the two guards and Nimrod. When he had gotten home he had just finished running for his life and knew he ("the killer" as they didn't know who he was specifically) was being hunted by Nimrod's army. He believed he would be dead soon anyways, so what was a birthright to a dead man.) I am familiar with that info, but didn't want to open that can of worms at this point.

"Beans are loaded with soluble fiber, which helps lower LDL (bad) cholesterol and reduces blood pressure. *Dr. James Anderson*, a noted researcher at the *University of Kentucky*, recommends a minimum of one cup of cooked beans daily to help prevent heart disease. The fiber in beans also helps to keep blood sugar levels stable, fights off hunger, and has been shown to reduce the insulin requirements of diabetics. Beans can help prevent constipation and the development of hemorrhoids and other bowel-related problems. Diets high in beans will help to lower one's risk of developing certain cancers." [3 (page 84)]

"Beans and garlic have often been boiled together to produce a primitive version of cough medicine. Beans are packed with vitamin C which has great antioxidant value.

Just one cup of beans can provide:

- 6 to 7 grams of fiber
- Potassium, iron, and thiamine
- 12 grams of complex carbohydrates or starches
- 17.9 grams of protein

"And that cup of beans has no cholesterol and virtually no fat. They usually provide two to four times more protein than grains. They have been called 'the poor man's meat.'" [3 (page 84-85)]

Beans and grains when mixed together create complete proteins and provide valuable nutrients to the body. An example is black beans and rice! When adding fibrous foods to your diet, be sure to drink plenty of fluids, this will help avoid the constipation issue.

Fresh or dried beans are a better choice than canned. If using canned beans, be sure to rinse them prior to use to remove as much salt as possible. It does take more time to prepare dried beans, but you can create many delicious dishes if you take the time. I have even made brownies using black beans. They boost the nutrient content and make the brownies healthier and tasty!

The mix of beans and grains creates a complex combination called for in *Ezekiel* 4:9. We touched on that in grains and here is the story of where this recipe came from. It is the *Our Father's* recipe!

"In *Ezekiel* 4, the Lord commanded *Ezekiel* to lie on his left side for 390 days and when he was finished, the Lord directed him to lie on his right side for 40 days. God said to *Ezekiel*, 'Also take for yourself wheat, barley, beans, lentils, millet, and spelt (or rye); put them into one vessel and make bread of them for yourself' (*Ezekiel* 4:9). *Ezekiel* was to eat this bread in the amount of twenty shekels over a day, along with water. That was about half a pound of bread. The Lord also commanded him to eat barely cakes that were baked over a fire that used human waste as fuel (see *Ezekiel* 4:12)." [3 (page 85)]

In reading in *Ezekiel*, we may miss the plea *Ezekiel* makes to God regarding the cooking over human waste. Human waste is unclean! Let's look at the context and the complete passage in *Ezekiel* 4:9-15.

Yechezk'El (*Ezekiel*) [4:9] "'Take wheat, barley, beans, lentils, millet and buckwheat; put them together in one bowl; and make bread from it. For as long as you lie on your side, 390 days, this is what you are to eat. [10] Each day the food you eat must weigh only three-quarters of a pound; you may eat it from time to time [during the day]. [11] You are also to drink a limited amount of water, two-thirds of a quart; you may drink it from time to time [during the day]. [12] [The bread] you eat so to be baked like barley cakes; you are to bake it before their eyes, using human dung as fuel.' [13] *ADONAI* said, 'This is how the people of *Isra'el* will eat their food – *unclean* – in the nations where I am driving them.' [14] I objected: 'No, *Adonai ELOHIM*! I have never defiled myself – from my youth until now. I have never eaten anything that died by itself or was killed by wild animals; no such disgusting food has ever entered my mouth.' [15] He answered, 'All right, I will give you cow dung to use instead of human dung, and you can prepare your bread on it.'" [1 (page 717)]

"Note that *Ezekiel* lived on this bread for a total of 430 days! The bread was a combination of grains (wheat, barley, millet, and spelt, or rye) and legumes and beans. It was a complete protein mixture. *Ezekiel's* bread can be found in many health food stores. Some of those products are sprouted breads, which are even more nutritious. When seed is sprouted into a new plant, the new sprouts are very nutrient rich. The protein content usually increases between 15 to 30 percent. The chlorophyll and fiber content also increases, and the sprout is usually a rich green color. Both the B vitamins and vitamin C are increased, and the sprouts contain living enzymes." [3 (page 86)]

"Lentils were commonly consumed in *Israel* during biblical times. Lentils are actually one of the oldest cultivated plants. Lentils have 7.5 percent protein, but they are deficient in the amino acids methionine, and cysteine." Methionine and cysteine can be added when used in combination with grains or rice. Lentils "are very low in fat and contain high amounts of soluble fiber that help to lower cholesterol and control blood sugar. Lentils are good in combination with other vegetables in soups, stews, and casseroles." [3 (page 87-88)]

"Another popular bean common to the *Middle East* is the garbanzo bean, also called the chickpea."

Chickpeas can be used in making hummus. "In *Israel*, people usually eat hummus by dipping a piece of flat bread (pita bread) into a shallow bowl of the mixture. Olive oil is sometimes added in small quantities. Hummus has been called 'the peanut butter of the *Middle East*.' Chickpeas are also used to make *falafel* (*Middle Eastern* meatballs) as well as many other dishes." [3 (page 88)]

Be sure to add these wonderful and tasty beans, legumes and lentils to your recipes. There are so very many types from which to choose. Here I have listed some of them: dried split-peas, kidney beans, pinto beans, chickpeas, black beans, pigeon-peas, black-eyed peas, lima beans, white beans, soy beans, and many more! Spruce up your soups and salads with these amazing gifts from the Creator of the Universe!

Fruits and Vegetables

B'resheet (*Genesis*) [1:29] "Then God said, 'Here! Throughout the whole earth I am giving you as food every seed-bearing plant ('herb' in NKJ) and every tree with seed-bearing fruit." [1 (page 4)]

Yehovah's initial plan for humankind was to eat from plants that He designed with seeds. These include herbs, vegetables, and fruits. We see this in *Genesis* 1:29. The only fruit not allowed were those coming from the *tree of the knowledge of good and evil.* (Genesis 2:17)

Even though Adam and Eve were disobedient, Yehovah did not stop the supply of fruits, herbs, nuts and grains. However, because of their rebellion, they had to leave the Garden and bring forth these foods from a cursed ground now shared with thorns and thistles. (Genesis 3:18)

Tilling the ground was now a much harder job. Even though it is more difficult to bring forth foods from the cursed ground, God is merciful and through Adam's effort, herbs, vegetables, and fruit would still come forth.

Seed-bearing is the important part. Able to recreate themselves and provide nourishment to the world! Herbs, vegetables, and fruits! So much from which to choose! Color, flavors, variety, textures, shapes, sizes and more!

"Many vegetables that are not commonly found in the *Middle East* are still valuable for our consumption today. In fact, the wider the variety of vegetables that we eat, the less likely we are to become bored with vegetables and the greater the nutritional benefit we will receive from them." [3 (page 93-94)]

"Many of the vegetables that have high amounts of phytonutrients – those nutrients that are most potent in protecting us from cancer and heart disease – are not mentioned in the *Bible*. They are not commonly available in *Mediterranean* nations, yet they are powerful allies for health." [3 (page 94)]

Some of those that were available in the Mediterranean area were probably leeks, cucumbers, melons and others in these families.

For our discussion, we will start with cruciferous vegetables. Broccoli, cauliflower, Brussel sprouts, Bok choy, collard greens, kale, mustard greens, watercress, turnip greens, radishes, rutabaga, horseradish, and cabbage. These vegetables help reduce the risk of cancer. [3 (page 94)]

"Cruciferous vegetables contain numerous anticancer compounds, including isothiocyanates, phenols, and sulfur-containing compounds such as sulforaphane and indoles, such as indole-3-carinol. These phytonutrients protect against cancer by stimulating the protective enzymes in the body – enzymes that are able to detoxify cancer-causing chemicals and rid them from the body. Indoles help prevent cancers that are dependent on hormones, such as breast cancer, by deactivating estrogens. Indole-3-carbinol is able to decrease estradiol, which is the most active form of estrogen, by converting the estradiol to estrone. Having less estradiol and more estrone is associated with a decreased incidence of both breast and uterine cancers." [3 (page 94)]

"Cabbage family vegetables are also able to increase the body's production of one of the important antioxidant enzymes in the body, glutathione peroxidase. They stimulate the liver to destroy cancer-causing agents. In addition, cruciferous vegetables contain folic acid, vitamin C and beta-carotene – all of which are important nutrients for good health. And finally, these vegetables provide a good source of nutritional fiber." [3 (page 95)]

"Carotenoids are found in yellow, orange, and red fruits and vegetables, as well as in dark green leafy vegetables. Carotenoids are actually red, yellow, and orange pigments – in dark leafy green vegetables, the color is concealed by the green of chlorophyll. There are more than six hundred different carotenoids. Beta carotene is perhaps the most familiar one." [3 (page 95)]

"Beta-carotene is converted in the body to vitamin A, a strong stimulant for the immune system. Beta carotene seems especially capable of stimulating T-helper cells. It also functions as an antioxidant. Diets rich in foods that contain carotenoids are associated with a decreased risk of both cancer and heart disease." [3 (page 95)]

"Red-pigment foods containing lycopene include tomatoes, watermelons, pink grapefruit, apricots, and carrots. Lycopene is an excellent antioxidant and also seems to have cancer-prevention properties. Studies involving prostate cancer have revealed these properties. Foods rich in lycopene also seem to have protective value against cancers of the colon, rectum, stomach, esophagus, and possibly other organs in the body." [3 (page 96)]

"Foods high in lutein include spinach, collard greens, kale, romaine lettuce, and leeks. Eating foods high in lutein seems to help prevent cataracts and loss of vision." [3 (page 96)]

"Other powerful carotenoids include alpha and gamma carotene, as well as zeaxanthin – all of which have greater antioxidant activity than beta carotene. It is very unlikely that a person can get all of these powerful antioxidants carotenoids in a single vitamin tablet. The best approach for eating carotenoids is to eat plenty of carrots, tomatoes, squash, sweet potatoes, spinach, kale, and other dark green leafy vegetables. The best antioxidant protection is provided as a person eats a wide variety of carotenoid foods on a daily basis." [3 (page 96)]

"Chlorophyll is responsible for the green pigment in plants. Generally speaking, the darker green the plant or vegetable, the more chlorophyll it contains." [3 (page 96)]

"Chlorophyll helps protect our DNA – our genetic blueprint – from various toxins. Two of these toxins are ones that have been linked to cancer – cigarette smoke and charred meat. In addition to chlorophyll's anticancer properties, it has antioxidant effects. Foods high in chlorophyll include spinach, kale, collard greens, beet-tops and parsley." [3 (page 97)]

"If you eat charcoal-grilled or fried foods, it is strongly suggested you consume one of these high chlorophyll foods to block any cancer-causing chemicals that are produced as a result of frying or charcoal grilling." [3 (page 97)]

As we saw with beans, "most vegetables and grains are incomplete proteins, which means they do not have all the essential amino acids. Soy is the exception. (Dairy products, meat, and eggs contain all the food-supplied essential amino acids required by the body.)" [3 (page 97)]

The essential amino acids are histidine, isoleucine, leucine, lysine, methionine, phenylalanine, theanine, tryptophan, and valine. A complete protein contains the eight essential amino acids. They are called essential because they cannot be produced in the body. They must be provided by the food we eat. So essential means essential for us! We need to get these amino acids from our foods. eat. [3]

To build a complete protein, we need to eat a mixture of the seeds, beans, nuts, and grains that have incomplete protein. We can combine grains with beans or pasta noodles with cheese or nuts. Creativity is required to get these wonderful amino acids combined for our required needs.

"Complete proteins such as meat, dairy, eggs, and soy have all eight essential amino acids. Grains tend to be low in the amino acid lysine. However, beans and legumes have high amounts of lysine. Beans have low amounts of methionine and cysteine – grains have a higher content of those two amino acids. When a person eats beans and grains together, all of the essential amino acids are provided. The protein in combination is complete." [3 (page 97-98)]

The prophet *Dani'el* understood the value of clean eating with God's eating plan.

Dani'el [1:8] "But *Dani'el* resolved that he would not defile himself with the king's food or wine he drank, so he asked the chief officer to be excused from defiling himself. [9] God caused the chief officer to be kind and sympathetic toward *Dani'el*; [10] however, the chief officer said to *Dani'el*, 'I'm afraid of my lord the king. After all, he has given you an allowance of food and drink; so if he were to see you boys looking worse than the others your age, you would be putting my own head in danger from the king." [11] Then *Dani'el* said to the guard whom the chief officer had put in charge of *Dani'el*, *Hananyah*, *Misha'el*, and *Azaryah*, [12] 'Please! Try an experiment on your servants – for ten days have them give us only vegetables to eat and water to drink. [13] Then see how we look and compare us with how the boys who eat the king's food look; and deal with your servants according to what you see.' [14] He agreed to do what they had asked and gave them a ten-day test. [15] At the end of ten days they looked better and more robust than all the boys who were eating the king's food. [16] So the guard took away their food and the wine they were supposed to drink and gave them vegetables." [1 (page 1241)]

"At the end of the ten days, their appearances appeared fairer and 'fatter in flesh than those who had been eating the king's delicacies. They continued to eat vegetables and water for the next three years!" [3 (page 99)]

"The actual word for their food is *pulse*, which is a mixture of vegetables and grains such as wheat, barley, rye, peas, beans, and lentils. Again, these grains and beans form a complete protein when eaten together, and if the substance included sprouted grains and beans, the foods would have been even higher in nutritional content." [3 (page 99)]

"At the end of the three years, the king found that these four young men were 'ten times better than all the magicians and astrologers who were in his realm' in matters of 'wisdom and understanding. (*Daniel* 1:20). Nothing about their diet had diminished their brain capacity in the least!" [3 (page 99)]

"No doubt at all that Jesus ate a diversity of garlic, onions, vegetables, beans, and lentils. He also ate incomplete proteins in combinations that resulted in complete protein supplied to His body." [3 (page 99)]

We are blessed in this world as fruits and vegetables are available throughout the world and in every season, some will be available somewhere! All have nutrients that are beneficial to our bodies and even some of the seeds can be helpful as teas or additions to salads. Enjoy the abundance – fresh apples, peaches, grapes, pears, berries, tomatoes, cucumbers, melons and avocado! I am sure everyone can list more of their favorites too!

Learn what is available locally and choose those! Fresh fruit and vegetables are the mainstay of a good meal. To use them all year long canning, a lost skill, helps keep a variety of foods on hand. Additionally, freezing and dehydration are other options.

Vegetables, herbs, and fruits can be prepared in the freshest season and used in winter when less fresh foods are available.

Finding a local market can be a great option to find local vegetables and fruits. Through local farms you will find seasonal produce when it is most nutritious. You want to choose the best quality product with no signs of decay.

Decayed fruits or vegetables can ferment in your stomach causing distress, food poisoning, and in severe cases, sepsis, sometimes called blood poisoning. This can be life threatening. Be sure to wash the produce thoroughly under running water before eating.

It is so important we do not cause our bodies problems of over acidity. Although fruit can help with a dyspeptic stomach, be sure not to eat too much at one time. Also, fruit should not be eaten on a very full stomach.

If someone does get indigestion, fasting is a good remedy to let the body rest. Eating only fruit for a few days can also bring relief, especially to people who work mostly with their brains. However, complete abstinence from food, with moderate eating after a time. This will allow the body to restore itself. *Yehovah's* original plan of herbs and fruits probably brought about the longer life spans talked about earlier.

What's for Dessert?

When we think of desserts we think of pies, cookies, ice cream, cake, and brownies! But what about in Biblical days and what might we consider now?

"What type of sweets did *Jesus* eat? What did he have for dessert? The answer to both questions is simple fruit." [3 (page 145)]

"Fruit was a main staple food of *Jesus*, just as it had been for the *Israelites* for thousands of years. Grapes, figs, and pomegranates are three fruits mentioned frequently in the *Bible*. They are fruits that have strong symbolic significance as well as practical uses. Other fruits mentioned in the *Bible* include apples, apricot, berries, melons, dates, and raisins." [3 (page 146)]

"The *Bible* has more references to grapes and grapevines than to any other fruit and plant except olives and olive trees." [3 (page 146)]

"Grapes are the first cultivated plant mentioned in the *Bible*. They can be traced all the way back to *Noah* (*Genesis* 9:20-21). After *Noah* left the ark, he planted a vineyard; he went from being a caretaker of animals to a caretaker of vines. Throughout the ages, from July to October each year, fresh, ripe grapes have been eaten along with bread as one of the mainstays of the daily diet of those living in *Israel*. Grapes become ripe first in the south of the land, beginning in July, and are ripe in the areas of the north of *Galilee* as late as October." [3 (pages 146-147)]

"Purple and red grapes are rich in anthocyanin, a form of flavonoid that functions as an antioxidant. A family of chemicals known as OPC's [Oligomeric Proanthocyanidins] include grape seed extract and pine bark extract. These phytonutrients are water soluble and clinical studies have suggested that they may be fifty times more potent than vitamin E and twenty times more potent than vitamin C in terms of antioxidant activity. OPC's are able to cross the blood-brain barrier, and thus have the ability to protect the brain and spinal nerves from free radical damage. Grape seed extract also helps repair connective tissue and protect the liver from damage from numerous toxins. Grape seed extract may reduce the pain and swelling from varicose veins, as well as revitalize aging skin and decrease bruising of the skin. Grapes have been shown to fight tooth decay and to stop viruses, and they are high in caffeic acid, a substance shown to be a strong cancer fighting agent." [3 (page 147)]

"Grapes are also a rich source of resveratrol, another powerful phytonutrient. Resveratrol is found in the highest concentrations in red grapes, especially those from cold, damp regions such as *France* and *Canada*. It is present in both the grape leaves and the grape skins. Resveratrol is found in the highest concentrations in red wine and purple grape juice. White grape juice, white grapes, and white wine have low concentrations of this phytonutrient." [3 (page 147)]

"Resveratrol is an antioxidant that helps protect the heart and blood vessels in several ways: it decreases the stickiness of platelets, and it has been shown to help boost good (HDL) cholesterol and block oxidation of bad (LDL) cholesterol. It helps decrease inflammation. Animal studies with resveratrol suggest it also may inhibit the development and progression of cancer. Finally, resveratrol functions as a Cox-2 inhibitor – when the Cox-2 enzyme is inhibited, cancer activity is reduced, as is inflammation. The benefits are especially important to those who suffer from arthritis." [3 (page 147-148)]

Resveratrol and phytonutrients are important to our overall health and wellbeing as we age. If you decide to supplement, I recommend researching a patented blend of polyphenols from a well-researched and reputable company. The combination of muscadine grape with resveratrol and extracts from red wine, purple carrot, black current, pomegranate, and chebulic myrobalan brings together a potent blend providing excellent benefits.

"Yet another phytonutrient in grapes is ellagic acid, which has both antimutagenic and anticarcinogenic properties. It has been shown to inhibit chemically induced cancers of the liver, lungs, skin, and esophagus in rodent studies. Ellagic acid also protects our DNA." [3 (page 148)]

"Grapes are high in boron, a mineral known to help ward off osteoporosis. They are also high in potassium and zinc, and the vitamins A, B, and C. And the good news for dieters is that a cup of raw grapes has only fifty-eight calories, only 0.3 grams of fat, and no cholesterol." [3 (page 148)]

"The *Israelites* in ancient times made grape honey, a product similar to our jams and jellies but without artificial preservatives or added sugar. You can make this today by following this simple recipe. Wash four cups of grapes and remove all stems. Place the grapes in a pan with a half cup of water, and boil the mixture for about twenty minutes, or until it thickens. Strain off the grape seeds. Store the mixture in sterilized jars and refrigerate them. The natural sugars in the grapes become concentrated – the sweeter the grapes were to begin with, the sweeter the grape honey will be." [3 (page 148)]

"Grapes were pressed to make not only wine, but also fresh juice and vinegar. Grapes were pressed into cakes of flour, as were raisins. Sour wine and vinegar made from grapes were given to Roman soldiers to prevent diarrhea and help make them strong in battle. As *Jesus* hung on the cross, He was given sour wine on a sponge of hyssop (*John* 19:28-30)." [3 (page 148)]

"In addition to fresh grapes and the juice from grapes, grapes were dried and eaten in the form of raisins. Researchers at *Tufts University* have developed a method for analyzing each food to determine its comprehensive antioxidant capacity. Samples of foods are blended into liquid chromatographs, and then they are analyzed as to how quickly and effectively free radicals are quenched when they are added to the mix. The foods highest in antioxidant capacity as a whole were fruits and vegetables. The top two individual foods were prunes and raisins!" [3 (page 149)]

"In the *Old Testament*, we read how *Abigail* gave *David* a great provision of food, including a hundred clusters of raisins (1 *Samuel* 25:18). Raisins were also brought to *King David* as he fled from *Absalom* (2 *Samuel* 16:1)." [3 (page 149)]

"Besides having a high concentration of antioxidants, raisins are a good source of iron, potassium, B vitamins, dietary fiber, and carbohydrates! A word of warning, however – raisins have a much higher concentration of sugar than does other fresh fruit. They also are subject to more pesticide residue." To stay on the safe side, choosing organic raisins and fruits is best. [3 (page 149)]

"The fig tree is the first fruit tree actually mentioned by name in the *Bible*. Figs are one of the seven plants mentioned in *Deuteronomy* 8:7-10, the passage of scripture in which God describes the abundance of the promised land. For centuries, various nations and cultures around the world have regarded figs as a powerful remedy for ailments ranging from cancer to constipation, scurvy to hemorrhoids, gangrene to boils, liver troubles to menopausal symptoms." [3 (page 149-150)]

"*Isaiah* also gave this advice to *King Hezekiah*: 'let them take a lump of figs, and apply it as a poultice on the boil, and he shall recover." (*Isaiah* 38:21) [3 (page 150)]

"Figs have been used throughout the ages to help fight skin cancers. Figs, as well as the extract from figs, contain benzaldehyde. Japanese researchers, especially, have experimented with benzaldehyde derived from figs as a treatment for cancer patients, and their results are impressive." [3 (page 150-151)]

"Figs have high amounts of fiber, magnesium, potassium, calcium, manganese, copper, iron, and vitamins C and B_6. Figs have been recommended for centuries to tone and nourish the intestines." [3 (page 151)]

"In *Bible* times, figs were usually eaten as dried figs and were often pressed into cakes. But here is a warning – dried figs are quite high in sugar, and they have a laxative effect. I do not recommend that a person eat an excessive quantity of figs at one time!" [3 (page 151)]

"Fresh figs range in color from deep purple black to golden yellow. When you purchase them fresh, they should be fragrant, firm, and without any soft or brown spots. Dried or fresh, figs keep best in the refrigerator. If you are buying dried figs, be sure to check what may have been added to them. Some people are allergic to sulfites, which are often used to preserve dried figs and other dried fruits." [3 (page 151)]

"Pomegranates have been growing in *Israel* for thousands of years. They are among the fruits brought back by the twelve spies sent out by *Moses*. Pomegranates are rich in color, but they are also considered to be one of the most difficult fruits to eat due to the large quantity of seeds inside each piece of fruit. According to *Jewish* tradition, there are 613 seeds in a fully mature pomegranate – the same number as the number of laws God gave to *Israel*." [3 (page 152)]

"The pomegranate has sweet juicy fruit, and one of the best ways to eat the fruit is fresh, slowly sucking the fruit from each seed. Pomegranate juice is also available. It is usually called 'grenadine.' A refreshing drink is made in the *Middle East* using pomegranate juice and carbonated mineral water. Pomegranates are high in potassium as well as vitamins B and C, copper, and magnesium. Pomegranates are a good source of fiber." [3 (page 152]

The seeds of the pomegranate are nutritious as well. They can be chewed as a crunchy treat! Enjoy in moderation! Sprinkle them on salads, in yogurt, cereals and more.

If you are on medications, like statins, check with your medical practitioner or pharmacist as a precaution. Some medications can be altered by certain foods or supplements possibly changing the absorption or breakdown of the medication.

What about apples? Did you know there are over 7,000 varieties of apples grown worldwide? In the United States there are about 2,500 varieties with about 100 grown commercially. For me, organic is the only way! I would eat an apple and end up with terrible indigestion. Then I tried an organic Gala apple. No problems at all! Seems I was probably having a reaction to the chemicals sprayed on the apples, but when organic, not a problem!

"Did Adam and Eve actually eat an apple from an apple tree? That question has been asked for hundreds of years. It is very unlikely, however, that the fruit was not the apple as we know it in the *United States* because there are no apple trees native to that area of the world." [3 (page 153)]

"It is neither likely that apples as we know them are the fruit called 'apples' in the *Song of Solomon*. It is much more likely that the fruit in questions was either pomegranates or bitter oranges. This does not at all mean, however, that we should avoid eating the apples with which we are familiar. The very opposite is true! Unpeeled apples are high in pectin, a special form of fiber that has been shown to lower cholesterol levels, bind and eliminate toxins from the G.I tract, and help relieve constipation. Fresh apples contain phytonutrients including ellagic acid, which, as noted previously, possesses significant anticancer properties. Those who eat apples regularly have far fewer colds and upper respiratory infections than those who do not. The old saying, 'An apple a day, keeps the doctor away' has a great deal of medicinal truth to it!" [3 (page 153)]

"The only way, however, to get the maximum nutrition from an apple is to eat the apple unpeeled. Most of the phytonutrients are destroyed by cooking the apples for applesauce or apple juice. Dr. Colbert and I recommend that you purchase organically grown apples to avoid the pesticides, chemicals, and waxes that are often found on apples." [3 (page 153-154)]

"Researchers at *Michigan State University* have called the apple 'the all-around health food.' Apples have been shown to:

- Lower LDL (bad) cholesterol and high blood pressure
- Fight viruses
- Stabilize blood sugar.
- Suppress the appetite without robbing the body of necessary nutrients, which is of help especially to those who are attempting to lose weight.
- Regulate bowel function, preventing constipation or helping treat diarrhea, depending upon a person's need.
- Help stop the growth of cancer cells." [3 (page 154)]

"A person who eats two or three apples a day can greatly boost the body's protection against heart disease. One study conducted in *France* concluded that a diet heavy in apples actually lowered heart-damaging cholesterol levels from 28 to 52 points, without any other significant changes in eating or exercising habits!" [3 (page 154)]

If Adam and Eve's fruit wasn't an apple, could the fruit they ate be an apricot?

Proverbs 25:11 says, 'A word fitly spoken is like apples of gold in settings of silver.' Should it be 'apricots of gold in settings of silver'?

"For centuries, the people in the mountainous countries of the *Himalayas* have traditionally eaten large amounts of a wild apricot known as the *kubani*. They attribute their good health and long life to this fruit." [3 (page 154)]

"Dried apricots may be even better for us than raw fruit. And there's good news for dieters – one apricot has only seventeen calories and a mere 0.4 grams of fat while providing more than half the recommended supply of vitamin A. Apricots are abundant in the *Holy Land*. They are high in carotenes including beta-carotene, potassium, magnesium, and iron. The apricot pits contain amygdalin, otherwise known as B_{17} or laetrile. Amygdalin is found in many other foods including the seed of apples, cherries, peaches, and plums. It is also found in millet and buckwheat. Amygdalin is a compound composed of two sugar molecules, hydrogen cyanide and benzaldehyde. According to some scientists, apricot pits can either cure or kill. A study at the *Mayo Clinic* showed that patients can actually develop symptoms of cyanide poisoning since laetrile is able to form cyanide in the body." [3 (page 155)]

"Cancer treatment with laetrile is illegal in the *United States*; those who seek this treatment generally go to clinics in *Mexico*. Some of the clinics there have reported great success in treating a wide variety of cancers. A large clinical study performed at the *Mayo Clinic* and sponsored by the *National Cancer Institute* using laetrile, however, did not find any beneficial effects of laetrile for those with advanced cancer." [3 (page 155)]

"Still other researchers claim that there are benefits from eating the raw, natural ground-up pits of apricots, as well as the pits and seeds from other seed-bearing fruits. Their recommendation is that fruit be eaten whole –skin, fruit, and seeds or pits – and that there are great health benefits in eating the whole of a fruit, as opposed to ingesting only one part of it. More studies need to be done in this area, specifically in the use of laetrile; we need to determine definitively the safety and effectiveness of laetrile." [3 (page 155)]

"Berries are also mentioned in Scripture, especially the fruit of the mulberry tree (see 2 *Samuel* 5:23-24; 1 *Chronicles* 14:14-15). The fruit of the mulberry tree resembled large blackberries. Black mulberries were commonly eaten fresh or were juiced. They have been used for centuries in the making of jam or jelly, and to make wine." [3 (page 156)]

"Berries such as blueberries and blackberries also have a high antioxidant capacity. In fact, blueberries and blackberries are third and fourth on the list of potent antioxidant foods (after prunes and raisins). Berries – especially blackberries, blueberries, raspberries, and strawberries – are rich in flavonoid phytonutrients. The phytonutrient called anthocyanin is actually responsible for the rich colors of the different types of berries. Berries also contain the important phytonutrient ellagic acid." [3 (page 156)]

"Melons are another of the foods that the *Israelites* craved from their days of living in *Egypt*. Some *Bible* historians believe that these melons were watermelons which continue to grow profusely along the banks of the *Nile* and in various other regions of *Egypt*. Others believe the melons were muskmelons, or what we know as cantaloupes in the *United States*." [3 (page 156)]

"The muskmelon has sometimes been called the 'Queen of Cucumbers.' Many people believe the cucumbers mentioned in the *Bible* are actually melons, including the 'garden of cucumbers in *Isaiah* 1:8. If you remove the seeds from cucumbers, you will likely find the fruit of a peeled cucumber is virtually indistinguishable from a melon as an ingredient in a fruit salad. It is the rind and the seeds of cucumbers that give them their distinctive taste – and their gaseous effect." [3 (page 156)]

"The good news is that melons of all types have good nutritional benefits! Cantaloupes are an important source of carotenoids – the beta carotene in cantaloupe is converted to vitamins A, which helps to stimulate the immune system. Beta carotene also works as an antioxidant, and it helps to stimulate T-helper cells, which are very important to immune function. Studies have repeatedly shown that diets high in carotenoids help decrease the likelihood of developing several types of cancer." Cantaloupe also has ingredients that act as anticoagulants (blood thinners), which may explain the correlation between cantaloupe and the prevention of cardiovascular disease. [3 (page 157)]

"Watermelon contains the powerful carotenoid lycopene, which is responsible for its red pigment. Food high in lycopene has been shown to help prevent prostate cancer. Watermelon has one of the highest water contents of all fruits – if you dislike drinking water you may try eating more watermelon to keep your body adequately hydrated. Watermelon is also an excellent diuretic. In eating watermelon and other water-rich fruits and vegetables you need to make certain that they have not been grown in an area that uses sewage as fertilizer. This is especially true when it comes to eating melons grown in developing countries. Many tourists have become ill from eating melons grown in areas where raw sewage was used to fertilize crops." [3 (page 157)]

Although not always easy to find, watermelon seed tea is a light, refreshing tea that is very hydrating and beneficial to the bladder and kidneys.

"Date palm trees have been growing in *Israel* since the earliest biblical times. The palm has always flourished in the desert, and it tends to be an indicator in the desert that water is near. Date palms still flourish along the *Seacoast of Israel*, in the *Galilee* region, and the deserts." [3 (page 157)]

"*Psalm* 92:12, 'The righteous shall flourish like a palm tree.' This is a reference to the longevity, fruitfulness, and usefulness of the palm. The date palm is a tree that has multiple beneficial uses – virtually every aspect of the tree has a direct use for humans." [3 (page 158)]

"Dates grow in clusters. A cluster may have as many as two hundred dates and weigh up to twenty-five pounds. Dates are very sweet and succulent. They are a rich source of minerals and fiber. Perhaps their only detriment is that they are high in sugar. In fact, their sugar content is about 60 to 70 percent. It was the fronds of the date palm that the people waved as they welcomed *Jesus* to Jerusalem, crying, 'Hosanna! Blessed is He who comes in the name of the LORD! The *King of Israel*! (*John* 12:13)" [3 (page 158)]

Dates are a delectable treat! I like to eat one as a snack just by itself, but they can be stuffed with cream cheese or almond butter for a richer option.

"The *Bible* has hundreds of references to plants, and we certainly cannot cover them all in a couple of chapters. Many fruits were not common to *Israel* but are very good for human health, such as pineapple and citrus fruits. Certainly, you need not limit your consumption of fruit to only those named in the *Bible*." [3 (page 158)]

"It is recommended that you eat a variety of fruits in your diet, making sure to eat at least two to four servings of raw fruit each day. Eating such a diversity of fruits will help you get all the different phytonutrients your body needs and give you maximum benefit from these phytonutrients in preventing cancer, heart disease, and a variety of other degenerative diseases. People who consume the most fruits and vegetables usually have lower rates of cancer, hypertension, heart disease, diabetes, and arthritis. The *U.S. Department of Agriculture* recommends a person eat three to five servings of vegetables a day, and two to four servings of fruit a day." [3 (page 158)]

"For thousands of years, serving honey has been a way of honoring guests. It generally was served after the main meal at the end of the day. A common dessert even today in the *Middle East* is 'honey cream.' A quarter to a half cup of honey is added to a pint of plain yogurt, sour cream, or heavy cream. Generally speaking, both honey and yogurt (or sour cream or heavy cream) are put in bowls on the table, and each guest mixes his own dessert to taste. On cold nights, the yogurt, or cream may be heated slightly; in the summer months, the yogurt or cream is chilled." [3 (page 161)]

"In the *Middle East*, nuts are far more commonly served as a dessert than they are as an appetizer. Nuts, such as almonds, pistachios, and walnuts, were plentiful in Jesus' day, and they were often used as ingredients in desserts. Nuts, we now know, are beneficial in regulating blood sugar and lowering cholesterol when consumed in moderation." [3 (page 161)]

"*Solomon* had a 'garden of nuts.' Many believe this was a grove of walnut trees, since walnuts were highly prized in ancient *Israel* for the oil they produced. Walnut oil was considered only slightly inferior to olive oil. The walnuts themselves were considered to be a delicious treat. King's frequently had groves of almond, walnut, and pistachio trees along with their olive and fig tree groves. Walnuts were so highly prized that they were called the 'royal' nut." [3 (page 161-162)]

"Nuts have been associated with cancer prevention, a lower risk of heart disease, and help for diabetes." [3 (page 162)]

"Nuts are rich in important minerals such as zinc, iron, copper, calcium, magnesium, and phosphorus. They are also high in protease inhibitors, substances some consider to be the most significant natural cancer blockers yet discovered. All kinds of nuts seem to have protease inhibitors – pistachios, peanuts, walnuts, almonds, Brazil nuts, cashews, acorns, chestnuts, and hazelnuts. Peanuts are not true nuts but are actually a legume." [3 (page 162)]

"Nuts are also loaded with polyphenols, which researchers are associating with cancer prevention. Polyphenols appear to tackle cancer cells before they begin to spread uncontrollably throughout the body." [3 (page 163)]

"For centuries in *Israel*, nuts have been a gift that signifies peace and goodwill. *Kibbet*, which means 'treat' in *Hebrew*, is a mixture of dates, figs, raisins, and nuts. It is often offered to visitors or is served at the end of a meal with honey, yogurt, and tea. A very common dish served at the *Passover* meal is *Haroset*. It is a dish that symbolizes the mortar that the *Hebrew* slaves used in building *Pharoah's* pyramid. *Haroset* is made by combining three-fourth cup of chopped almonds, walnuts, or other nuts with three cups of chopped apples, a half cup of raisins, a half teaspoon of cinnamon, and three-fourths cup of grape juice or red wine." [3 (page 163)]

"*Jesus* ate a great deal of fruit, some nuts, and some honey. We do well to eat more fresh, whole fruit daily, and occasionally to treat ourselves to nuts and a little honey mixed into yogurt or drizzled on fruit." [3 (page 164)]

Milk and Honey

Milk, eggs and butter should not be classified with flesh meats. These three categories can certainly be beneficial in some areas. Milk and honey are mentioned together several times in scripture. The first time *Yehovah* spoke to *Moshe* was from the *Burning Bush*. *Yehovah* shared His Name and stated His intent. "I have come down to rescue them [the *Israelites*] from the Egyptians and to bring them up out of that country to a good and spacious land, a land flowing with milk and honey…" [1 (page 73)]

"A land 'flowing with milk' was a land with such lush pasturelands that the cattle, sheep, and goats could graze to their hearts delight, and in so doing produce an abundance of milk. A land 'flowing with honey' was a land with such lush flowering vegetation, including fruit trees, that the blossoms provided abundant nectar for honeybees. Most of us would enjoy living in such a land!" [3 (page 71)]

The milk at the time of the Bible would have been much like what we call raw milk today. Raw milk is unpasteurized and straight from the source. Today raw milk has been unavailable in many areas of our country unless purchased to use with animals. Dairy cows today are not nourished in the same way as in biblical times. If you are going to drink cows milk I recommend you purchase milk from grass fed cattle that have been as chemical free as possible.

We think of milk from dairy cattle, but the Hebrews primarily used the milk of sheep and goats. It is unlikely that the *Israelites* drank milk as we do in the Western world. Humans, especially in the Western cultures, continue to drink the milk of another animal into adulthood. However, the milk of the dairy cow is designed to nourish the life of a calf, not a human. In most parts of the world, the baby is nourished by its own mother until weaned. At that time, no milk is required. Each mother is designed to nourish her individual baby. Recently I read that the nutrients in the mother's milk can vary daily depending on the needs of that particular infant. If at all possible the mother should breast feed her infant until the time for weaning. The benefits for the child are many, including a stronger immune system and less risk of ear infections. There are benefits for the mother too!

"The milk used by the *Israelites* was generally consumed in the form of butter, cheese, or yogurt. We read in *Deuteronomy* 32:14 about 'curds from the cattle, and milk of the flock.' In *Proverbs* 30:32, we read that 'the churning of milk' produces butter.' Cheese is mentioned in 1 *Samuel* 17:18. *Jesse*, the father of *David*, gave him ten cheeses to take to the captain of the *Israelite* army." [3 (page 72)]

"Many *Bible* scholars believe that the 'butter' of the *Bible* was actually a type of curdled milk, cultured in a way very similar to yogurt. Curdled milk, in some translations, also refers to cheese." [3 (page 72)]

"Butter, milk, and cheese are all high in saturated fat. Butter contains 81 percent fat. Cheese typically has about 75 percent saturated fat. Whole milk, even though it contains only 4 percent saturated fat, draws 48% of its calories from the fat." [3 (page 72)]

"Eating saturated fats from dairy products raises LDL (bad) cholesterol levels. Conversely, decreasing or avoiding dairy fat and eliminating fatty cuts of meat from the diet nearly always result in lower LDL (bad) cholesterol." [3 (page 72)]

"Cheese in *Bible* times often had garlic, parsley, thyme, dill, and olive oil added to it. This is something you can make today. Start with a half-pound of fresh curd cheese (or farmers cheese, cream cheese, or yogurt cheese). Add four cloves of garlic, two tablespoons of olive oil, and a tablespoon each of thyme, dill, and fresh parsley. If you don't have fresh herbs, use only one teaspoon each of dried thyme, dill, and parsley. Add salt to taste. This mixture is excellent on nutty, whole-grain breads." This can also be made with fat-free cream cheese or yogurt cheese for a lower saturated fat option. [3 (page 75)]

"*Jesus* ate yogurt, and some cheese and butter, generally on special occasions. In His day, dairy products fell mostly into the category of condiments rather than main dishes or beverages. We should limit our consumption of dairy to nonfat and low-fat products, especially yogurt with live cultures. We should eat butter and cheese sparingly and rarely." [3 (page 79)]

Again, if consuming milk and dairy products, I encourage you to use products from animals that have been grass-fed and finished and processed as little as possible with additional stabilizers, food colorings and other additives.

Honey is a nectar that nourishes and brings our tastebuds to life! It is a natural sweetener and is the symbol of blessing and abundance. As we saw, in *Exodus* 3:8, the *Promised Land* is described as a "land flowing with milk and honey." This symbolized the fertility and prosperity of God's promise to the *Israelites*.

"Perhaps because it is so sweet, honey is a major symbol for the abundance of God's blessing in the *Bible*. Instead of processed sugar, people in *Bible* times used natural honey as a sweetener or ate the honeyed pulps of fresh fruit. It is known from experience that honey, rich in sugar, was a high-energy fuel for the body." [3 (page 159)]

Proverbs 24:13 warns, "Eat honey my son, for it is good, and the honeycomb is sweet to your taste." There is also a cautionary message warning not to overeat honey as it can make one feel sick. Temperance, or moderation, is a good rule with honey or other sweets.

"An ancient Egyptian scroll lists approximately nine hundred treatments for a wide variety of illnesses and injuries. More than five hundred of the treatments have honey as a primary ingredient." [3 (page 160)]

"The Greek and Romans knew that honey rubbed into wounds served as a rapid and effective healer. Honey actually can kill dangerous bacteria on the inside as well as outside of the body. International travelers often take honey with them; it seems to work many times when nothing else does to put a stop to diarrhea. Researchers have found that honey also may be effective in combatting pathogenic bacteria which can cause food poisoning such as salmonella, shigella, E. coli, and even cholera!" [3 (page 160)]

The *Hebrew* culture valued honey and used it to sweeten drinks and foods just like we do today. Honey is a great alternative to sugar which wasn't available in ancient *Israel*. Honey can also be consumed by itself or added to lemon as a remedy for coughs and sore throats. In his book Folk Medicine, published in 1958, D.C. Jarvis suggested that honey should be used as a treatment for coughs, cramps, burns, and congestion. He also wrote, 'A tablespoon of honey at the evening meal' was an effective way of fighting insomnia." [3 (page 160)]

Bees work hard to bring us this delightful treat! Today, honey can come from both wild and domesticated bees. Be aware that all honey is not chemical free. It is good to choose local honey provided by people in your area. Local honey can benefit with allergies and other respiratory issues. The taste and color of honey varies depending on the flowers nourishing the bees. It is important that the flowers are healthy! If not healthy, the flower will be passed over as it can't provide what the bee is looking for.

Honey can fill in the gaps that might occur in daily food intake. Bacteria cannot live in the presence of honey and honey is also an excellent source of potassium. Honey provides iron, copper, manganese, calcium, sodium, potassium, phosphorus, magnesium and more. These minerals are all derived from the soil in which the plants grow. Honey will vary in mineral content based on the mineral resources in the soil. This is a reason it is harmful to use chemicals and poisons on plants and lawns. Although the amounts of the nutrients in the honey are small, they are sufficient for a normal individual. Darker honeys contain more minerals like manganese, iron, and copper. Honey also provides some vitamins like Vitamin C. Honey can sooth the stomach, calm a cough, possibly relieve the pain of arthritis and can be a laxative too. A very versatile food.

A note of caution comes from *The Center for Disease Control*. "Caution parents of young children not to give honey to a child under the age of one years. The reason is that botulism bacterial spores can stick to honey. The immune system of adults is mature and strong enough to fight off such attacks, but very young children are not able to do so." [3 (page 160)]

"A single serving of honey, about one tablespoon, has sixty-four calories and seventeen carbohydrate grams. Because honey is high in calories and carbohydrates, we do well to heed the advice of *Proverbs* 25:16: 'Have you found honey? Eat only as much as you need, lest you be filled with it and vomit.'" [3 (page 161)]

Milk and honey are symbols of God's hand and provision. The food that He fed the *Israelites* in the wilderness, the manna, was heaven sent and tasted like honey. I imagine *Yeshua* and His followers enjoyed honey, along with dairy products like butter or yogurt and other fruits and nuts. Personally, I am a great fan of grass-fed butter on a slice of freshly baked sourdough bread with a splash of honey local from our area! Yum!

Garlic, Onions, and Leeks

The Hebrews, like us, also loved garlic and onions! Both garlic and onions are healing herbs and boost the immune system and the flavor of foods!

"Garlic, onions, and leeks – all technically members of the lily family – are closely related. They have been used in both cooking and medicine for thousands of years." [3 (page 89)]

"Garlic was used by the *Israelites* as food and medicine long before *Moses* led the children of *Israel* out of *Egypt*." ... "Garlic is credited with having given strength to pyramid builders and courage to the *Roman* legions. It was used in both world wars as a potent antiseptic." [3 (page 89)]

Personally, we use garlic in just about everything we eat! It is a staple in dishes like spaghetti, chili, pepper and onions on rice, soups, omelets and wherever we can slip them in! We have also used slices of garlic on wounds as an antibacterial healing "ointment".

"The *Chinese* have been using garlic for its medicinal qualities for at least three thousand years. The father of medicine, *Hippocrates*, used garlic, as did *Aristotle*. Although he is not widely known for his research into garlic, *Louis Pasteur* actually confirmed garlic could kill bacteria." [3 (page 89)]

"At least sixty-seven different varieties of garlic and onions have been identified as growing in the *Middle East*. Garlic has many different health benefits, including a number of benefits to the cardiovascular system." [3 (page 89-90)]

- An antibiotic medication
- Helps slow blood coagulation.
- It has antioxidant properties.
- Mild antihypertensive effects
- May lower cholesterol levels
- Antimicrobial activity
- Mildly beneficial against some intestinal parasites, fungi, bacteria, and viruses
- And many more benefits. [3 (page 90)]

"Eaten raw or taken as a syrup, garlic has been a popular remedy for colds, sore throats, and coughs. It has been prescribed by healers of various types as a diuretic and for intestinal disorders and rheumatism." [3 (page 91)]

I have placed garlic bulbs in honey to infuse the honey with garlic. This creates a great throat and can be used by itself or with various foods and teas.

"In ancient times, onions were considered a food that gave great energy and endurance. Slaves and laborers –many of them *Israelites* in *Egypt* – were fed diets rich in onions to keep the people strong for hard manual labor." [3 (page 91)]

"Onions have been used externally as an antiseptic and pain reliever and taken internally as a tonic to ease intestinal gas pains and to alleviate the symptoms of hypertension, high blood sugar, and high cholesterol. Through the centuries, onions have especially been used to treat kidney and bladder problems. Modern herbalists believe onions to be a good expectorant and an excellent diuretic." [3 (page 92)]

One of our tactics when battling a cold or some type of respiratory issues is we slice onions into quarters and place them on a plate in the bedroom near the bed. It is amazing how it reduces coughing and helps with breathing issues.

We like to make onion soup and baked onions too! Additional tasty ways of adding the healing benefits of onions to your lifestyle. You can also make a tea using the onion peels themselves. This is rich in antioxidants like quercetin. The tea helps with inflammation and may even lower blood pressure.

"*George Washington* once quoted as saying, 'My own remedy is always to eat, just before I step into bed, a hot roasted onion, if I have a cold." [3 (page 92)]

"A great many research studies have demonstrated that onions raise HDL (good) cholesterol and lower LDL (bad) cholesterol. Onions slow blood clotting, regulate blood sugar, and may help prevent cancer. A single tablespoon of cooked onions can help nullify some of the adverse effects of eating a meal that is high in fat." [3 (page 92)]

"Up to 150 different chemicals have been isolated in the onion. Many of these chemicals are still to be studied. Raw onions seem to have more nutritional and therapeutic value than cooked onions. Cooking seems to reduce the onion's blood-cleansing and cholesterol-reducing powers, but these results still need to be tested further." [3 (page 92)]

"Of the 150 chemicals in onions, sulfur is a major one that induces enzyme systems in the liver that detoxify harmful compounds and help block tumor growth in animals. Onions possess antibiotic properties that are effective against a variety of bacteria, fungi, and parasites. They also contain flavonoids, which are antioxidants that quench free radical reactions." [3 (page 92)]

"Onions are also high in vitamins, especially B_1 (thiamine), B_2 (riboflavin), and C." [3 (page 93)]

"A milder, sweeter version of the onion is the leek. In cooking, leeks are extremely versatile. Leeks have a more delicate flavor than either garlic or onions, and they form the base for many traditional dishes in ancient Israel. One such dish was a popular porridge made from the white bulb of the leek, rice (or other whole grain), crushed almonds, and honey as a sweetener." [3 (page 93)]

"Leeks were prescribed in quantity for infertile women. They were also prescribed by ancient people for obesity, kidney complaints, coughs, and intestinal disorders." [3 (page 93)]

As you can see, it is a very good thing to add garlic and onions in their many forms to a healthy lifestyle. They can be added to everything from salads, soups, and stews to baking onion bread or garlic bread. Enjoy these wonderful healers!

Herbs and Tastebud Treats

We are so blessed to be provided a variety of herbs and spices from *Yehovah Yireh*, Our Provider. These herbs and spices flavor food and can be used medicinally as well. Let's take a look at a few used now and in Bible times. The first is coriander.

"The people called the food manna. It was like coriander seed, white; and it tasted like honey cakes." *Sh'mot* (*Exodus*) 16:31 [1 (page 93)]

"Coriander is better known to many people today as cilantro. It has been called 'the healer from heaven.' Coriander is an annual plant of the parsley or carrot family. The fruit of the plant consists of grayish-white globular seeds, which have a pleasant, aromatic oil. Coriander has been used to flavor pastries, meats, candies, salads, curries, soups and even wine." [3 (page 105)]

Coriander seeds are nutty and citrusy. They have a floral and earthy flavor when toasted. The leaves, the cilantro part, is similar to parsley and citrus, but can taste soapy to some people,

"Coriander has been used for centuries to treat minor stomach ailments, including indigestion, flatulence, and diarrhea. It has been applied topically to ease muscle and joint pain." [3 (page 106)]

"A good yogurt-based condiment for use with grilled chicken, lamb, or fish can be made by adding a clove of garlic, one tablespoon of vinegar, a half teaspoon of salt, and a half teaspoon of cumin to a cup of chopped coriander leaves and eight ounces of yogurt. Blend this and chill it before serving." [3 (page 106)"]

Hyssop is the next herb we will learn about. Hyssop is used in savory dishes, meats, and salads as it has a pleasant bitter floral taste with slight piney notes. The anise hyssop variety leans toward a licorice taste. It can also be used with sweets like syrups and custards.

"Many *Bible* scholars believe that hyssop was a type of marjoram, part of the mint family. Hyssop grew abundantly in *Israel* and the *Sinai Peninsula* during Bible times, and it still is used extensively in the *Middle East* for flavoring and in medicinal teas." [3 (page 106)]

"Hyssop is known to help prevent blood from coagulating. It is an age-old decongestant. It has also been shown in modern experiments to halt the growth of the herpes simplex virus, which causes cold sores and genital herpes. *Dr. James Balch* states that hyssop promotes the expulsion of mucus from the respiratory tract, relieves congestion, regulates blood pressure, and dispels gas." [3 (page 106)]

Mint is next. My grandmother would make the best tea in summer, adding a fresh sprig of her own mint for a refreshing flavor. Mint flavors and scents are favorites of mine.

"Although the taste of mint is very pleasant to most people, mint is listed among the herbs that many *Bible* scholars believe were 'bitter herbs' in *Exodus* 12:8 and *Numbers* 9:11. Other bitter herbs are believed to be the leaves of endive, chicory, lettuce, watercress, sorrel, and dandelion – all of which were eaten as something of a 'salad' in *Bible* times. The two main species of mint that grow throughout the *Middle East* are peppermint and spearmint." [3 (page 106)]

"The *Romans* and *Greeks* used mint to keep milk from spoiling. They routinely offered mint after meals as a digestive aid. Modern herbalists recommend peppermint for menstrual cramps, morning sickness, colds, flu, headache, and insomnia. Mint is also an antiseptic. Mint soothes the muscles of the digestive tract and uterus. It has been shown to be good for nausea, as well as to stimulate menstruation. Women who have a history of miscarriages should avoid peppermint as a treatment for morning sickness." [3 (page 107)]

Drinking peppermint tea can help with digestion, reducing edema and relieving nausea. Even inhalation of the peppermint essential oils can ease nausea and can help with fatigue while providing an energy boost. Regarding pregnancy, some think peppermint might be a uterine stimulant inducing labor, if used in large amounts. Generally, inhaling peppermint oil can be a benefit during the transition phase of delivery.

Among the well-known herbs we use today too is parsley. It is a great addition to stews, soups, and salads or even a lovely garnish. Also, parsley can be used as a bitter herb dipped in salt water as part of the Passover meal. The salt water represents the tears shed during slavery.

"The *Bible* identifies a group of plants as 'scented herbs' (*Song of Songs* 5:13). Parsley is thought to have been one of these herbs. It grows profusely in *Israel*. It is one of the first herbs to appear in the spring, which is perhaps why it is part of most traditional *Passover* meals. Parsley is a rich source of vitamins A and C. Two of the chemicals in parsley, apiol and myristicin, act as a mild laxative and strong diuretic. Its diuretic action may help control high blood pressure. In *Germany*, parsley tea is often prescribed for that purpose." [3 (page 107)]

"Scientific research has shown that parsley blocks the formation of histamines, the chemical that triggers allergy attacks. It may help those who suffer from hay fever or have an outbreak of hives. *Dr. James Balch* states parsley relieves gas, stimulates normal activity of the digestive system, and freshens breath. It also helps bladder, kidney, liver, lung, stomach, and thyroid function. It is good for bed-wetting, hypertension, edema, bad breath, gas, and kidney disease." [3 (page 107)]

Horseradish is another of the bitter herbs. If you have ever used horseradish, you are aware it is great to open your sinuses. At Passover, horseradish is served with an apple date dish called *charoset*. This sweet apple mixture is placed with the horseradish in a matzah as a wonderful sandwich awakening all your senses! The horseradish, called maror, represents the time the Hebrews were in bondage in Egypt. The charoset is a sweet symbol of the mortar used while in slavery, but also the hope of freedom.

Horseradish has many benefits like helping with digestion, boosting the immune system as it is high in vitamin C. It also reduces inflammation and fights bacteria. Rich in antioxidants, horseradish helps clear respiratory congestion. It can be used for condiments, but also as a poultice. Herbs have so many uses and benefits.

Many additional herbs are used in Middle Eastern cooking even though some might not be mentioned in the Bible. Some of these are aloe, balsam, cassia, cinnamon, cumin, frankincense, mustard and saffron. We know that having trust as small as a mustard seed is a blessing. Other blessings from the mustard herb that is packed with nutrients. They have fiber and are antioxidants.

Saffron is a powerful antioxidant and is anti-inflammatory too. An exciting benefit of saffron is it is mood enhancing and can help bring a sense of well-being. It might be a help in filling the nutrient gaps that may negatively affect mood.

"*Jesus* ate a diet loaded with vegetables, especially garlic, onions, leeks, beans, and lentils – these vegetables were often a main dish and were routinely enhanced with herbs and spices common to *Israel*." [3 (page 108)]

"We can eat as Jesus ate by adding more vegetables to our diet, and by eating these fresh, whole vegetables raw, lightly steamed or lightly fried in olive oil." [3 (page 108)]

It is so fun to experiment with various herbs and plants. Sometimes my experiments are successful; and sometimes not so much! When that happens, my kind husband will say "You don't need to make this again.." Such a kind way to let me know my experiment is a flop! So on to try again!

Oils and Fats

"The fats we tend to eat in America today are not the same fats that Jesus ate. Unfortunately, we suffer as a result. Americans as a whole are eating way too many saturated fats, hydrogenated fats, and refined, highly processed polyunsaturated fats. They are also consuming too many fried foods." [3 (page 109)]

Keep in mind that quality matters in fats and oils just as with all other foods. The less processing and added chemicals and heat, the better.

"Saturated fats are primarily found in dairy products, meats, lard, many fried foods, and eggs. Whole milk, ice cream, creamers, visible and marbled fats in hamburger meat and steaks, and chicken skins are special culprits in this category. Hydrogenated fats are found primarily in margarine, shortening, and peanut butters." [3 (page 109)]

What about beef tallow and lard? Any idea the difference? Recently we have heard quite a lot about beef tallow and many tout it as a healthier choice then whatever was being used previously. That may be true, but as with everything, the source makes the difference. Yes, this is a fat that comes from beef, so it is on the clean list. However, you might remember we were warned not to eat fat! So, caution and moderation with these fats and oils as with all other food.

Beef tallow is being used for cooking at high heat and making lotions for the body! The quality of the produced product will only be as good as the health of the cow and the type of processing. The health, food, and environment of the source, the cow, makes a difference for the cows and for the consumer. If you plan to use beef tallow, I recommend looking for organic, grass-fed grass finished sources.

Beef tallow has a high smoke point and a firmer texture making it beneficial to use when using high heat for baking and frying. Beef tallow from grass fed cows does provide some nutrients, one being CLA, or conjugated linoleic acid. These nutrients are for the benefit of the animal, not necessarily for humans consuming it second hand.

Lard on the other hand is made from the fat of pigs. Already on the "unclean" list, it is not a product that should be consumed. As will all pork products, we encourage these to be eliminated from food plans.

And then there are the vegetable fats that are solid at room temperature. To make them solid, the fats must go through a process called hydrogenation. This takes a liquid vegetable oil and creates a solid product at room temperature. This is not a natural process. The process saturates the molecules by changing their properties and solidifying the product. This process takes a catalyst like nickel, palladium, or platinum to speed up the reaction. Just reading about this lets us know these hydrogenated products will not build good health.

So, what can we use? There are fats that can be used at higher temperatures but are in more natural state and not damaged by chemical processing. The first is Ghee.

Ghee is called a clarified butter. It is made from butter, but the water and the milk solids have been removed. Ghee is a pure butterfat and offers the flavor of butter but can be used at higher heats. If sautéing or frying, ghee might be a good choice.

Although really a fruit, coconut oil can be a handy choice to have around. Not only can you cook at higher temperatures with it, but it is great as a hand lotion, to soothe burns and just as a snack! It can also be used in drinks like coffee! I like to use it as a replacement for butter in baking! It makes yummy cookies!

Coconut oil is naturally solid at room temperature. This consistency is the recommended way to use coconut oil. The liquified version has gone through processing, so isn't the best choice. Again, I suggest organic raw coconut oil especially when using it for foods.

When lower temperatures are required or for salad dressings and dips, olive oil is the choice. Olive oil is also from the olive fruit! My choice is the first cold pressed, extra virgin olive oil from a single source. Organic is best! If you like a peppery flavor, a spoonful of olive oil can be a nice treat!

"When the *Israelites* were still wandering in the wilderness, they received a promise from God that they would be led to a 'land of olive oil' (*Deuteronomy* 8:8). Indeed, they were!" [3 (page 111)]

"The olive tree is one of the longest living trees – many live longer than a thousand years, and some trees alive in Israel today are estimated to have been alive two thousand years ago when Jesus walked the earth. A few of these ancient olive trees are in the area of the *Garden of Gethsemane*." [3 (page 112)]

"Not only are olive trees long lived, but they are also among the most resilient of trees. Through the ages, wars have ravaged the land of *Israel*, and many of the olive orchards have been cut down. The olive tree, however, seems to have the unique ability to grow back even when it appears to be dead." [3 (page 112)]

"Bread made during the time of *Jesus* was a 'flat bread' similar to pita bread, and it was made using olive oil. The best breads were made with the purest flour and the purest olive oil, and these were brought to the temple of *Jerusalem* as an offering. Three handfuls of meal were usually required to make a loaf of flat bread." [3 (page 112)]

"The olive tree was first cultivated in the Mediterranean countries more than six thousand years ago. Many believe it was first cultivated in *Greece*. Today, *Spain* and *Italy* produce more that 50 percent of the world's olives and olive oil. *California* is the leading state in olive production in the *United States*. During the days of *Jesus*, olives were eaten both raw and cooked, but most olives were pressed into oil." [3 (page 113)]

Don't you imagine the olive tree was one of the trees in the Garden of Eden? As important as it is, I would think it was a special tree from the beginning! I love olives by themselves, but the oil is a treat and so versatile.

"Olive oil was extracted from olives using large wooden presses. In the *Old Testament* times, some olive oil was extracted by the treading of olives by feet. Some olive oil was also extracted by pressing the fruit with a round milestone." [3 (page 114)]

"Not only was olive oil used for cooking, but it was also used as an ointment for making medicines, as part of cosmetics, and as a component of soap. Even today, castile soap is made of pure olive oil." [3 (page 114)]

"Symbolically, olive oil was used for anointing. Prophets were anointed with oil when they assumed their duties (1 *Kings* 19:16). Throughout the Scriptures, the anointing by olive oil typically symbolized the impartation of the Holy Spirit." [3 (page 114)]

"From ancient times olive oil was used in the making of bread and as an ingredient in many other dishes. Olive oil was also used as the butter for bread. Even today, olive oil to which cracked pepper or other spices and herbs have been added is called '*Italian* butter' – morsels of bread are dipped into the oil at the time of eating. (By the way, *Italians* consume one hundred times more olive oil than *Americans* consume). [3 (page 115)]

"All olive oil is not equal. It comes in different grades depending on the pressing from which the oil is derived. In the pressing of olives, whole undamaged olives are pressed mechanically several times without heat. In fact, the temperature of olive oil extraction ranges from 58 to 110 degrees Fahrenheit. Extra virgin olive oil is oil from the first pressing of olives; the oil is extracted, filtered, and undergoes no-further refining. It is the highest quality oil. Very strict guidelines exist for a product to be named 'extra virgin.' Virgin olive oil is from the end of the first pressing or the second pressing." [3 (page 115)]

"For maximum health benefits, olive oil that is consumed should be extra virgin or virgin olive oil. If a bottle of olive oil is not labeled as 'extra virgin' or 'virgin,' then the oil has been refined in some way. If olives have been damaged and started to spoil, the olive oil is of lesser quality and must be refined. The same for pressings of the fruit that occur after the second pressing. In the refining process, olive oil is degummed, refined, bleached, and deodorized. It is heated above 300 Fahrenheit, which chemically changes the oil and causes it to lose many of its health effects." [3 (page 116)]

"Just one tablespoon of olive oil has the following:

- Calories: 119
- Vitamin E: 3 - 30mg
- Monounsaturated fatty acids (oleic): 56 - 83%
- Polyunsaturated fatty acids (linoleic): 3.5 - 20%
- Saturated fatty acids: 8.0 – 23.5%." [3 (page 116)]

"Olive oil is composed primarily of monounsaturated fat, specifically oleic acid, which makes up about 75 percent of the fat in olive oil. Oleic acid has been shown to lower cholesterol levels. Olive oil also contains a saturated fat called palmitic acid, which comprises about 10 percent of olive oil and the polyunsaturated fat, linoleic acid, which also averages 10 percent. Several other saturated fatty acids, as well as another monounsaturated fatty acid, comprise the fat content of the remaining 15 percent." [3 (page 116)]

"The monounsaturated fat as well as the low amount of saturated fat in olive oil make the oil very stable, which gives it a long shelf life. Olive oil does not require refrigeration, unlike polyunsaturated fat that readily become rancid." [3 (page 116)]

"We need fatty acids for health! The average person has approximately sixty to one hundred trillion cells in the body, and every one of those cells is surrounded by a fatty cell membrane. It is the cell membrane that allows nutrients to enter the cell and that allows waste to be expelled from the cell. In the brain, cell membranes allow for the quick and efficient flow of electrical impulses, which is directly related to clear thinking and memory. The essential fatty acids help maintain membrane development and improve cell membrane function. Extra virgin olive oil is a great aid to cell membrane development and health." [3 (page 117)]

"Olive oil has been shown to help decrease LDL (bad) cholesterol levels and increase HDL (good) cholesterol levels. In contrast, polyunsaturated fats such as sunflower, safflower, corn, and soybean oil lower good cholesterol and lower bad cholesterol. However, they also caused an increase in oxidation of LDL cholesterol. *Dr. Daniel Steinberg*, at the *University of California*, actually found that olive oil blocks the oxidation of LDL cholesterol." … "the group that had consumed olive oil was found to have half the oxidation of their LDL cholesterol. Oxidized cholesterol is much more likely to form plaque and thus clog arteries. Anything a person can do to keep LDL cholesterol from oxidizing is valuable!" [3 (page 117)]

"Another significant landmark study in this area was conducted in 1950's by *Dr. Keyes* and his colleagues. They followed twelve thousand middle-aged men in seven different countries for thirty years. The mortality rates for coronary heart disease were significantly lower for *Greek* men, when compared to *Northern European*, *Japanese*, and *American* groups. The island of *Crete* has one of the lowest incidences of heart disease and cancer. Approximately 45 percent of the calories in the people's diet comes from fat, and about 33 percent of these calories are from olive oil. Residents of *Crete* consume more olive oil per person than any other nation. They sometimes drink olive oil by the glass! In a fifteen-year period, 38 out of 10,000 *Cretans* died of heart disease, as compared to 773 out of 10,000 Americans. In other words, the *United States* had twenty times as much heart disease as *Crete*." [3 (page 118)]

"Most other *Mediterranean* nations also have low rates of heart disease, even though the people in these nations eat more fat than *Americans*. The difference is that 75 percent of their fat calories come from monounsaturated fats (olive oil). In *Italy*, physicians usually recommend olive oil to patients after they have had heart attacks. One of the reasons for this is the beneficial properties of olive oil on platelet function. Olive oil helps decrease the stickiness of platelets, thus helping prevent coronary thrombosis and blood clots." [3 (page 118)]

"Olive oil also functions in the body to stimulate the gallbladder to contract. This helps to eliminate biliary sludge and even small gallstones. *Dr. Colbert* recommends you should consult your physician, however, before consuming olive oil for this purpose. Olive oil helps relieve constipation since it functions as a mild, natural laxative. One to two tablespoons at bedtime are usually recommended as a dose to help relieve constipation." [3 (page118)]

"Olive oil also has other nutritional components – generally known as minor components nutritionally. These include antioxidants such as vitamin E, beta carotene, lecithin, chlorophyll, and squalene, which help deliver oxygen to tissue. It also contains phytosterols, which help lower cholesterol levels, as well as polyphenols, which have antioxidant properties and immune-enhancing properties. Many other phytonutrients are found in olives, all of which have health promoting effects." [3 (page 119)]

There are benefits from the roots and the leaves of the olive tree as well.

"Olive leaf extract – which is obtained not from the olives but from olive leaves – is rich in phytochemicals, the most effective of which is oleuropein. According to *James Balch, M.D.*, olive leaf extract has been shown to be effective against virtually all viruses and bacteria on which it has been tested. It has been shown useful in treating sore throat, sinusitis, skin diseases, as well as fungal and bacterial infections. It may also prove helpful for chronic fatigue syndrome, inflammatory arthritis, psoriasis, as well as diarrheal disease." [3 (page 119)]

"Roots of olive trees were used in construction. Growing up in a carpenter's home, Jesus was likely very familiar with the use of olive wood in the construction of cabinets, doors, and pieces of furniture. In 1 *Kings* 6, we read that *King Solomon* ordered that the cherubim of the temple, the inner and outer doors, and the posts of the sanctuary all be made of olive wood." [3 (page 119)]

"One of the best ways to incorporate extra virgin olive oil into the diet is to use it on salads as a dressing. Combine it with Balsamic or apple cider vinegar. It is also a good idea to use olive oil instead of butter or polyunsaturated fats in cooking." [3 (page 119)]

"Jesus very likely consumed extra virgin oil on a daily basis. We can follow His example by using olive oil instead of butter, other oils, and salad dressing. Olive oil is the best choice for both cooking and eating." [3 (page 120)]

I enjoy organic olive oil by the spoonful just to be sure I get its many benefits! It makes a wonderful replacement for butter on sourdough or other breads! Add this wonderful oil to your food and table.

Wine and Juice

"During the days of Jesus, wine was a regular part of most everyone's diet, just as bread and water were consumed routinely. Wine was most commonly made from grapes, but it was also made from figs, dates, and even pomegranates." [3 (page 125-126)]

"The wine produced in *Israel* during the days of *Jesus* was primarily red wine. Red wine is by far the most common wine produced throughout history. Red wine has been used in medicine for thousands of years. *Hippocrates*, the father of medicine, used wine around 400BC to treat numerous ailments including headaches, mood swing, and cardiac irregularities. He also used it as a means to aid digestion, as a sleeping aid, and as a nerve tonic." [3 (page 131)]

"The consumption of moderate amounts of red wine has been shown to decrease the risk of developing ischemic stroke. An ischemic stroke is caused by a blood clot, and the flavonoids of red wine – especially quercetin, catechin, epicatechin, and resveratrol – all decrease the clotting tendency of the blood. Red wines have fifty to one hundred times more resveratrol than white wines. Resveratrol is a substance found in grape skins. It helps prevent fungus from growing on the grape skin. In the human body, resveratrol increases HDL (good) cholesterol and functions as an antioxidant, inhibiting the oxidation of LDL (bad) cholesterol and reducing the amount of plaque that builds up in a person's arteries. Oxidized cholesterol is a main cause of atherosclerosis. Resveratrol also helps prevent blood clots." [3 (page 132-133)]

"Another potent flavonoid in red wine is quercetin, which functions as an antioxidant and an anti-inflammatory. It also prevents blood clots by decreasing platelet clumping. More than a thousand different ingredients and nutrients have been found in red wine. It is especially rich in phenolic compounds.... Red wine also has more than one hundred different flavonoids – flavanols, anthocyanins, catechins, and the oligomers and polymers of the catechins. Flavonoids have antioxidant and anti-inflammatory properties. Apart from quercetin and resveratrol, some of the most common flavonoids in red wine are catechin and epicatechin. Flavonoids as a whole inhibit platelet aggregation, which decreases the risk of blood clots and thereby decreases the likelihood of heart attacks and strokes. It is a combination of flavonoids and phenolic compounds that provides protection against cardiovascular disease and stroke." [3 (page 133)]

"The properties of red wine also seem to have some beneficial properties against cancer. Quercetin, especially, has been found to have powerful anticancer properties. Red wine also helps stimulate digestion. We read in Paul's letter to Timothy: 'No longer drink only water but use a little wine for your stomach's sake and your frequent infirmities.' (*1 Timothy* 5:23). Moderate amounts of red wine stimulate acid secretion in the stomach without injuring the mucosal lining. (Note: If a person has gastritis or ulcer disease, by all means avoid *all* forms of alcohol.)" [3 (page 134)]

"Not only does wine help to improve digestion, but it helps prevent gastroenteritis and traveler's diarrhea. *Dr. Martin Weisse*, of *West Virginia University* found that drinking one to two glasses of wine with a meal may also help prevent food poisoning and dysentery. In his research study, red wine outperformed bismuth salicylate, which is the active ingredient in *Pepto-Bismol*. Both red and white wines were found to be more effective in killing bacteria associated with dysentery than other forms of alcohol." [3 (page 134-135)]

"In the late nineteenth century, a cholera epidemic broke out in *Paris*. Those who drank wine generally avoided the dysentery associated with cholera. Wine is effective in preventing kidney stones. Of twenty-one beverages studied, wine was most strongly associated with the decreased formation of kidney stones in a study conducted by a *Harvard* research team." [3 (page 135)]

"Physicians for centuries have prescribed one to two glasses of wine at bedtime for both insomnia and anxiety. Alcohol, however, is a central nervous system depressant, and since alcoholics are prone to depression, we do not recommend any alcohol for anyone with depression. Depression may actually lead to a person becoming an alcoholic." [3 (page 135)]

"Consumption of wine must only be in moderation. When we speak of a 'glass of wine,' we generally are talking about four ounces of wine, or half a cup. That amount is the average amount in a traditional wine glass… Keep in mind that a standard portion of wine – a glass – is only half a cup. In drinking one or two glasses of wine with a meal, a person should be drinking no more than eight ounces, or one measuring cup worth." [3 (page 136)]

"From cover to cover, the *Bible* has strict admonitions against excessive drinking of alcohol. Repeatedly, we find that those who drink in excess experience terrible consequences." [3 (page 137)]

"Medically speaking there are also pitfalls to excessive consumption of alcohol. Heavy consumption of alcohol is associated with an increased risk of certain cancers, especially cancer of the tongue, larynx, esophagus, stomach, pancreas, and liver – all of which are more common to heavy drinkers." [3 (page 139)]

"In Jewish tradition, teens are considered to have come of age at thirteen. They are expected to drink small glasses of wine along with adults as part of their religious services. The rate of alcoholism among Jews, interestingly, is among the lowest rates of alcoholism in the world." [3 (page 139)]

"Should you have a personal conviction against drinking any form of alcohol, there are several alternatives you should consider. One alternative is to take an extract of the beneficial properties of red wine available in supplement form. This supplement, available in a capsule [or liquid] is marketed under many different brand names…. The capsules have been standardized as to their content and they provide the important phytochemicals found in red wine." [3 (page 142)]

We don't drink alcohol, but do use resveratrol, polyphenol supplements. One is from muscadine grapes and the other from pomegranates.

"The second alternative to red wine is to purchase nonalcoholic red wine products. These have all the beneficial effects of red wine without the adverse effects associated with alcohol. Finally, purple grape juice – preferably natural grape juice that has had no sugar added – has many of the same health benefits of red wine. The problem with the consumption of grape juice is that it tends to be overconsumed – more than four ounces – and people often choose grape juice drinks that have been diluted and have a great deal of added sugar." [3 (page 142)]

The grape juice we use is *Kedem* Grape Juice made of concord grapes. It is 100% grape juice and has no added sugar, coloring or flavoring. We use it when remembering what *Yeshua* did for us on the cross through communion and served with the broken bread.

"Jesus certainly drank water and red wine and may have drunk various juices and herbal teas as well. In addition to water and wine, a number of teas and juices were likely consumed in Jesus' time. We know, for example, that berries were juiced, as were pomegranates. Mulberries were also crushed to make a refreshing beverage. A number of teas were also made and were generally used for medicinal purposes more than as a beverage at meals. Mint tea was certainly common then, as it is today. Jesus certainly may have consumed these juices and teas – there is no record of His having done so, however, in the *Bible*." [3 (page 143)]

Again, a word of caution to remember moderation when adding wine or other alcoholic drinks to your lifestyle.

Two- Piece Fish Dinner

Not only were wheat and grains a big part of meals in Jesus time, but we remember the story of the loaves and fishes too! (*Matthew* 14:13-21).

"Fishing was a major industry along the *Jordan River* and the *Sea of Galilee* throughout Bible times. The *Hebrews* were highly skilled fishermen, and several of *Jesus'* chosen apostles were fishermen by trade. A number of *Jesus'* teachings and miracles related to fishing." [3 (page 35)]

It is thought that *Yeshua* had fish daily as fish was the most common meat eaten at the time of His life. The fish eaten would have been clean, fresh, and unpolluted fish. [3] However, he would get all the Omega-3 fatty acids, vitamins, minerals and proteins required for his health through nuts, seeds, green vegetables, soy, beans, lentils, blueberries and more. So again, the Original Plan was certainly still enough! With that said, let's look at fish!

"Fish were so plentiful in the markets of *Jerusalem* that one gate into the old city of *Jerusalem* was named the *Fish Gate*. [3 (page 36)]

"The *Law of Moses* gave specific commands related to fish that were acceptable for human consumption" (*Leviticus* 11:9-12) … "Scales can be scraped from the skin of a fish without tearing the skin from the flesh. Bony tubercles are not considered scales. Fish that have types of scales that are unclean include swordfish, sturgeon, sharks, lump fish, and *European* flat fish. Fish without any scales include catfish, sculpins, and monkfish." [3 (page 37-38)]

"Clean fish with fins and scales are extremely beneficial for human consumption. A major multiple-risk factor intervention trial study that involved more than thirteen thousand men in the *United States* revealed that the risk of dying from a heart attack was approximately 40 percent less for those who ate the most fish." [3 (page 39)] "Most fish have high-quality protein and are a good source of essential nutrients such as zinc, copper, magnesium, B vitamins, and iodine, as well as other minerals." [3 (page 40)]

"Fish consumption has many beneficial properties. It has been shown to:

- Thin the blood
- Protect arteries from damage.
- Inhibit formation of blood clots
- Lower LDL (bad) cholesterol
- Lower blood pressure
- Reduce triglycerides.
- Reduce the risk of strokes and heart attacks.
- Reduce the risk of lupus.
- Fight inflammation
- Ease symptoms of Rheumatoid Arthritis
- Help regulate the immune system.
- Relieve migraine headaches.
- Soothe bronchial asthma.
- Combat early kidney disease.
- Inhibit growth of cancerous tumors in animals." [3 (page 40)]

"Many people believe that all fat is bad for a person. This is not so. Our bodies need certain kinds of fat – especially fats called essential fatty acids. These are called 'essential' because our bodies cannot manufacture these fats directly. We need to acquire them from food sources. However, what we do not need are foods high in saturated fat." [3 (page 40-41)]

"Fish is low in saturated fat. The fat content of fish varies widely, however. Fish are nutritionally divided into three groups.

- Lower-fat fish – fewer than 5 grams of fat in a 3.5 ounce serving.
- Fatty Fish – 5 to 10 grams of fat in a 3.5 ounce serving.
- High-fat Fish – more than 10 grams of fat in a 3.5 ounce serving." [3 (page 41)]

"Lower-fat fish include cod, flounder, haddock, halibut, perch, pollack, red snapper, sea bass, rainbow trout, and yellow fin tuna.

"Fatty fish include freshwater bass, bluefish, mullet, orange roughy, and blue fin tuna.

"High fat fish include herring, mackerel, pompano, salmon, and sardines. These fish are very high in the essential omega-3 fatty acids." [3 (page 41)]

"Diets high in fish oil were associated with a lower death rate from coronary heart disease…Fish oil contains two very important fatty acids that people are generally able to produce on their own. However, some people lose their ability to produce these because of disease or other reasons. The richest sources of these fatty acids are in fatty, cold-water fish such as mackerel, sardines, salmon, herring, and pompano." [3 (page 41)]

"The omega-3 fats make up approximately 15 to 30 percent of the oils in these fish. Omega-3 fatty acids are also found in lower-fat fish, only in smaller concentrations. [3 (page 41)]

"Omega-3 fatty acids have many health benefits. They help lower cholesterol and triglyceride levels. They improve blood sugar control and also improve neurotransmitter communication necessary for good brain-function, including increased memory function.

Specifically, fish oils make brain cell membranes more flexible, creating better communication between synapses and thus improving brain function. There is an old saying that what's good for the heart is good for the brain, and fish has been commonly called 'brainfood' for centuries." [3 (page 42)]

"Fish oils help atherosclerosis, thereby helping to prevent coronary artery disease and heart attacks. They help lower triglycerides up to 65 percent. And fish oil can help lower blood pressure." [3 (page 42)]

"Fish oils help decrease inflammation from rheumatoid arthritis and lupus. They actually act like an anti-inflammatory medication. Fish oils decrease inflammation substances significantly within a period of just a month. Leukotriene B_4 is an inflammatory substance that is one of the most powerful mediators of pain and inflammation in the body. One can decrease leukotriene B_4 levels with powerful medication such as prednisone, but the downside is that these medications are associated with dangerous side effects. Or a person can decrease leukotriene levels with fish oil. 'I'll choose fish oil any-day'" [3 (page 42)]

"Fish oil has been shown to be beneficial in providing relief to migraine sufferers and to patients with psoriasis, asthma, glaucoma, diabetes, and many other degenerative conditions. Fish oils decrease inflammation substances significantly within a period of just a month." [3 (page 42)]

"Fish oil may also be important in preventing certain cancers. Fish oil promotes good eicosanoids, which are immune enhancers – they decrease inflammation and the proliferation of cancer cells. Some animal studies have demonstrated that fish oil was able to block the growth and metastases of tumors." [3 (page 42)]

"*Jesus* certainly obtained His daily dose of fish oil from the wide variety of fish He had in His diet. We have options of obtaining benefits of fish oil from fish, or from fish oil supplements. Fish oil is readily available as capsules or in liquid forms or cod liver. 'I (*Dr. Colbert*) believe that the healthiest option is to take fish oil capsules and eat fatty fish a few times a week.'" [3 (page 43)]

As with all supplementations, products manufactured as close to nature as possible with enzymes present are the best options. There are few regulations or standards in the supplement industry. Looking at both the food sources, supplement sources and processes of manufacturing helps one become educated in what you are actually putting in your body. This is an area where I say, 'Buyer Beware!' (See Appendix for a source of Kosher Nutritional Products and Kosher Home Care Products)

"Fishermen have known for centuries that the quality and quantity of fish they catch are directly related to the purity of the waters in which the fish spawn and live out their lives. In purchasing fish, one of the most important things to know is where the fish has been harvested. Farm-raised or pen raised salmon have a higher risk of being contaminated with industrial pollutants if they are grown in waters near industrialized areas. Fish from the *Great Lakes* as well as freshwater fish may have been grown in polluted waters or near industrialized areas of the nation, and other fish such as swordfish, tuna, and pike are more likely to contain fat-soluble pollutants such as pesticides, PCB's, and mercury." [3 (page 44)]

"Unfortunately, even the high-fat fish such as pompano, mackerel, salmon, and herring – if caught in polluted waters such as those common in the Northeast – can be home to fat-soluble pollutants such as pesticides, PCB's, and mercury. But the high fat content in these fish actually causes these fish to accumulate more toxins. Lower fat fish, such as sole and flounder usually have less pollutants, as do fish harvested from clean areas in the northern *Pacific*. Salmon that is harvested off the coast of *Alaska* is much less likely to be polluted by industrial waste and PCB's than salmon from the northern *Atlantic*. The waters off *Mexico*, *Argentina*, and *Chile* are extremely pure, as are the seas surrounding *New Zealand* and *Iceland*." [3 (page 44)]

"You should also know that fish raised on 'fish farms' often have lower levels of omega-3 fatty acids. Cold-water salmon feed on algae, plankton, krill, and other foods that are high in omega-3 fatty acids." [3 (page 45)]

"Do not eat raw fish. Raw fish should be avoided. Raw fish often contains tapeworms and other parasites and smoking that fish may not kill all of them. It is important to cook fish adequately to destroy any parasites that may be in the flesh of the fish." [3 (page 45)]

"Fish should be refrigerated immediately after purchase, and frozen fish should be stored no longer than a month." … "Frying cancels out the beneficial effects of the omega-3 fatty acids. You may grill fish on a non-charcoal grill, bake it, broil it, or poach it." [3 (page 45)]

"*Jesus* ate a wide variety of fresh, clean-species fish, probably on a daily basis. He benefited from the essential fatty acids they provided. He most likely ate fish that was grilled, baked, broiled, and poached. We can follow His example by adding more fish to our diet and by taking fish oil supplements. We must make sure that our fish comes from unpolluted waters, that it is fresh, and that we have stored and cooked it in a way that maintains maximum nutritional benefit." [3 (page 46)]

Poultry – The Chicken and the Egg

"*Deuteronomy* 14:20 states, 'You may eat all clean birds.' These birds include chicken, geese, turkeys, ducks, and doves. During the time of *Jesus*, Jews consumed domestic fowl such as chickens, geese, pigeons, partridges, duck, and quail. We do not have specific references for *Jesus* eating poultry. He did, however, refer to chicks and hens in a statement recorded in *Matthew* 23:37." [3 (page 66)]

Chickens and other fouls would need to be killed humanely, just as other clean animals. The process would be quick, as painless as possible and the blood drained out on the ground.

Before purchasing poultry, take a look at where the birds came from and how they were raised. Were they given antibiotics or other drugs? Were they pasture raised or raised in overcrowded buildings? Many questions, but they are necessary. I believe the documentary "*Food, Inc.*" delves into the horrors some of these animals go through.

Free range chickens raised in natural grassy areas where they can get some exercise, insects and fresh air is best! Individual families and small family farms were the original design. Now we have these large industries whose bottom lines are profits, not health. If you can get your eggs from local farms or coops that allow their chicken to run around the year, that is best.

The first time I realized there was a difference in eggs I was surprised! I was living in West Palm Beach, Florida and saw a carton of eggs that touted "Eggs from Happy Chickens that have Known Roosters!" So, do you think it would be better to get eggs from happy chickens? I believe it makes all the difference in the chicken's world at least! The hens that have "known" roosters have a possibility of raising chicks too!

Milk, eggs, and butter are not classified with flesh meats, however, they are beneficial as sources of many nutrients and proteins.

"Eggs were also consumed during Bible times. The use of eggs was actually fairly common during the time of *Jesus*. Eggs were prepared in several ways, including boiling and frying. Some people cooked fish under a layer of eggs. I (*Dr. Colbert*) recommend that you purchase eggs from free-range chicken. Free-range chickens, as noted before, are not given hormones, antibiotics, or pesticides, and they usually feed on grass or grain – all of these factors enhance the nutritional value of the egg." [3 (page 67-68)]

"If a blood spot is found on a fertilized egg, that is possibly a sign that a chicken embryo has started to form. Eggs that have blood spots are forbidden under kosher food-laws." [3 (page 68)]

"Many people avoid eggs because they fear a problem with cholesterol. Actually, egg yolks are one of the best-known sources for choline, which is the raw material used in the body's production of acetylcholine, one of the most important neurotransmitters associated with brain function and memory. In addition to choline, eggs contain folic acid, B vitamins, antioxidants, and unsaturated fat. What most people don't understand is that egg yolks are high in lecithin – an agent that emulsifies, or breaks up, the cholesterol of the egg yolk." [3 (page 68)]

"A study of *Harvard University* in April 1999 showed that eating one egg a day is unlikely to increase one's risk of either heart disease or strokes. In fact, consuming one egg a day may even help to prevent heart disease." [3 (page 69)]

"The best way to avoid the pathogenic bacteria that tend to be associated with eggs is to make sure that you eat cooked eggs. We recommend that you never add raw eggs to a health drink or shake. I also recommend that you avoid Caesar salad dressings that are made with raw eggs. If a recipe calls for a raw egg, it's best to substitute pasteurized egg white, such as *Egg Beaters*." [3 (page 69)]

"Make sure you cook the egg until the yolk is firm. Those who eat their eggs sunny side up, over easy, or with a yolk that is runny, are at a higher risk of salmonella. Eggs should be stored in the coldest part of the refrigerator and kept in their original containers. Do not keep eggs for more than three weeks." [3 (page 69)]

Enjoy your eggs and chicken too! Just be sure to get the healthiest and cleanest source for these and all your food choices.

Rumanints: Beef, Lamb, Deer, Goat

Ruminants are hoofed animals with a four-chamber stomach which allows the grasses and plants time to properly digest and extract the maximum nutrients from their food. As they graze they chew the plants, swallow the mixture and then regurgitate and rechew the mixture. This is called 'chewing their cud!' Ruminating animals in the 'clean' category are in the families of cattle, sheep, goat, bison, antelope and deer. These animals also have the split hooves specified in scripture. Remember, to be clean it has to have both qualifications. (Leviticus 11:3, Deuteronomy 14:6)

Nowadays, beef is very easy to obtain. Grocery stores carry an abundance of cuts of beef, lamb, poultry and sometimes goat. Turkey is generally available, and some stores might have deer as well. If you are fortunate enough to live near farms and local processing centers, you might be able to get your meat directly from the farms or in small stores in the area. Hopefully a farmer in your area has grass-fed and pastured animals raised in the healthiest manner with the least amount of stress.

As these ruminating animals were designed to eat grasses and plants, it is best to obtain the meat from a producer that does not use chemicals or sprays. The nutrients the animals need is straight from the ground, air, sunshine and clean water. My understanding is that properly raised animals don't have the problems of E-Coli that the cattle raised on corn and chemicals do. Corn, not a proper food for ruminants, causes digestive problems for the animal and therefore is not necessarily healthy for people either.

Grass-fed and finished cows are less stressed and, many times, the babies are allowed to mature slower. After all, cow's milk is really for the calves! The saturated fat content of grass-fed and finished cows is lower than those commercially grown.

Commercially grown in industrial farms, the cows do not have the luxury of raising their young. In the dairy industry, many times the babies are removed from the mothers very soon after birth and placed in an area like a nursery. The milking mothers need to get back to work, so their babies get milk but probably not exclusively from their mother. The milk from all the cows on the line go into large collection containers then are processed and sold for various purposes. In grocery stores we see the end result as cartons of milk, cottage cheese, cheese, yogurt, sour cream and more.

In the 1800's Ellen G. White cautioned against eating meat and dairy products and those cautions are valid today. Even in the 1800's she was aware that the health of the cattle was waning and producing products that were not healthy. She pointed out that animals can be diseased without the evidence showing. The meat of the diseased animal can bring disease with it and harm the person eating it. If you choose to eat meat, the best choices are those pasture raised, grass-fed, and grass finished on organically grown grass. Like humans, animals benefit from sunshine, fresh air, and fresh, pure water!

"Beef in *Jesus'* day was scarce and of a different type from that found in today's fast-food hamburgers. Red meat simply was not abundant in the Jewish diet." [3 (page 47)]

"Red meat was nearly always a specialty food reserved for feasts, weddings, holidays, banquets, and parties. Lambs were slaughtered annually for the keeping of the *Passover Feast*." [3 (page 47)]

"It is very likely that *Jesus* ate beef since we know that many people celebrated His presence in their homes, and we also know from Scripture that He attended weddings, where beef was often included as a feast food. Beef consumption, however, would not have been a daily or weekly practice for *Jesus*." [3 (page 48)]

"For the most part, animals were not kept for their meat. Sheep and goats were valued as a source of fiber, from their wool or hair, and a source of milk. Cattle were prized for their ability to be beasts of burden. When red meat was eaten, the meat was more likely to be from a lamb or goat than from a cow or ox." [3 (page 48)]

"What we do know with certainty about the meat that *Jesus* ate is this:

1. *Jesus* did not eat pork or any other unclean meat.
2. *Jesus* did not eat meat fat.
3. *Jesus* did not eat the blood of slaughtered animals.
4. Jesus ate meat sparingly." [3 (page 48)]

In *Leviticus* 7:23-25, "The Lord clearly forbade consumption of all types of fat. He was referring not to plants here, or to the fats found in fish, but to the fat from animals declared clean for sacrifice to the Lord." [3 (page 51)]

"What is referenced is what we call today 'midriff fat,' or the fat surrounding the kidneys and intestines. This fat was burned as a part of the sacrifices offered in the tabernacle and the temple. The regulation does not refer to the marbled fat in clean meats, such as beef." [3 (page 51)]

"All animal fat is saturated fat – it has been closely linked to elevated cholesterol as well as heart disease." [3 (page 52)]

"We have absolutely no mention of *Jesus* ever sitting down to a juicy steak dinner or grilling a greasy hamburger to put between two pieces of pita bread. But we do read about *Jesus* sitting down to meals of fish and bread. We would be wise to follow that example." [3 (page 52)]

I agree with Dr. Don Colbert who "recommends that a person eat as little animal or dairy fat as possible. When eating meat, trim any visible fat from the meat before cooking it. The same goes for poultry fat and skin." [3 (page 52)]

"Free-range cattle have lower fat content in their meat since they exercise by walking and feeding on the open range. In other words, they are not cooped up in small pens or in overcrowded feed lots. Free-range beef does not have the overabundance of pesticides, antibiotics, or hormones that are usually fed to feed-lot animals." [3 (page 53)]

"In making our dietary choices, we should also be aware of the diseases that are associated with red meat. According to the *Centers for Disease Control* (CDC), food-borne pathogens cause approximately seventy-six million illnesses and approximately five thousand deaths each year in the United *States*! Unfortunately, the cause of many of these illnesses is due to contamination of meat by bacteria that comes from the animals' own intestinal tracts. Fecal contamination of red meat and poultry is all too common." [3 (page 53)]

As you can see, even though a kind of animal that was considered 'clean', it may be very 'unclean' due to lifestyle, corn, chemicals, various injections, and drugs given throughout the life of the animal. As I mentioned, the best choices are those pasture raised, and 'fed and finished' on chemical free, organically grown grass on the range.

"The slaughter of animals in the *Bible* was quite different from what goes on today. First, animals were not killed in any kind of 'processing plants' mode. There was no assembly-line approach. It was the common procedure for one animal to be selected from a flock or herd as described in *Deuteronomy* 12:21: 'You may slaughter from your herd and from your flock which the Lord has given you.'" [3 (page 60)]

"The actual method of slaughter is known as the *shehitah*. Jews consider this method to have been given to *Moses* as part of the 'oral torah' – the verbal law that God gave to *Moses* on *Mount Sinai*. The *shehitah* method of slaughter was intended to cause the least amount of pain to an animal, and to result in the extraction of the most amount of blood. The animal's throat was to be cut rapidly with a to-and-fro cut. The movement was intended to take only a fraction of a second and resulted in severing of the trachea, esophagus, two vagus nerves, both carotid arteries, and the jugular vein. The blade of the knife was to be adequately long and was kept extremely sharp and free of any nick or irregularity." [3 (page 60)]

"An animal's neck was to be clean and free of mud, pebbles, dirt, and sand prior to its being killed. The cut was to be made without any hesitation, with a continuous stroke, and with no pressure applied – the sharpness of the blade did the cutting. After the cut was made, the cut was to be examined by the slaughterer, who was called the *shochet*, to make sure the trachea and esophagus had been properly and thoroughly severed. The process is one that requires significant skill and expertise – it was also to be done with piety and respect for the fact that God had created the animal that was being killed. Slaughtermen had to pass a rigid exam and be certified by *Rabbinic* authorities. If any of these procedures were not followed, the meat was to be considered unfit for consumption." [3 (page 61)]

"After the slaughter, the animal's lungs and other internal organs were examined. Animals that have been injured in a fall or that have been torn by wild animals or poisoned, will generally have a defect to their internal organs. Such animals were considered unfit for consumption. Using this biblical method, no animal suffered more than necessary. No harmful hormones were released into the tissues and meat. The maximum amount of blood was drained from the animal." [3 (page 61)]

Although not stated in scripture, the process of koshering, or making fit, can be done in two ways.

"The first method of koshering is a 'soak and salt' method. This is actually the method that gives definition to the word *kosher*. In this process, meat is thoroughly washed under cold running water, and then the meat is immersed in cool water for thirty minutes. After the soaking, the meat is covered on all sides by a layer of medium coarse salt, which helps absorb blood from the meat. The meat is placed on a surface, at an incline, so the blood will drain. It is kept in salt for one hour and then thoroughly rinsed again under running water. The meat is heavily rinsed three times or undergoes three thorough soakings, each time in clean water. The triple rinsing and soaking remove all salt and blood." [3 (page 62)]

"The other method of koshering is by broiling. In this method, raw meat is thoroughly washed and lightly salted. It is then placed on a grill and broiled – this method allows the blood to drain away as the meat is cooked. The meat may be turned over, so it broils evenly. After the meat is broiled, it is rinsed with cool water to wash any residual blood that may remain on the surface of the meat. Many supermarkets offer kosher meats. Again, the price may be a little higher, but your health is worth it." [3 (page 62)]

If red meat is going to be eaten, I agree with Dr. Colbert that you do the following:

1. "Cut down on the intake of animal proteins. Eat far fewer portions of red meat per month.
2. Make sure all the red meat that you do eat is trimmed of the fat. Choose 'extra lean' and 'range-fed' meats, and if possible, choose kosher meat.
3. Store the meat in the coldest part of the refrigerator and use it within two to five days of purchase. Ground beef and sausage should be tossed out after two days. Frozen meats should be defrosted either in a refrigerator or in a microwave oven.
4. Cook ground beef to temperatures of at least 160 degrees Fahrenheit. Cooked meat should not be left outside the refrigerator for longer than two hours. If you are having a cookout or a picnic, make sure that any leftover hamburger patties are refrigerated as soon as possible. If they are left out for even a few hours, the bacteria multiply rapidly! Be sure to reheat all leftovers that include meat to their proper temperature. That includes heating pizza to 160 degrees Fahrenheit." [3 (page 65-66)]

You may be wondering if I include meat in my diet. Over the years I have moved more toward a vegetarian diet, but still do have some local organically grown grass-fed and finished beef; locally raised, organic free-range chicken; and wild deer upon occasion. I do get locally raised lamb, as well, for Passover and other special times. However, I have learned to cook more vegetarian dishes and soups and we love salads! Fruit salads, vegetable salads, salads with grains, salads with Feta cheese, and more. I strive to get organically grown vegetables as much as possible. We also enjoy making dishes with peppers of all colors, onions, garlic and either rice or pasta! Yummy!

For years growing up, I did eat foods that I would now consider off-limits! Ham, pork chops, bacon were family favorites as we did not realize the truth. And, as a result, I suffered with all kinds of digestive problems. Not once did anyone question what I was eating. Then I heard a talk by Dr. Ted Broer. He explained the dietary laws in a fun way and I realized those unclean foods should not come near my lips! A wonderful benefit of that decision is my stomach problems sort of just went away! I was sold on the idea that Father Truly Knows Best!! I encourage you to try stepping away from eating things that are not food and traveling The Way of The King, *Yehovah*! Blessings will follow!

CHAPTER EIGHT

CONCLUSION AND SUMMARY

For now, we have come to an end. Certainly, I have not uncovered all the information that could be presented in focusing on how great our Creator and Father is and how He brought everything together in amazing ways! The systems He put in place at least six thousand years ago, work in concert still today.

Our focus was to point out the relevance of the Hebrew *Torah* in our lives today and look at whether or not Our Lord and Savior, *Yeshua* Jesus decided to change His laws during His stay on earth. I don't believe He did and believe I have shown not only that He didn't change His mind, but that He had specific reasons for the decisions He made.

Throughout our history, perhaps our lack of understanding of how our bodies function and how we can make choices to improve or damage our physical health has put blinders on how we see things. Our physical health impacts our mental and emotional health and in turn, affects our spiritual life too!

Our bodies are created in such a remarkable way, different in many ways from the animal world. These differences are part of the image of God humans were given from the beginning.

In his book *The Design and Origin of Man*, *Stuart Burgess* shares several areas that make the human a unique design and separated from any other being on the planet. Some of those areas that set us apart are as follows:

Upright Stature: "God made man upright." (*Ecclesiastes* 7:29) "There are thousands of species of land mammals and, apart from humans, they are all quadrupeds (4-legged). The fact that humans are the only bipedal (2-legged) land mammal means that humans are unique and very different from creatures like apes." [1 (page 24)]

Skillful Hands: "If I forget you, O Jerusalem, let my right hand forget her skill!" (*Psalm* 137:5) "The human hand is one of the most precise and wonderful mechanical devices in creation and vastly more impressive than any mechanical device that man has made. The amazing skill of human hands can be seen in a wide range of applications such as writing, surgery, art, and the playing of musical instruments." "The over-design of human hands is just what would be expected from a Creator who intended man to be a creative being and steward over creation." [1 (page 38)]

Fine Skin: "I will praise you, for I am fearfully and wonderfully made." (*Psalm* 139:14) "Human skin has a unique structure of astonishing complexity and detail. In just one square centimetre of skin there are typically 10 oil glands, 100 sweat glands, thousands of intricate sensors, an intricate network of nerves and a constant supply of blood." "The amazing sensitivity of human skin shows that humans have been designed to be creative and to experience pleasure." [1 (page 48)]

Facial Expressions: "I will put off my sad face and wear a smile." (*Job* 9:27) "Humans have an amazing and unique ability to make many types of intricate facial expressions. Humans have around 50 facial muscles that allow every part of the face to be moved with precision. About half of these facial muscles are needed for essential tasks like eating but the other half of the muscles of the face have the sole purpose of making facial expressions. In contrast, apes do not have facial muscles dedicated for making expressions. The ability to make facial expressions shows that man has been created to be an emotional being with a need to communicate feelings to other people." [1 (page 57)]

Language and Speech: "And whatever Adam called each living creature, that was its name." (*Genesis* 2:19) "The human being is supremely well designed to communicate through language and speech. In the English language, there are over a million different words, and these can be used to articulate a vast range of ideas and messages. Many precise design features are required for speech such as a deep throat, delicate muscles, agile tongue, and special speech processing areas in the brain. These features are unique to humans and show that man has been uniquely created to be a spiritual being who is capable of expressing thoughts and emotions." [1 (page 64)]

Unique Childhood: "Let the little children come to me, and do not forbid them; for of such is the kingdom of God." (*Luke* 18:16) "Childhood is one of the most wonderful aspects of human life. Children have beautiful looks and are capable of very innocent behaviour. There are several unique aspects to human childhood including long duration, an exceptionally high brain growth rate and a very high capacity for learning. Childhood enables humans to develop as emotional beings and to learn the skills and knowledge needed for adult life." "The uniqueness of childhood provides wonderful evidence that humans are not related to apes but have been created to be spiritual beings." [1 (page 71)]

Unique Reproduction: "Therefore a man shall leave his father and mother and be joined to his wife, and they shall become one flesh." (*Genesis* 2:24) "One of the most profound differences between humans and animals is that of reproduction. Apart from humans, all creatures have specific mating seasons, and the only purpose of sexual union is that of procreation. In contrast, humans have fertile periods throughout the year and the purpose of sexual union is to help create an intimate bond in marriage as well as to procreate. Both women and men have a unique sexual design that shows that humans are special spiritual beings." [1 (page 76)]

Unique Genome: "He does great things which we cannot comprehend." (Job 37:5) "The human genome contains around 3 billion units of information that specify every single physical design feature in the human body. The DNA molecule that stores the information of the genome contains an astounding level of precise and optimal design. A single copy of the human genome is able to replicate itself with an astonishing level of accuracy. The human genome has unique features such as 23 pairs of chromosomes. In contrast, apes have 24 pairs of chromosomes. The wonderful structure and uniqueness of the human genome reveals a supremely intelligent Designer." [1 (page 80)]

Unique Brain: "And God gave Solomon wisdom and exceedingly great understanding." (*1 Kings* 4:29) "The human brain is truly awesome in complexity and there are many aspects of its design that are not understood by man. The human brain has around 100 billion brain cells and 100,000 billion connections. The billions of cells in the brain are precisely arranged and connected to perform immensely complex tasks. The vast number of connections between brain cells gives humans a phenomenal capacity for learning and memory. The abilities of the human brain are vastly beyond what is required for survival and show that human beings have been specially made to be spiritual beings capable of extreme levels of intellectual activity." [1 (page 91)]

Spiritual Being: "And the LORD God formed man of the dust of the ground and breathed into his nostrils the breath of life; and man became a living soul." (*Genesis* 2:7, AV) "The most profound difference between humans and animals is that only humans are spiritual beings. Man is unique in consisting of two distinct parts: a physical body and an invisible soul. Even though there may be a relatively small difference between the genome of humans and chimpanzees, there is an infinite difference between the spiritual status of humans and chimpanzees. Whereas chimpanzees generally act by instinct, humans have powers of choice in every area of their lives. The fact that humans have rational thought, emotions, desires, and moral values demonstrates that humans are spiritual beings made in the image of God." [1 (page 100)]

Now we can see that in so many ways we are unique and created in an image and body that functions totally differently than any other creature. With that, it makes perfect sense that our Creator would provide knowledge and wisdom to us in ways different from the animals.

One way He provided a reminder of His plan for us on this planet was through the *Torah*. As we saw the information included in the *Torah* had been taught and handed down to God's followers throughout the ages. It came through Noah and his offspring and continued on. However, many did not worship God and began following other ways. By the time the Israelites were delivered from Egypt, they needed a reminder, and Moses was the conduit to bring the information.

As we observed, the wisdom of the *Torah* provided a way God's people could live a better life and the goal was they would teach others.

The purpose of this book is to point out the relevance of the Hebrew *Torah* and all God's Word in Health and Lifestyle today; and to determine if, in fact, Jesus did away with the *Torah* (Law) especially the Dietary Laws. Only as we look through the eyes of *Hebrew* culture can we actually see the overarching legacy of the lessons in *Torah* and embrace its Wisdom for our lives. I believe we can conclude that our loving God, *Yehovah*, provided a plan and components of light burdens and an easy yoke called *Torah*. (*Matthew* 11:30)

Just like we were specially designed and created in the beginning, God's plan for our health was designed and instituted from the very beginning of His Creation and is still relevant today.

We call this plan the Creator put in place Original Medicine. It was based on His original design and functions for His creation. He looked at all we would need and planned everything in order.

- Fresh, pure air
- Pure, unadulterated water.
- The sun's healing energy
- Live, natural foods – Fruits, Herbs, Vegetable
- Regular exercise
- Rest
- Moderation
- Belief and trust in His Divine Power [2]

He wants us to follow *Torah*, not as a heavy burden of works, but out of love and relationship for our God, *Yehovah*, and Creator, *Elohim*. In following *Torah*, we are following Original Medicine as well.

Although not written on tablets of stone in the beginning, the *Word* was spoken and carried on through the faithful until Noah. Noah carried the ways of life in *Yehovah* with him and started a new generation of followers after the flood. Then it continued on with the faithful until *Yehovah* wrote it in stone for the *Israelites* at *Mt. Sinai*. Through the *Tanakh*, the Old Testament, which includes *Torah*, *Writings*, and the *Prophets*, *Yehovah* journeyed with His Chosen people teaching, encouraging, and disciplining them through the years. If they followed His *Torah*, they would find blessings and health. If not, the consequences were not so good.

And then came to earth the very *Word* who had spoken the World into existence. In Section Two – *Did Jesus (Yeshua) Do Away with Torah, including Dietary Laws?* we see He would focus the people back to *His Word* in *Torah* as it was meant to be. Not with harsh rules and procedures, but those things that would be good for the people and bring them into a relationship with him. Traditions of men and added doctrines cloud God's *Word* and create a picture of a harsh and demanding, wrathful God. Health comes through God's grace and love, not harsh rules.

As we saw, *Yeshua Jesus* continued to follow the *Torah* the *Godhead* had implemented. Again, not heavy burdens, but a light yoke instead. He did not delete anything from the *Word* that God had given from the beginning. Instead, he addressed the false teachings and traditions that had been added by Pharisees and other leaders over the years. Nowhere did he give his stamp of approval to eating unclean (detestable) animals or add unclean (detestable) animals to the clean (permissible) list. There is nowhere noted in Hebrew scripture that show he did away with the very own teachings he had put in place to provide an abundant, healthy life for all who would choose to follow.

In this section of the book, we took a look at various scriptures of the *Words* of Jesus in both *Hebrew* and *Greek* establishing what Jesus taught based on the *Hebrew* culture and writings. There were mistranslations, or at least, misunderstandings based on the two very different cultures. As we looked at verses in *Matthew* 15, *Matthew* 23, and *Mark* 7, we discovered the beauty of *Torah*, the importance Jesus placed on the *Word* from the Father, and what he taught his students over their time together.

In Chapter Three we looked at scriptures speaking about Peter (*Kefa*), Paul (*Sha'ul*), and James (*Yaakov*) to reveal whether or not *Torah* was disregarded in their lives after Jesus' resurrection. Did they give their approval to God's Messianic congregations to serve and eat what *Torah* called 'unclean' animals? Absolutely not!

What we found was none of these people turned away from following *Torah*. They did not see a separation in following *Torah* as they journeyed with *Yeshua* Jesus. They found clarification and a deeper understanding.

In Chapter Four, we looked at the details of 'Clean' and 'Unclean' and the job description of those animals deemed 'unclean'. Avoiding those animals and situations deemed unclean was a protection for the overall health of the individual and the community. Those animals called "unclean' were not creations that were flawed, but creations for specific purposes that made them able to consume toxic waste and still live. Their jobs on earth are important and necessary for the health of the earth in total!

And then Chapter Five – *Disease, Pharmaceuticals and Medicine, Clean or Unclean?* – Oh, how sad God's *Word* has been ignored in foods and pharmaceuticals. It is as though the Adversary himself is putting together concoctions that destroy health and the planet. One should not even wonder why there is so much sickness and disease. Not only do these poisons cause physical damage, but mental and emotional damage too. God's Word has everything we need but has been absconded with and sorcery has become the acceptable and trusted answer. Deception, destruction, and death are the outcomes of following the current, established medical industries.

We have seen how wonderful the human body is and how people have thought of human function over the years. The manual provided us by our original Creator lays out a plan for creating health and vitality as well as avoiding that which can destroy health. We are like no other created thing! The Owner's Manual is a great help to us! Obedience is the call!

A more in depth look at the bounty offered us through the many fruits, nuts, herbs, and vegetables provides us insight into the importance of eating those items that are created to be foods. They provide us the nutrients and frequency we need to keep our human vehicle in tip top working order. The abundance of variety and foods we can consume are far and away greater and denser than those we need to avoid. Our Maker knew just what we needed for proper function and energy.

So now we conclude. I believe I have shown that *Yeshua* Jesus made no attempt to delete the *Torah*, including the Dietary Laws, during His ministry here on earth. He did separate His Words from those traditions and added rules of men. He showed that legalism was not His way. Peter, James, and Paul sent that same message. There is such joy in following His Word and living according to His precepts.

I hope through this book, I have conveyed the importance of His *Torah* and His Dietary Laws. If we can someday move the pharmaceutical and food industries to value His Way, perhaps our world will become a much healthier and happier place to live. For now, our individual decisions to follow His Ways in obedience can bring us abundance, joy and health for ourselves and our families.

I have been inspired through this journey and hope it will inspire others too! Blessings to all and thanks be to God, the Creator and Maker of us all.

AFTERWORD

I don't even know where to start. This has been a lifelong journey that I wasn't even aware of until connecting with Original Medicine. I certainly never expected to be working on a book, especially a book looking at how the *Torah* could have such an impact on my life and the lives of others.

It makes me sad to think that the majority of Christian denominations overlook or deny the value of *Torah*. I now believe it is part of Satan's plan to blind even God's people from understanding the importance of Dietary teachings and Original Medicine. Through whatever means he has used, he has misdirected people and as a result, we live in a world of sickness and disease.

I hope through this work I may have a chance to encourage at least a few to revisit these Words of God and understand that we can live differently and have an abundant, long life!

There are many sources that helped me weave this tapestry of information. I recommend each and every book and article mentioned in the End Notes and Bibliography! We are not alone in bringing the Word. Many others are waking up in their own ways to Truth as well.

I hope you find this book a refreshing look at God's Word and an eye-opening understanding of some of the ways the message has been misunderstood and therefore taught incorrectly.

Original Medicine is a way back to *Yehovah* God and to His Wisdom, Knowledge, Understanding and Discernment. He did not leave us lost and alone. He provided for us in such loving ways. His Ways. As I learn new information I realize the journey will be life long and exciting! The blessings are many!

Thank you for this opportunity to share my quest with you!

ADDITIONAL HELPFUL INFORMATION
TERMS, GLOSSARY, END NOTES, AND SCRIPTURE
ENERGY AND ELECTRICAL TERMS USED IN CHAPTER SIX

ATP: The body's high energy molecule made up of adenine, ribose and three phosphates. ATP is found in cells of living things. It uses chemical energy that comes from the breakdown of food and releases the energy to fuel cellular processes. It drives metabolic reactions that would not automatically occur; it moves muscles and other mechanical processes, and transports substances across membranes. It does not store energy, it delivers energy for actions in various cells where needed.

Amino Acid Core (ACC) – "The center structure of an amino acid." [6 (page 3)]

Amino Acid: An organic chemical that functions as building blocks of proteins and nine are essential to life. The body makes eleven amino acids from foods. The essential amino acids are: leucine, histidine, lysine, isoleucine, methionine, threonine. Tryptophan, valine and phenylalanine.

Ampere: The measure of the amount of electric charge in motion. The electric current. Equal to the quantity of current passing through a circuit that has the resistance of one Ohm.

Anion – "The smallest particle of energy discussed in Biologic Ionization. Its energy exists in the ratio between its center and outer shell. This ratio of energy can exist in value from 1 unit, called the Milhouse (absolute) unit, to as much as 499 Milhouse units. The anion has a positive core and a dominant negative electromagnetic field around it moving in a clockwise direction." [6 (page 3)]

Anionic Elements – "Calcium, Potassium, Chlorine." [6 (page 3)]

Atom: The building block of all matter. It is the smallest unit of a chemical element. It has a nucleus containing protons (positive) and electrons (neutral), and the nucleus is surrounded by negatively charged particles.

Cation – "The next smallest complete energy package next to an anion. Its Milhouse (absolute) unit value can be from the smallest of 500 to its maximum of 999. Above 999, it has an unstable ratio which causes it to split and form 1 anion and 1 cation. It could even form several anions. The cation has a negative charge core and a dominant positive charged shell which rotates in a counterclockwise direction." [6 (page 4)]

Cell - Alpha Cell; "a fully functioning healthy cell. **Delta Cell**: is a worn-out cell and is functioning very poorly. It functions extremely inefficiently. **Omega Cell is** a dead cell." [6 (page 4)]

Dyne: A unit of force specified as the centimetre-gram-system (CGS) of units of power or force.

Electron: Negatively charged particles that circulate around the nucleus of an atom. The number is equal to the positive protons on the nucleus.

Element – "Pure substance, and or the building blocks for all compounds in organic and inorganic matter." [6 (page 4)]

Energy – "An electromagnetic force that can be either **Heat**, **Electricity**, or **Matter**. Energy is always given off when resistance is encountered. Energy cannot be created or destroyed but is instead converted from one form to another. As an example, when wood is burned the by-products would be heat, light, and electricity, plus the matter that is left, called ash, and that matter which is given off as smoke. The absolute unit of energy measure is the **millhouse unit**." [6 (page 4-5)]

ERG: A unit of energy originating from centimetre-gream-system of units. Also called an ergon which means action, work, or task. The unit of energy, work, expended in overcoming a resistance. Ex. Ergonomics is the study of work efficiency.

Frequency – "Refers to periodic motion of electrons about atoms or molecules. Specifically, it refers to the time it takes for one revolution or period. It is the common denominator or energy exchange ration necessary for a living system to continue to function properly." [6 (page 5)]

Health – "The harmonious function of the body; controlled by reason and judgment which is under the direction of the power of God's Spirit." [6 (page 5)]

Illness – "Refers to a loss of Reserve Energy; or, to put it another way, the first day more energy is not obtained from food eaten than is used during the day's activities. This is the first day Reserve Energy is being lost, so it is the first day that illness begins biochemically." [6 (page 5)]

Joule: A unit of energy, work, or heat expressed as watts (power) for seconds (time).

Line of Least Resistance – "Refers to the path of flow of electricity between two points where there is the smallest amount of interference to the flow, or the greatest amount of conductance potential. It can also be thought of as the line of greatest current flow." [6 (page 6)]

Loss of Energy – "Refers to the breakdown process where the molecular structure that makes up an amino acid is coming apart." [6 (page 6)]

Mass – "Quantity of matter. Substance that can be handled, touched, and weighed." [6 (page 6)]

Micronage – "Refers to the way the anions and cations are stacked together to make the frequency that makes the species. [6 (page 6)]

Milhouse Units – "The absolute units in the Biologic Ionization Principles." [6 (page 6)]

Milli-Micronage – "Refers to the path of the electron in orbit so that when light strikes it, it gives color, tints, and hues." [6 (page 6)]

Milli-Milli-Micronage – "The smallest subdivision within the frequency structure. It dictates identity." [6 (page 6)]

Mil-li-volt – unit of electrical potential equal to one-thousandth part of a volt.

Mil-li-volt-meter – Instrument used for measuring voltage in terms of millivolts.

Mil-li-watt – a unit of power equal to one-thousandth part of a watt.

Mineral – "Refers to the individual elements in pure state. It is used generally to refer to all the elements, minerals, as well as non-mineral." [6 (page 6)]

Neutrons: A particle of an atom with a neutral charge. Neutrons are about the same mass as a proton.

Nutrition – "Refers to how the nutrients that are contained in the food are utilized. A good diet does not always ensure good nutrition. Individual body chemistry makes the difference as to whether food is healthful or toxic to a person." [6 (page 6)]

Ohm – "the unit of electrical resistance, equal to the resistance of a circuit in which an electromotive force of one volt maintains a current of one ampere." [7 (page 520)]

Organic – "Refers to any substance that contains carbon in its molecular structure. [6 (page 6)]

pH – "A measure of resistance. A pH of 7 means that there is an equal resistance between anions and cations." [6 (page 7)]

Positron: Also called an electron. A particle with the same charge and mass as an electron. It is an antiparticle and when it collides with an electron, low energy annihilation produces two photons. Photons have no mass.

Proton: The positive charged particle in the nucleus of the atom. Opposite to the negative charge electron in atoms.

Reserve Energy – "Refers to the amount of energy left. It is like a savings account. The lower the reserve, the weaker the liver, and the poorer the health." [6 (page 8)]

Van Allen Belt – "A belt of magnetic radiation energy surrounding the earth about 100 miles above its surface. It is this belt that the sun's anions hit to produce the rotation of the earth. Also known as the *magnosphere*." [6 (page 8)]

Volt: Energy per charge. One volt is the electrical force which causes a current of one ampere to flow against resistance of one Ohm.

Watt: In the metric system, it is a unit of power equal to one joule per second. Especially used to measure electrical power.

GLOSSARY OF HEBREW WORDS

"Ab•ba" – "An affectionate way to say "father", hence, "Dear father", "Dad", or even, "Daddy". Aramaic, then incorporated into ancient Hebrew." [1 (Page 1813)]

Abomination – (Strong's #8262, 8263), "means utterly detestable filth". [5 (Page 9)]

"*A*cha****rit*** *Ha*ya****min***" – "Literally, 'the end of the days.' The end times or 'latter days,' when the '*olam hazeh* is coming to a close and the '*olam haba* is about to begin. 1 Corinthians 10:11) + [1 (page 1813)]

*"A•****dam"*** – "The first man; the word means "man" or "Human" generally; from the Hebrew root a*lef-dalet-men* (*a-d-m*), "red", from which also comes the word *a-da-**mah*** (earth)." [1 (Page 1813)]

*"A•do•****nai"-*** "Literally, "my Lord", a word the Hebrew Bible uses to refer to God. When in large and small capital letters in the CJB (*A•DO•**NAI***), it represents the tetragrammaton, the Hebrew name of God, consisting of the four letters Yud-Heh-Vav-Heh (Y-H-V-H), sometimes rendered in English as Jehovah or Yahweh, but usually as LORD, sometimes as God." [1 (Page 1813)]

"*A•DO•**NAI***" – "The Lord our God" [1 (Page 1813)]

Adonai – "Lord". Hebrew epithet of *Yehovah*. Later used as a replacement for the name of *Yehovah*. Whenever a Pharisee sees the word *Yehovah* in Scripture, he reads it as if it was written *Adonai*. See *Ban on Divine Name*. [2 (Page 93)]

"*A•ha•**ron*** (Aaron)" – "*Moshe's* brother; traditionally the first *cohen gadol*." [1 (Page 1815)]

"*A•Lef* (Aleph)" – "1st letter of the Hebrew alphabet" [1 (Page 1815)]

"*A•men*" – 'It is true', 'so be it', 'may it become true.' "Spoken after a prayer or statement to indicate agreement. (1) Most translators take *Yeshua's* '*Amen*' as referring forward to what he was about to say: 'Truly, I say to you…' 'But there is no other instance of *amen* pointing forward in early church literature, and the context does not require it. *Yeshua* uses *Amen* to refer back, either seriously or ironically, to what he or someone else has said, or to what has just happened. *Matthew* 5:18 ('Yes indeed!') (2) Occasionally, the term tells the congregation to say *Amen* at the end of a prayer. *Matthew* 6:13" [1 (Page 1815)]

Anomians – violators of *Torah*. [9 (page 304)]

asiyat hatorah – "practical application of the *Torah's* teachings" [1 (page 1750)]

*"Av•ra•****ham*** (*Abraham*)" – "First of the three patriarchs of the Jewish people. *Matthew* 1.1+" [1 (Page 1815)]

Ba-ash – "stink; to be offensive morally." (*1 Samuel* 13:4) [5 (Page 51)]

Ban on Divine Name – "Pharisaic Law, instituted sometime in the 2nd century CE. According to the ban, it is forbidden to say the name "Yehovah" even in prayer or when reading from the *Torah*. As a rule, Pharisees replace the name "Yehovah" with the epithet Adonai (Lord)." [2 (Page 94)]

Biblical Hebrew **–** Language of the *Tanach* (*Tanakh*) (*Old Testament*). Biblical Hebrew was spoken in ancient Israel. After the return from Babylonia, Biblical Hebrew was gradually replaced with Aramaic and what became known later as *Mishaic Hebrew*." [2 (Page 94)]

B'li•ya•al (*Belial*) – "Another name for Satan, the Adversary. The Hebrew means 'without profit, worthless.'" [1 (page 1821)]

B'rakhah -khot – "Blessing(s), benediction(s). The word comes from *berekh* ('knee') and shows the connection between worship and kneeling. To 'make a *b'rakhah*' is to say a blessing, to bless." [1 (page 1822)]

"B'rit" – "Covenant, contract. The major biblical covenants are those God made through *Noach* (*Genesis* 9), *Avraham* (*Genesis* 17), Moshe (*Exodus* 19-24), David (*2 Samuel* 7), and Yeshua (*Jeremiah* 31; *Matthew* 26:28 +). The first is with all humanity, the next three relate primarily to the Jewish people and the last, though made with the Jewish people, brings all humanity into relationship with all the covenants." [1 (Page 1815)]

"*B'**rit Ha**•da•**Shah***"- *New Covenant*, *New Testament*. The term is used in the Introduction but not in the text of the *Complete Jewish Bible*. The New Covenant, however, is mentioned in *Matthew* 26:28; *Mark* 14:24; *Luke* 22:20; *1 Corinthians* 11:25; *Galatians* 4:24; and throughout *Hebrews* 7:22-10:31; as well as in the *Tanakh* at *Jeremiah* 31:30-33 (31-34)" [1 (Page 1822)]

"*B'rit•mi•lah*" – "Literally, "covenant of circumcision" (see *Genesis* 17). The term can mean either the act or the ceremony of covenantal circumcision, which is normally performed on the eighth day of a male Jew's life and required of any male Gentile who converts to Judaism. *Luke* 1:59+" [1 (Page 1822)]

"co•**hen**", pl. "*co•ha•**nin***" – "Priest (in the Temple or tabernacle). *Matthew* 2:4+" [1 (Page 1822)]

"*co•**hen** ga•**dol***", pl. "*co•ha•**nim** g'do•lim*" – "High priest. *Co•**hen** ha•ga•dol* means "the High priest". *Matthew* 26:3" [1 (Page 1822)]

"***Da***•*Let* (Daleth)" – "4th Letter of the Hebrew alphabet". [1 (Page 1822)]

Defilement – "spiritual term" – "evil, lust and corruption of our sinful hearts." [4 (Page 107)]

Ecclesia – "the called out", "the body of Christ, who is the Head of this corporate body of believers." [originally Hebrew Messianic believers and followers of Yeshua] [4 (Page 57, 216)]

"*El•**yon***" – "God Most High" [1 (Page 1824)]

"*El•Shad•**dai***" – "God Almighty" [1 (Page 1824)]

Emissary – apostle, [1 (Page xivii)]

Erga nomou (Greek) "legalistic observance of *Torah* commands" [1 (Page 1)]

Eruv – Man-made rules for activities allowed or not allowed on Shabbat. *Eruv* does not allow for carrying objects from a private place to a public or semi-public place.

Euphemistic (*Euphemism*) – "the substitution of an agreeable or inoffensive expression for one that may offend or suggest something unpleasant. Also, the expression so substituted." https://www.merriam-webster.com/dictionary/euphemism

Execution stake – Cross, [1 (Page xivii)]

*Hal*le*lu*yah!* (Hallelujah!) – A command in the plural, "Praise Yah!" (Yah is the name of God; see Ps. 68:5[4]. Sometimes rendered "Praise the Lord!" Rev. 19:1ff [2 (page 1829)]

Haluq – (*Haluk, Chaluk*) – One of two garments worn daily by Jewish men. The first garment is a long linen undershirt. This garment was worn at home but not in public. This is the garment the soldiers gambled for in John 19:23. The Haluq was worn under the tallit.

HaShem – "is the Hebrew word which many pious Jews use instead of the *yod-hey-vav-hey* (*YHVH*) name, in casual conversations, and literally means *The Name*. When they encounter this name during prayers or when reading from the *Torah*, they visualize *YHVH* and say *Adonai*. *Hashem* is used 7488 times in the *Tanach*. (*HaShem* by Rabbi Dr. Hillel ben David (Greg Killian), http://www.betemunah.org/hashem.html, 8/17/21)

"*Ha•**vah*** (Eve)" – "The first woman. *2 Corinthians* 11:3; *Titus* 2:13." [1 (Page 1830)]

Hebraisms – "Hebrew thought patterns translated literally into another language such as Greek." [2 (Page 96)]

Hebraisms – Thought patterns, expressions, word puns. See 'word puns'. [3]

"*Heh*" – "5th Letter of the Hebrew alphabet". [1 (Page 1830)]

Hilasterion – Hebrew – Translated "atonement, propitiation, mercy seat". [4 (Page 50)] [At-one-ment]

Holy (hō'lē) – Associated with the Divine Power. Consecrated to God . Devoted to the service of God.

Hugiaino – Greek verb – literally to "be in health"," to be well in body", and to have sound health". Translated in English as "hygiene". [4 (Page 48)]

Immersion – baptism, [1 (Page xivii)]

Kanaph (Kanaf, Kanafim plural) – The fringe or ribbons on the four corners of the tallit. They are mentioned in *Malachi* 4:2 as wings or healing.

Kaphar – Hebrew – translated "atonement", "to cover, as in cover sin". Also used in *Genesis* 6:14 to refer to "pitch" or bitumen used to cover Noah's ark so that the waters of judgement could not destroy him and his family. [4 (Page 50)]

Karaite – Name given to Jews who adhere to the Hebrew Scripture as the sole source of divine instruction. Also, called a Hebrew Scripturalist. [2 (page 97)]

Katallage – Greek – "reconciliation". See *Hilasterion,* [4 (Page 50)]

*"Ke•**fa*** (*Cephas*, Peter)" – Name given by *Yeshua* to *Shim'on Bar Yochanan;* it means 'rock' in Aramaic, as does the Greek equivalent, petro. *Matthew* 4:18+" [1 (Page 1833)]

Kashrut – Kosher Laws, Clean and Unclean. Today called 'Dietary Laws'. [1 (Page 142)]

Kehillah (pl. *kehillahs* or *kehillot*) Hebrew: a community, a congregation. A type of Jewish community in eastern Europe. Any Jewish community, especially, a secular Jewish communal organization, or the secular dimension of a religious one. (https://www.wordsense.eu)

Libertines – "Freed Slaves" [1 (page 1567)]

Ma'asim – "Literally: "works, deeds". Pharisaic term referring to precedents of the Rabbis that provide a source for Pharisaic rulings. Also, rulings made based on these precedents." [2 (Page 97)]

Ma'asim – Literal meaning – "actions, deeds". Greek translated *ma'asim* as "ergon" which was translated "works" in English. [3]

Man-Made Laws – See *Takanot* [2 (Page 98)]

*"Mat•tit•**yah**, ya•hu* (*Matthew, Matthias, Mattathias*)" – (1) One of *Yeshua's* twelve *talmidim*, author of one of the Gospels, also known as *Levi* (*Matthew* 9:9); usually rendered in English as "*Matthew…*" [1 (Page 1837)]

"*ma•**tzah***", pl. "*ma•**tzot***" – "Unleavened bread. The "first day for *matzah*" would be the day on which, when evening comes, the *Seder* (Passover) is held." [1 (Page 1837)]

Messianic community – Assembly (today translated "church") [1 (Page xivii)]

"*mid•**rash***" – "Allegorical interpretation or homiletical application of a text. The hearer is expected to understand that the maker of the *midrash* is not expounding the plain meaning or the text but introducing his own ideas. *Galatians* 4:24." [1 (Page 1838)]

Midrash – "One of the pillars of the Oral Law written down from the 2nd to the 9th Centuries CE. *Midrash* is generally arranged as a running commentary on biblical verses, as opposed to the *Mishnah* and *Talmud* which are arranged by topic." [2 (Page 98)]

Minhag – Customs – "The Rabbis believe that if something is done by an entire Jewish community for an extended period of time, then the custom becomes binding upon the community. Ex. *Kippah*, *Kippot* or skull cap. [2 (page 94)]

"*mik•**veh***" – "Bath or pool with a flow of fresh water; used in Orthodox Judaism to this day for ritual purification. *Ephesians* 5:26; *Titus* 3:5." [1 (Page 1838)]

Mishnah – "One of the pillars of the Oral Law, the Mishnah contains the discussions in the Pharisaic academies up until the time it was written down in about 200 CE by Rabbi Judah the Prince." [2 (Page 98)] "***mitz•****vah***", pl. "mitz•**vot**" – a. literally, 'command', 'commandment'; more broadly: general principle for living, good deed. *Matthew* 5:19+. b. faithful performance of the biblical commandments. [a 1 (Page 1839); b 1 (page 1750)]

"*Mo•she* (Moses)" – "(1) Deliverer of *Isra'el* from Egypt, agent through whom *Isra'el* received the *Torah*. Matt. 8:4+. (2) In the time of *Yeshua* and after, the "seat of *Moshe*" was not only a metaphor for authority of the *Torah*-teachers but an actual chair on which they sat when they taught. An example from the third century c.e., discovered in the ruins of *Korazin* [city on the shore of Lake Kinneret, two miles north of *K'far-Nachum*. Page 1834] is on display at the Isra'el Museum in Yerushalayim. *Matthew* 23:2." [1 (Page 1839)]

*Mo•tza•'****ei****-Shab•****bat*** – "Literally, the 'going out of the *Sabbath*,' i.e., Saturday night. By biblical and Jewish reckoning, days begin at sunset; so, where the text tells us that the believers met on 'the first day of the week' it means Saturday night, not Sunday. *Acts* 20:7; *1 Corinthians* 16:2 [1 (page 1839)]

Negel vasser - hand washing vessel. [9 (page 304)]

Nenomothetêtai – Greek - is a compound word made up of: '*Nomos'* can be translated 'law', but in the book of *Hebrews* it always means *Torah;* and *"tithêmi",* a common word meaning 'put' or 'place' *Nenomothetêtai* is used in *Hebrews* 7:11 and *Hebrews* 8:6 [1 (Page 1)]

Nephesh – Hebrew – "breathing creation". English translation "living being". [4 (Page 48)]

"***nid•****dah*" – (1) Menstrual uncleanness; (2) the time of the same. [1 (Page 1841)]

"No•ach (Noah)" – "Builder of the ark; survivor of the Flood, and ancestor of all humanity since then (*Genesis* 5-11) …" [1 (Page 1841)]

*"nti•****lat****-ya•****da****•yim*" – Ceremonial handwashing prescribed by the Oral *Torah*, to be done before meals and at other times in order to be ritually pure; it continues to be a norm in Orthodox Judaism. *Matthew* 15:2+." [1 (Page 1841)]

*"o****lam*** *ha****ba***" – "The world to come, the age to come." [1 (page 1842)]

"*o****lam*** *ha****zeh***" – "This world, this age" [1 (page 1842)]

Oral Law – Body of information which the Pharisees claim was revealed to Moses orally on Mt. Sinai. The Oral Law was written down in the form of the *Mishnah*, *Talmud*, and *Midrash.* [2 (Page 99)]

"***Papias***" – (c.60-130CE) – "Church Father" who lived in Asia Minor. He studied under John who wrote the *Gospel of John*. Papias reports matter-of-factly that the *Gospel of Matthew* was written in Hebrew and that the translations of this book into other languages were known to be bad translations." [2 (Page 99)]

"***Pe•****sach*" (Passover) – The feast that celebrates the Exodus of the Jewish Nation from Egypt under the leadership of Moshe. It is along with *Shavu'ot* and *Sukkot*, one of the three pilgrim festivals when Jews were to come to *Yerushalayim*. *Matthew* 26:2+." [1 (Page 1843)]

Pharisees – "Jewish sect founded in the 2nd Century BCE. The primary doctrine of the sect is the belief in the "Oral Law", a secret revelation that Moses allegedly received at Mt. Sinai. Modern "Orthodox" Judaism is the direct continuation of ancient Phariseeism and medieval Rabbanism." [2 (Page 99)]

Piggul – "unclean, to stink. *Leviticus* 1:10. [5 (Page 51)]

Ruach – Hebrew, "in-breathed", "in-spired" "We as humans were inbreathed with God's own likeness, image and nature; therefore, God's likeness, image and nature should be revealed through every advance, discovery and step that we achieve." [4 (Page 49, 216)]

"***Ru***•*ach Ha*•***Ko***•*desh*" – "The Holy Spirit, referred to four times in the *Tanakh* as such, and many times as the Spirit of God. *Matthew* 1:18+." [1 (Page 1845)]

Sadducees - "Jewish movement in the late Second Temple times who adhered to the *Tanach* alone. Some later Sadducees denied the future resurrection of the dead." [2 (Page 100)]

"**Se**•der"– The ceremonial evening meal with which *Pesach* begins in Jewish homes. *Matthew* 26:17+." [1 (Page 1845)]

"***se***•*lah*" – "Pause in the music accompanying a psalm or prayer." [1 (Page 1845)]

Septuagint – "Greek translation of the *Tanach* (*Old Testament*). The original *Septuagint* was translated in the 3rd Century BCE. However, the Septuagint translation underwent many revisions and with the exception of a few fragments from the *Dead Sea Scrolls*, the version we have today is from 4th Century CE Christian hands." [2 (Page 100)]

"*Shab*•***bat***, pl. *Shab*•*ba*•***tot***" – Sabbath, *Matthew* 12:1+." [1 (Page 1846)]

Shabbat – means 'rest'. "Lasts from sundown Friday to sundown Saturday (day 7 in Hebrew lunar calendar.) "There was evening and there was morning". "Each new day starts at sunset." [1 (Page 5)]

Shabbat-walk: Approximately one-half mile per *Josephus*. It is the distance from *Yerushalyim* to the Mount of Olives.[1 (page 1559)]

"*Sha*•***lom***"- Peace, tranquility, safety, well-being, welfare, health, contentment, success, comfort, wholeness, and integrity. "*Shalom!*" is a common greeting. *Matthew* 10:12+." [1 (Page 1846)]

"*Sha*•***lom*** *a'lei*•***khem***" – "Peace be upon you [plural]! "A common greeting. *Matthew* 10:12+." [1 (Page 1846)]

"*Sha*•*'ul* (Saul)" – "Also known as Paul" (Acts 13:9). "Yeshua, the Messiah's emissary to the Gentile world, who presented *Isra'el's* New Covenant faith in God and his Messiah in a way that does not require Gentiles to convert to Judaism. Act 7:58+; named for *Sha'ul Ben-Kish* (Saul, the son of Kish), *Isra'el's* first king. *Acts* 13:21." [1 (Page 1846)]

"*Sha*•*vu*•*'**ot***" – "*The Feast of Weeks,* since it comes seven weeks after *Pesach* (Passover); also called Pentecost (from Greek *pentekostos*, 'fifty'), since one counts fifty days after *Pesach.* One of the three *regalim* ("pilgrim festivals") when Jews were expected to celebrate before God in *Yerushalayim*; the other two are *Pesach* and *Sukkot*. *Acts* 2:1+." [1 (Page 1846)]

Shegets, Shagots – "to be filthy, to loathe, to pollute, to be hateful, detestable, abominable." *Leviticus* 11:11-13, 20, 23, 41-42; *Isaiah* 66:17. [5 (Page 52)]

"Shem-Tov's Hebrew Matthew" – A Hebrew version of the *Gospel of Matthew* preserved as an appendix in a 14th Century Jewish polemical work written by *Shem-Tov Ibn Shaprut*. Long believed to be a translation from the Greek or Latin, this Hebrew version of *Matthew*, has recently been shown to contain original reading that would not be found in a translation from Greek or Latin." [2 (Page 101)]

Shigguts – "translated as abomination, means disgusting, filthy, and idolatrous, or an idol." *1 Kings* 11:5, 7 and *2 Kings* 23:13 it refers to idols, two false faiths." [5 (Page 51)]

*Sh'iki****nah*** – Divine Presence, the manifest glory of God present with people. [2 (page 1848)]

Sozo – "Salvation" in Greek. Save, make whole, heal, deliver from danger. Includes freedom from spiritual, emotional and physical sickness." [4 (Page 235)]

"*Suk•**kot*** (Succoth)" – "*The Feast of Booths* (*Tabernacles*), celebrating the forty years when the people of Isra'el lived in *suk•kot* (booths, tents, shacks, [tabernacles]; singular *suk•kah*) in the desert between Egypt and *Eretz-Yisrael*. It is one of three pilgrim festivals when Jews were expected to go up to *Yerushalayim*. *John* 7:2." [1 (Page 1850)]

"Tahor - (clean) term used to describe spiritual or moral state of being rather than physical." [1 (Page 142)]

Takanot – 'Enactments'. Hebrew word to describe laws enacted by the Pharisees. [2 (Page 101)]

"*tal•**mid***", fem. *Tal•mi•**dah***, pl. *tal•mi•**dim***" – "Disciple, student. The relationship between a talmid and his rabbi was very close: not only did the *talmid* learn facts, reasoning processes and how to perform religious practices from his rabbi, but he regarded him as an example to be imitated in conduct and character (see *Matthew* 10:24, 25; *Luke* 6:40; *John* 13:13-15; *1 Corinthians* 11:1). The rabbi, in turn, was considered responsible for his *talmidim*. (*Matthew* 12:2; *Luke* 19:39; *John* 17:12). *Matthew* 5:1+." [1 (Page 1850)]

Talmud – "Collection of discussions from the Pharisaic academies primary on meaning of the *Mishnah*. Also known by the Aramaic name *Gemara*." [2 (Page 101)]

Tamai (unclean): "used only in relation to moral and religious deficiencies that contaminate the soul and character of man, particularly incest and idol worship, and to characterize the absence of ritual purity. Also, translated 'defilement'. The creatures designated as *tamai* were not only forbidden as food, but also for sacrificial purposes. The English words *clean* and *unclean* are therefore to be understood as purity and defilement in a spiritual-ritual sense." [1 (Page 142)]

Tame – (Strong's #2930, 2931) contaminate, foul, and/or impure. [5 (Page 9)]

"*Ta•**nakh***" – Acronym formed from the first letters of the three parts of the Hebrew Bible: *Torah*, *Nevi'im* [Prophets], and *K'tuvim* [writings], hence the *Old Testament*;

rendered 'scripture' or 'it is written' in most translations or the *New Testament.* The reason the *New Testament* writers cite the *Tanakh* so frequently is that they understand it as God's authoritative word to humanity. *Matthew* 4:4." [1 (Page 1850)]

Tefillin (*t'fillm*) – "[A]– Two black leather boxes containing scrolls with Bible passages on them. During synagogue prayers, men affix one to their hand and arm and the other to their forehead, in obedience to *Deuteronomy* 6:8. *T'fillin* are called phylacteries in most translations. [1 (page 1851)]

"*telos*" – Greek - usually means "goal, purpose, consummation," not "termination." The Messiah did not bring the *Torah* to an end. Rather, as the CJB's *B'rit Hadashah* renders it, "The goal at which the *Torah* aims is the Messiah, who offers righteousness to everyone who trusts." [1 (Page 1)]

"***To•****rah*" – "Literally, 'teaching', but usually translated 'law' because Greek uses *nomos* ('law') to render Hebrew *Torah.* (1) *The Five Books of Moses*, the *Pentateuch* (*Genesis*, *Exodus*, *Leviticus*, *Numbers*, and *Deuteronomy*), called the Written *Torah. Matthew* 5:17… (4) Uncapitalized, *torah* can be understood generically as 'law' or 'principle'. *Romans* 7:21-8:2." [1 (Page 1852)]

Tow'ebah – "disgusting, an abhorrence or idolatry." Several references including *Leviticus* 18:22, 20:13 (sodomy); *Deuteronomy* 7:25-26; 12:31; 13:14 (idols); *Deuteronomy* 25:16 (false weights and measures, etc.) [5 (Page 51)]

Traditions of the Elders – "Another name for *Takanot*." [2 (Page 102)]

"*t'shu•****vah***" – "Literally, 'turning'. In the context of behavior, it means repentance since the sinner who "does *t'shuvah*" is turning from sin to God. *Matthew* 13:15+." [1 (Page 1852)]

"*tza•****ra•****'at*" (leprosy) – A contagious disease and source of ritual uncleanness evidenced by skin lesions; death with in *Leviticus* 13-14. Generally believed not to be Hansen's disease, which is the modern meaning of "leprosy." [1 (Page 1852)]

"*tza•****tzit***", pl. "*tzi•tzi•****yot***" – "Specially made fringes worn on the four corners of a man's *tallit*, fulfilling the *mitzvah* in *Numbers* 15:37-41. In ancient times, including the first century, the *tallit* was a cloak or robe included in normal male attire. After clothes stopped being made with "corners", Judaism created the modern *tallit* (prayer shawl) so that the *mitzvah* could be performed. *Matthew* 9:20+ [*Malachi* 3:20 (4:2) "But to you who fear my name, the sun of righteousness will rise with healing in its wings; and you will break out leaping like calves released from the stall."] [1 (Page 897, 1853)]

tzedakah – "literally 'righteousness,' but since ancient times also used to mean 'charity'." [1 (page 1853)]

Upo nomon (Greek) – "in subjection to the system which results from perverting the *Torah* into legalism." [1 (Page 1)]

Washing the Hands – "Pharisaic Law requiring a ritual washing of the hands and an accompanying blessing before each meal." [2 (Page 102)]

Word Press – "Use of similar sounding Hebrew words to create a beautiful literary texture or sometimes to emphasize a point." [2 (Page 102)]

Word Puns – Poetical style – generally only in Hebrew. Words with similar sounds, but different meanings. [3]

Yatsar – Hebrew – "formed" "to press or squeeze into shape", or "to mold" as a potter." "Man, as a vessel of clay and dust, was uniquely formed on the Great Potter's wheel for a very special purpose." …" He [Man] possessed a unique capacity for worship and intimate fellowship with God." [4 (Page 49)]

Yehovah – "Name of the God of Israel. In Hebrew written *YHWH*." [2 (Page 102)]

Yehovah – "Hebrew Name of God. Name used in the Bible 6828 times and is the name of the Creator. Hebrew name of God in a 10th Century manuscript of the Bible (British Library, Or 1880, *Leviticus* 23:26). This is one of the many early Masoretic manuscripts that preserve the Hebrew pronunciation of God's holy name." [3]

"*Ye•ru•sha•**la**•yim*" (Jerusalem) – Capital of *Eretz-Yisrael* [Land of Israel, Page 1825] since the days of King David. Psalm 48 calls it "the city of our God…beautiful for situation, the joy of the whole earth." *Matthew* 21+." [1 (Page 1856)]

"*Ye•**shu**•a"* (Jesus) – "Variant of '*Y'hoshua*' (Joshua)…In the *Tanakh* nine (people) and a city have the name Yeshua, usually transliterated as 'Jeshua' or 'Jeshuah'. In the Septuagint and the New Testament, the name was brought over into Greek as *Iêsous and thence into English as 'Jesus'. It means "Y-H-V-H Saves"* (*Matthew* 1:21) and is also the masculine form of *yeshu'ah* (*'*salvation*'*) ... *"* [1 (Page 1856)]

Yeshua – "Most Hebrew names are made up of a number of smaller words which together form a short Hebrew sentence. The name Yeshua is formed from the two Hebrew words '*Yehovah'* (or *Yahweh*) and *yoshia* which together mean 'Yehovah saves'. Two manuscripts of Hebrew *Matthew* preserve Yeshua's Hebrew name as Yehoshua." *The Naming of Jesus in Hebrew Matthew* [6 (Page 6)]

Yeshu – A shortened version of Yeshua preserved in Hebrew *Matthew*. *The Naming of Jesus in Hebrew Matthew* [6 (Page 6)]

Yetzer hara – evil inclination. [1 (Page 1615)]

"*Yo•cha•**nan***" (John, Jona) – "The English name John is derived from Hebrew *Yochanan*, which means 'God gives grace.' (1) Yochanan the Immerser; (2) *Talmid* of Yeshua, son of Zavdai, brother of Ya'akov #4, and author of several New Testament books." *Matthew* 4:21+." [1 (Page 1858)]

"*Yom-Kip•**pur***" – The Day of Atonement. The Greek says, literally, 'the fast,' but a Jewish fast day in the fall spoken of with definite article can refer only to *Yom-Kippur*. *Acts* 27:9." [1 (Page 1858)]

"*Yud*" "(*Yodh*, jot)" – The 10th and smallest letter in the Hebrew alphabet. *Matthew* 5:18." [1 (Page 1859)]

"*Yud-Heh-Vav-Heh*" (*YHVH*) "The four-letter Hebrew name of God. (See *ADONAI*)" [1 (Page 1859)]

ADDITIONAL SCRIPTURES MENTIONED

Chapter One: Scripture References

Sh'mot (*Exodus*) [20: 8]" Remember the day, *Shabbat*, to set it apart for God. [9]You have six days to labor and do all your work, [10]but the seventh is a *Shabbat* for *ADONAI* your God. On it you are not to do any kind of work – not you, your son or daughter, not your male or female slave, not your livestock, and not the foreigner staying with you inside the gates to your property."

Sh'mot (*Exodus*) [31:16] "'The people of *Isra'el* are to keep the *Shabbat*, to observe *Shabbat* through all their generations as a perpetual covenant. [17]It is a sign between me and the people of *Isra'el* forever; for in six days *ADONAI* made heaven and earth, but on the seventh day he stopped working and rested.'" (Page 115)

D'varim (*Deuteronomy*) [30:6] "'Then *ADONAI* your God will circumcise your hearts and the hearts of your children, so that you will love *ADONAI* your God with all your heart and all your being, and thus you will live.'" (Page 265)

Yirmeyahu (*Jeremiah*) [4:4] "'People of *Y'hudah* and inhabitants of *Yerushalayim*, circumcise yourselves for *ADONAI*, remove the foreskins of your heart! Otherwise, my fury will lash out like fire, burning so hot that no one can quench it, because of how evil your actions are'" (Page 614)

Mal'akhi (*Malachi*) [3:6] "'But, because I, *ADONAI*, do not change, you sons of *Ya'akov* will not be destroyed.'" (Page 895)

Messianic Jews (*Hebrews*) [13:8] "*Yeshua* the Messiah is the same yesterday, today and forever." (Page 1749)

The Revelation of Yeshua The Messiah to Yochanan (John) (*Revelation*) [1:8] "'I am the *Alef* and the *Tav*,' says *ADONAI*, God of heavens armies, the One who is, who was and who is coming."

Chapter Two: Scripture References

Sh'mot (*Exodus*) [20:12] "Honor you father and mother, so that you may live long in the land which *ADONAI* your God is giving you." 2(page 99)

Sh'mot (*Exodus*) [21:17] "Whoever curses his father or mother must be put to death." 2 (page 101)

Vayikra (*Leviticus*) [15:19] "'If a woman has a discharge, and the discharge from her body is blood, she will be in her state of *niddah* for seven days. Whoever touches her will be unclean until evening. [20] Everything she lies on or sits on in her state of *niddah* will be unclean. [21] Whoever touches her bed is to wash his clothes and bathe himself in water; he will be unclean until evening. [22] Whoever touches anything she sits on is to wash his clothes and bathe himself in water; he will be unclean until evening. [23] As soon as he touches the bed or something she sat on, he will be unclean until evening. [24] If a man goes to bed with her, and her menstrual flow touches him, he will be unclean for seven days; and every bed he lies on will be unclean.

[25] "'If a woman has a discharge of blood for many days not during her period, or if her discharge lasts beyond the normal end of her period, then throughout the time she is having an unclean discharge she will be as when she is in *niddah* – she is unclean. [26] Every bed she lies on at any time while she is having her discharge will be for her like the bed, she uses during her time of *niddah*; and everything she sits on will be unclean with uncleanness like that of her time of *niddah*. [27] Whoever touches those things will be unclean; he is to wash his clothes and bathe himself in water; he will be unclean until evening.

[28] "'If she has become free of her discharge, she is to count seven days; after that she will be clean.[29] On the eighth day, she is to take for herself two doves or two young pigeons and bring them to the *Cohen* at the entrance of the meeting tent of meeting. [30] The *cohen* is to offer the one as a sin offering and the other as a burnt offering; thus, the *cohen* will make atonement for her before *ADONAI* on account of her unclean discharge.

[31] "'In this way you will separate the people of *Isra'el* from their uncleanness, so that they will not die in a state of uncleanness for defiling my tabernacle which is there with them.'" [2 (page 150)]

Vayikra (*Leviticus*) [20:9] "A person who curses his father or mother must be put to death; having cursed his father or mother, his blood is on him." [2(page 156)]

B'midbar (*Numbers*) [15:37] "*ADONAI* said to *Moshe*, [38] 'Speak to the people of *Isra'el*, instructing them to make, through all their generation, *tzitziyot* on the corners of their garments, and to put with the *tzitzit* on each corner a blue thread. [39] It is to be a *tzitzit* for you to look at and thereby remember all of *ADONAI'S mitzvot* and obey them, so that you won't go around wherever your own heart and eyes lead you to prostitute yourselves, [40] but it will help you remember and obey all my mitzvot and be holy for your God. [41] I am *ADONAI* your God, who brought you out of the land of Egypt in order to be your God. I am *ADONAI* your God.'" [2 (page 193)]

D'varim (*Deuteronomy*) [5:16] "Honor your father and mother, as *ADONAI* your God ordered you to do, so that you will live long and have things go well with you in the land *ADONAI* your God is giving you." [2(page 233)]

D'varim (*Deuteronomy*) [12:32] "Everything I am commanding you; you are to take care to do. Do not add to or subtract from it." [2(page 245)]

Tehillim (*Psalm*) [118:22] "The very rock that the builders rejected has become the cornerstone! [2 (page 1028)]

Psalm 118:22 Note: "This is a significant passage v. 22 is quoted in four passages in the *B'rit Hadashah* (*Luke* 20:17; *Acts* 4:11; *1 Peter* 2:4, 7). And there are two additional passages that quote this verse along with v. 23 (*Matthew* 21:42; *Mark* 12:10-11). The leaders' ('builders') rejection of *Yeshua* the Messiah becomes proof of his claim to Messiahship." [2 (page 1028)]

Mishlei (*Proverbs*) 30:6 "Don't add anything to his words, or he will rebuke you, and you be found a liar." 2 (page 1113)

Yesha-Yahu (*Isaiah*) 29:13 "The *Adonai* said: 'Because these people approach me with empty words, and the honor they bestow on me is mere lip-service; while in fact they have distanced their hearts from me, and their 'fear of me' is just a *mitzvah* of human origin –" 2 (page 533)

Dani'el (*Daniel*) 2:44 "In the days of those kings the God of heaven will establish a kingdom that will never be destroyed, and that kingdom will not pass into the hands of another people. It will break into pieces and consume all those kingdoms, but it, itself, will stand forever – 45 like the stone you saw, which, without human hands, separated itself from the mountains and broke to pieces the iron, the bronze, the clay, the silver and the gold. The great God has revealed to the king what will come about in the future. The dream is true, and its interpretation is reliable." 2 (page 1244)

Dani'el (*Daniel*) 7:13 "I kept watching the night visions, when I saw, coming with the clouds of heaven, someone like a son of man. He approached the Ancient One and was led into his presence. 14 To him was given rulership, glory, and a kingdom, so that all peoples, nations and languages should serve him. His rulership is an eternal rulership that will not pass away; and his kingdom is one that will never be destroyed." 2 (page 1253)

Mal'akhi (*Malachi*) 4:2 "But to you who fear my name, the sun of righteousness will rise with healing in his wings; and you will break out leaping, like calves released from the stall." 2 (page 897)

Mattityahu (*Matthew*) 3:2 "'Turn from your sins to God, for the Kingdom of Heaven is near!' 3 This is the man *Yesha'yahu* was taking about when he said, 'The voice of someone crying out: In the desert prepare the way of *ADONAI*! Make straight paths for him!" 2 (page 1386)

Mattityahu (*Matthew*) 4:17 "From that time on, *Yeshua* began proclaiming, 'Turn your sins to God, for the Kingdom of Heaven is near!" 2 (page 1388)

Mattityahu (*Matthew*) 11:13 "For all the prophets and the *Torah* prophesied until *Yochanan*.14 Indeed, if you are willing to accept it, he is *Eliyahu*, whose coming was predicted." 2 (page 1405)

Mattityahu (*Matthew*) 12:12 "'How much more valuable is a man than a sheep! Therefore, what is permitted on *Shabbat* is to do good.' 13 Then to the man he said, 'Hold out your hand.' As he held it out, it became restored, as sound as the other one. 14 But the *P'rushim* went out and began plotting how they might do away with Yeshua. 15 Aware of this, he left that area. Many people followed him; and he healed them all 16 but warned them not to make him known. 17 This was to fulfill what had been spoken through *Yesha'yahu* (*Isaiah*) the prophet." 2 (page 1407)

Mattityahu (*Matthew*) 14:35 "When the people of the place recognized him, they sent word throughout the neighborhood and brought him everyone who was ill. 36 They begged him that the sick people might only touch the tzitzit on his robe, and all who touched it were completely healed." 2 (page 1412)

Mattityahu (*Matthew*) 16:15 "'But you,' he said to them, 'who do you say I am?' 16 *Shim'on Kefa* answered, 'You are the *Mashiach*, the Son of the living God.' 17 '*Shim'on Bar-Yochanan*,' *Yeshua* said to him, 'how blessed you are! For no human being revealed this to you, no, it was my Father in heaven. 18 I also tell you this: you are *Kefa* [which means 'Rock.'] 'and on this rock I will build my Community, and the gates of *Sh'ol* will not overcome it. 19 I will give you the keys of the Kingdom of Heaven. Whatever you prohibit on earth will be prohibited in heaven, and whatever you permit on earth will be permitted in heaven.' 20 Then he warned the *talmidim* not to tell anyone that he was the Messiah." [2 (page 1415)]

Mattityahu (*Matthew*) 21:42 "*Yeshua* said to them, 'Haven't you ever read in the *Tanakh*, 'The very rock which the builders rejected has become the cornerstone! This has come from *ADONAI*, and in our eyes, it is amazing!'?" [2 (page 1422)]

Luke 1:26 "In the sixth month, the angel *Gavri'el* was sent by God to a city in the *Galil* called *Natzeret*, 27 to a virgin engaged to a man named *Yosef*, of the house of *David*: the virgin's name was *Miryam*. 38 Approaching her, the angel said, '*Shalom*, favored lady! *ADONAI* is with you! 29 She was deeply troubled by his words and wondered what kind of greeting this might be. 30 The angel said to her, 'Don't be afraid, *Miryam*, for you have found favor with God. 31 Look! You will become pregnant, you will give birth to a son, and you are to name him *Yeshua*. 32 He will be great; he will be called Son of *Ha 'Elyon*. *ADONAI*, God, will give him the throne of his forefather David; 33 and he will rule the House of *Ya'akov* forever – there will be no end to his Kingdom.'" [2 (page 1470)]

Yochanan (*John*) 2:1 Note: *Tuesday* is Greek: the third day, equivalent to Hebrew *yom shlishi*. [2 (page 1523)]

Yochanan (*John*) 7:15 "The *Judeans* were surprised: 'How does this man know so much without having studied?' they asked. 16 So *Yeshua* gave them an answer: 'My teaching is not my own, it comes from the One who sent me.'" [2 (page 1532)]

Yochanan (*John*) 14:6 "*Yeshua* said, 'I AM the Way – and the Truth and the Life; no one comes to the Father except through me. 7 Because you have known me, you will also know my Father; from now on, you do know him – in fact, you have seen him." [2 (page 1545)]

1 *Yochanan* (*John*) 1:1 "The Word, which gives life! He existed from the beginning. We have heard him, we have seen him with our eyes, we have contemplated him, we have touched him with our hands!" [2 (page 1770)]

Romans 10:4 "For the goal at which the *Torah* aims is the Messiah, who offers righteousness to everyone who trusts. 5 For *Moshe* writes about the righteousness grounded in the *Torah* that **the person who does these things will attain life through them**. 6 Moreover, the righteousness grounded in trusting says: **'Do not say in your heart, 'Who will ascend to heaven?'** – that is, to bring the Messiah down – 7 or, **'Who will descend into *Sh'ol*?'** – that is, to bring the Messiah up from the dead. 8 'What then does it say?' **'The word is near you, in your mouth and in your heart.'** – that is, the word about trust which we proclaim, namely, 9 that if you acknowledge publicly with your mouth that *Yeshua* is Lord and trust in your heart that God raised him from the dead, you will be delivered. 10 For with the heart one goes on trusting and thus continues toward righteousness, while with the mouth one keeps on making public acknowledgement and thus continues toward deliverance. [11] For the passage quoted says that *everyone* **who rests his trust** on him **will not be humiliated**. [12] That means that there is no difference between Jew and Gentile – *ADONAI* is the same for everyone, rich toward everyone who calls on him, [13] since everyone who calls on the name of *ADONAI* will be delivered. [2 (page 1620)]

Chapter Three: Scripture References

Acts [1:8] "But you will receive power when the *Ruach HaKodesh* comes upon you: you will be my witnesses both in *Yerushalayim* and in all *Y'hudah* and *Shomron*, indeed to the ends of the earth!" [3 (page 1558)]

Acts [8:1] "and *Sha'ul* gave his approval to his (Stephen) murder. Starting with that day, there arose intense persecution against the Messianic Community in *Yerushalayim*; all but the emissaries were scattered throughout the regions of *Y'hudah* and *Shomron*. [2] Some godly men buried Stephen and mourned him deeply. [3] But *Sha'ul* set out to destroy the Messianic Community – entering house after house, he dragged off both men and women and handed them over to be put in prison. [4] However, those who were scattered announced the *Good News* of the Word wherever they went.

[5] "Now Philip went down to a city in *Shomron* and was proclaiming the Messiah to them;
[6] and the crowds were paying close attention to what Philip said, as they heard and saw miraculous signs he was doing. [7] For many people were having unclean spirits driven out of them, shrieking; also, many paralytics and crippled persons were being healed; [8] so that there was great joy in that city. [9] But there was a man named *Shim'on* in the city who for some time had been practicing magic and astonishing the nation of *Shromron*, claiming to be somebody great. [10] Everyone gave heed to him, from the lowest to the highest, saying, 'This man is the power of God called 'The Great Power.' [11] They followed him because for a considerable time he had amazed them with his magic.

[12] "But when they came to believe Philip, as he announced the Good News concerning the Kingdom of God and the name of *Yeshua* the Messiah, they were immersed, both men and women. [13] Moreover, *Shim'on* himself came to believe; and after being immersed, he attached himself closely to Philip; and he was amazed as he saw the miraculous signs and great works of power that kept taking place.

[14] "When the emissaries in *Yerushalayim* heard that *Shomron* had received the *Word of God*, they sent them *Kefa* and *Yochanan*, [15] who came down and prayed for them, that they might receive the *Ruach HaKodesh*. [16] For until then he had not come upon any of them; they had only been immersed into the name of the Lord *Yeshua*. [17] Then, as *Kefa* and *Yochanan* placed their hands on them, they received the *Ruach HaKodesh*. [18]
Shim'on saw that the Spirit was given when the emissaries placed their hands on them, and he offered them money. [19] 'Give this power to me, too,' he said, 'so that whatever I place my hands on will receive the *Ruach HaKodesh*.' [20] But *Kefa* said to him, 'Your silver go to ruin – and you with it, for thinking the free gift of God can be bought!' [21]
You have no part at all in this matter; because in the eyes of God, your heart is crooked.

22 So repent of this wickedness of yours and pray to the Lord. Perhaps you will yet be forgiven for holding such a thought in your heart. 23 For I see that you are extremely bitter and completely under the control of sin!’ 24 *Shim’on* answered, ‘Pray to the Lord for me, so that none of the things you have spoken about will happen to me.’ 25 Then, after giving a thorough witness and speaking the Word of the Lord, *Kefa* and *Yochanan* started back to *Yerushalayim* announcing the Good News to many villages in *Shomron.* 26 An angel of *ADONAI* said to Philip, ‘Get up, and go southward on the road that goes down from *Yerushalayim* to *‘Azah*, the desert road.’ 27 So he got up and went. On his way, he caught sight of an *Ethiopian*, a eunuch who was a minister in charge of all the treasure of the *Kandake*, or queen, of *Ethiopia*. He had been to *Yerushalayim* to worship; 28 and now, as he was returning home, he was sitting in his chariot, reading the prophet *Yesha’yahu.* 29 The Spirit said to Philip, ‘Go over to this chariot, and stay close to it.’ 30 As Philip ran up, he heard the *Ethiopian* reading from *Yesha’yahu*, the prophet. ‘Do you understand what you’re reading?’ he asked. 31 ‘How can I.’ he said, ‘unless someone explains it to me?’ And he invited Philip to climb up and sit with him. 32 Now the portion of the *Tanakh* that he was reading was this: ‘**He was like a sheep led to be slaughtered; like a lamb silent before the shearer, he does not open his mouth. 33 He was humiliated and denied justice. Who will tell about his descendants, since his life has been taken from the earth?’”** [a] (a Isaiah 53:7-8; 3 Page 580) 3 (page 1570, 1571)

Acts 9:1 “Meanwhile, *Sha’ul*, still breathing murderous threats against the Lord’s *talmidim*, went to the *cohen hagadol* 2 and ask him for letters to the synagogues in *Dammesek*, authorizing him to arrest any people he might find, whether men or women, who belonged to ‘*the Way*,’ and bring them back to *Yerushalayim.* 3 He was on the road and nearing *Dammesek*, when suddenly a light from heaven flashed all around him. 4 Falling to the ground, he heard a voice saying to him, ‘*Sha’ul*! *Sha’ul*! Why do you keep persecuting me?’ 5 ‘Sir, who are you?’ he asked. ‘I am *Yeshua*, and you are persecuting me. 6 But get up, and go into the city, and you will be told what you have to do.’ 7 The men traveling with him stood speechless, hearing the voice but seeing no one. 8 They helped *Sha’ul* get up off the ground; but when he opened his eyes, he could see nothing. So, leading him by the hand, they brought him to *Dammesek.* 9 For three days he remained unable to see, and he neither ate nor drank. 10 There was a *talmid* in *Dammesek*, *Hananyah* by name; and in a vision the Lord said to him, ‘*Hananyah*!’ He said, ‘Here I am, Lord?’ 11 The Lord said to him, ‘Get up and go to *Straight Street*, to *Y’hudah’s* house; and ask for a man from *Tarsus* named *Sha’ul*; for he is praying, 12 and in a vision, he has seen a man named *Hananyah* coming in and placing his hands on him to restore his sight.’ 13 But *Hananyah* answered, ‘Lord, many have told me about this man, how much harm he has done to your people in *Yerushalayim*; 14 and here he has a warrant from the head *cohanim* to arrest everyone who calls on your name.’ 15 But the Lord said to him, ‘Go, because this man is my chosen instrument to carry my name to the nations, even to their kings, and to the sons of *Isra’el* as well. 16 For I myself will show him how much he will have to suffer on account of my name.

17 “So *Hananyah* left and went into the house. Placing his hands on him, he said, ‘Brother *Sha’u*l, the Lord – *Yeshua*, the one who appeared to you on the road as you were coming here – has sent me so that you may see again and be filled with the *Ruach HaKodesh*.’ 18 In that moment, something like scales fell away from *Sha’ul’s* eyes; and

he could see again. He got up and was immersed; [19] then he ate some food and regained his strength. *Sha'ul* spent some days with the *talmidim* in *Dammesek*, [20] and immediately he began proclaiming in the synagogues that *Yeshua* is the Son of God. [21] All who heard him were amazed. They asked, 'Isn't he the man who in *Yerushalayim* was trying to destroy the people who call on his name? In fact, isn't that why he came here, to arrest them and bring them back to the head *cohanin*?' [22] But *Sha'ul* was being filled with more and more power and was creating an uproar among the Jews living in *Dammesek* with his proof that *Yeshua* is the Messiah. [23] Quite some time later, the non-believing Jews gathered together and made plans to kill him; [24] but their plot became known to *Sha'ul*. They were watching the gates day and night in order to do away with him; [25] but under cover of night, his *talmidim* took him and let him down over the city wall, lowering him in a large basket.

[26] "On reaching *Yerushalayim*, he tried to join the *talmidim*; but they were all afraid of him – they didn't believe he was a *talmid*. [27] However, *Bar-Nabba* got hold of him and took him to the emissaries. He told them how *Sha'ul* had seen the Lord while traveling, that the Lord had spoken to him, and how in *Dammesek Sha'ul* had spoken out boldly in the name of *Yeshua*. [28] So he remained with them and went all over *Yerushalayim* continuing to speak out boldly in the name of the Lord. [29] He talked and debated with the Greek-speaking Jews, but they began making attempts to kill him. [30] When the brothers learned of it, they brought him down to *Caesarea* and sent him away to *Tarsus*. [31] Then the Messianic Community throughout *Y'hudah*, the *Galil* and *Shomron* enjoyed peace and was built up. They lived in the fear of the Lord with the counsel of the *Ruach HaKodesh*; and their numbers kept multiplying.

[32] "As *Kefa* traveled around the countryside, he came down to the believers in *Lud*. [33] There he found a man named *Aeneas* who had lain bedridden for eight years, because he was paralyzed. [34] *Kefa* said to him, '*Aeneas*! *Yeshua* the Messiah is healing you! Get up and make your bed!' [35] Everyone living in *Lud* and *Sharon* saw him, and they turned to the Lord. Now in *Yafo* there was a *talmidah* named *Tavita* [36] (which means 'gazelle'); she was always doing *tzedakah* and other good deeds. [37] It happened that just at that time she took sick and died. After washing her, they laid her in a room upstairs. [38] *Lud* is near *Yafo*, and the *talmidim* had heard that *Kefa* was there, so they sent two men to him and urged him 'Please come to us without delay.' [39] *Kefa* got up and went with them. When he arrived, they led him into the upstairs room. All the widows stood by him, sobbing, and showing all the dresses and coats *Tavita* had made them while she was still with them. [40] But *Kefa* put them all outside, kneeled down and prayed. Then, turning to the body, he said, '*Tavita*! Get up!' She opened her eyes; and on seeing *Kefa*, she sat up. [41] He offered her his hand and helped her to her feet; then, calling the believers and the widows, he presented her to them alive. [42] This became known all over *Yafo*, and many people put their trust in the Lord. [43] *Kefa* stayed on in *Yafo* for some time with a man named *Shim'on*, a leather tanner. [3 (page 1572-1574)]

Acts [10:40] "but God raised him up on the third day and let him be seen." [3 (page 1575)]

Acts [15:4] "On arrival in *Yerushalayim*, they were welcomed by the Messianic community, including the emissaries and the elders; and they reported what God had done through them. [5] But some of those who had come to trust were from the party of the *P'rushim*;

and they stood up and said, 'It is necessary to circumcise them and direct them to observe the *Torah* of *Moshe*.'" [3 (page 1582)]

Acts [15:27] "So we have sent *Y'hudah* and *Sila*, and they will confirm in person what we are writing. [28] For it seemed good to the *Ruach Hakodesh* and to us not to lay any heavier burden on you than the following requirements: [29] to abstain from what has been sacrificed to idols, from blood, from things strangled, and from fornication. If you keep yourselves from these, you will be doing the right thing. Shalom!" [3 (page 1584)]

Acts [20:7] "On *Motza'ei-Shabbat*, when we were gathered to break bread, *Sha'ul* addressed them." [3 (page 1591)]

Amos [9:11] "'When that day comes, I will raise up the fallen *sukkah* of David. I will close up its gaps, raise up its ruins and rebuild it as it used to be, [12] so that *Isra'el* can possess what is left of *Edom* and of all the nations bearing my name.' says *ADONAI*, who is doing this." [3 (page 827)]

Divrei-Hayamim Bet (2 Chronicles) [20:7] "You, our God, drove out those living in the land ahead of your people *Isra'el* and gave it forever to the descendants of *Avraham, your* friend." [3 (page 1355)]

1 Corinthians [4:17] "This is why I have sent you Timothy, my beloved and trustworthy child in the Lord. He will remind you of the way of life I follow in union with the Messiah *Yeshua* and teach everywhere in every congregation." [3 (page 1636)]

1 Corinthians [5:1] "It is actually being reported that there is sexual sin among you, and it is sexual sin of a kind that is condemned even by pagans – a man is living with his stepmother!" [3 (page 1636)]

1 Corinthians [6:18] "Run from sexual immorality! Every other sin a person commits is outside the body, but the fornicator sins against his own body. [19] Or don't you know that your body is a temple for *Ruach HaKodesh* who lives inside you, whom you receive from God? The fact is you don't belong to yourselves; [20] for you were bought at a price. So, use your bodies to glorify God." [3 (page 1638)]

1 Corinthians [9:19] "For although I am a free man, not bound to do anyone's bidding. I have made myself a slave to all in order to win as many people as possible. [20] That is, with Jews, what I did was put myself in the position of a Jew, in order to win Jews. With people in subjection to a legalistic perversion of the *Torah*, I put myself in the position of someone under such legalism, in order to win those under this legalism, even though I myself am not in subjection to a legalistic perversion of the *Torah*. [21] With those who live outside the framework of *Torah*, I put myself in the position of someone outside the *Torah* in order to win those outside the *Torah* – although I myself am not outside the framework of God's *Torah*, but within the framework of *Torah* as upheld by the Messiah. [22] With the 'weak' I became 'weak', in order to win the 'weak.' With all kinds of people, I have become all kinds of things, so that in all kinds of circumstances I might save at least some of them. [23] But I do it all because of the rewards promised by the Good News, so that I may share in them along with the others who come to trust." [3 (page 1642)]

1 Corinthians 15:3 "For among the first things I passed on to you was what I also received, namely this: the Messiah died for our sins, in accordance with what the *Tanakh* says; 4 and he was buried; and he was raised on the third day, in accordance with what the *Tanakh* says; 5 and he was seen by *Kefa*, then by the *Twelve*; 6 and afterwards he was seen by more than five hundred brothers at one time, the majority of whom are still alive, though some have died. 7 Later he was seen by *Ya'akov* then by all the emissaries; 8 and last of all he was seen by me, even though I was born at the wrong time. 9 For I am the least of all the emissaries, unfit to be called an emissary, because I persecuted the Messianic Community of God." [3 (page 1649)]

1 Corinthians 16:2 "Every week, on *Motza'ei-Shabbat*, each of you should set some money aside, according to his resources, and save it up; so that when I come, I won't have to do fundraising." [3 (page 1652)]

1 Corinthians 16:10 "If Timothy comes, see that he has nothing to be afraid of while he is with you; for he is doing the Lord's work, just as I am. 11 So let no one treat him with disrespect. Help him on his way in peace, so that he will return to me, for the brothers and I are expecting him." [3 (page 1652)]

D'varim (***Deuteronomy***) 4:2 "In order to obey the *mitzvot* of *ADONAI* your God which I am giving you, do not add to what I am saying, and do not subtract from it." [3 (page 230)]

D'varim (***Deuteronomy***) 5:19(22) "These words *ADONAI* spoke to your entire gathering at the mountain from fire, cloud, and thick mist, in a loud voice; then it ceased. But he wrote them on two stone tablets, which he gave to me. 20(23) When you heard the voice coming out of the darkness, as the mountain blazed with fire, you came to me, all the heads of your tribes and your leaders, 21(24) and said, 'Here, *ADONAI* our God has shown us his glory and his greatness! We have heard his voice coming from the fire, and we have seen today that God does speak with human beings, and they stay alive." [3 (page 233)]

D'varim (***Deuteronomy***) 6:4 "*Sh'ma, Yisra'el*! *ADONAI Eloheinu*, *ADONAI echad* (Hear *Isra'el*! *ADONAI* our God, *ADONAI* is one); 5 and you are to love *ADONAI* your God with all your heart, all your being and all your resources. 6 These words, which I am ordering you today, are to be on your heart; 7 and you are to teach them carefully to your children. You are to talk about them when you sit at home, when you are traveling on the road, when you lie down and when you get up. 8 Tie them on your hand as a sign, put them at the front of a headband around your forehead, 9 and write them on the doorframes of your house and on your gates." [3 (page 235)]

D'varim (***Deuteronomy***) 7:15 "*ADONAI* will remove all illness from you – he will not afflict you with any of Egypt's dreadful diseases, which you have known; instead, he will lay them on those who hate you.!" [3 (page 237)]

D'varim (***Deuteronomy***) 12:29 "When *ADONAI* your God has cut off ahead of you the nations you are entering in order to dispossess, and when you have dispossessed them and are living in their land, 30 be careful, after they have been destroyed ahead of you, not to be trapped into following them; so that you inquire after their gods and ask, 'How did these nations serve their gods? I want to do the same.' 31 You must not do this to *ADONAI* your God! For they have done to their gods all the abominations that *ADONAI* hated!

They even burn up their sons and daughters in the fires for their gods. [13:1 (12:32)] Everything I am commanding you; you are to take care to do. Do not add to it or subtract from it. [3 (page 245)]

Ephesians [2:11] "Therefore, remember your former state: you Gentiles by birth – called the Uncircumcised by those who, merely because of an operation on their flesh, are called Circumcised – [12] at that time had no Messiah. You were estranged from the national life of *Isra'el*. You were foreigners to the covenants embodying God's promise. You were in this world without hope and without God." [3 (page 1681)]

Ephesians [5:18] "Don't get drunk with wine, because it makes you lose control. Instead, keep on being filled with Spirit – [19] sing psalms, hymns, and spiritual songs to each other; sing to the Lord and make music in your heart to him; [20] always give thanks for everything to God the Father in the name of our Lord *Yeshua* the Messiah." [3 (page 1685)]

***Sh'mot* (*Exodus*)** [6:6] "Therefore, say to the people of *Isra'el*: 'I am *ADONAI*, I will free you from the forced labor of the Egyptians, rescue you from their oppression, and redeem you with an outstretched arm and with great judgements. [7] I will take you as my people, and I will be your God. Then you will know that I am *ADONAI* your God, who freed you from the forced labor of the Egyptians." [3 (page 77)]

***Sh'mot* (*Exodus*)** [15:18] "*ADONAI* will reign forever and ever." [3 (page 92)]

***Sh'mot* (*Exodus*)** [19:18] "*Mount Sinai* was enveloped in smoke, because *ADONAI* descended onto it in fire – its smoke went up like the smoke from a furnace, and the whole mountain shook violently. [19] As the sound of the *shofar* grew louder and louder, *Moshe* spoke, and God answered him with a voice." [3 (page 98)]

***Sh'mot* (*Exodus*)** [32:9] "*ADONAI* continued speaking to *Moshe*: 'I have been watching these people; and you can see how stiff-necked they are." [3 (page 115)]

***Sh'mot* (*Exodus*)** [33:3] "'You will go to a land flowing with milk and honey; but I myself will not go with you, because you are such a stiff-necked people that I might destroy you on the way.' [4] When the people heard this bad news, they went into mourning; and no one wore his ornaments. [5] *ADONAI* said to *Moshe*, 'Tell the people of *Isra'el*, 'You are a stiff-necked people! If I were to go up with you for even one moment, I would exterminate you! Now, keep your ornaments off; then I will decide what to do to you.'" [3 (page 116)]

***Yechezk'el* (*Ezekiel*)** [20:34] "I will bring you out from the peoples and gather you out of the countries where you were scattered, with a mighty hand, with a stretched-out arm and with poured-out fury; [35] then I will bring you into the desert of the peoples and judge you face to face." [3 (page 738)]

***Yechezk'el* (*Ezekiel*)** [20:41] "'I will accept you with your sweet aroma when I bring you out from the peoples and gather you out of the countries where you were scattered; and through you I will manifest my holiness in the sight of the nations.'" [3 (page 738)]

***Yechezk'el* (*Ezekiel*)** [37:27] "My home will be with them; I will be their God, and they will be my people." [3 (page 770)]

Galatians [1:15] "But when God, who picked me out before I was born and called me by his grace, chose [16] to reveal his Son to me, so that I might announce him to the Gentiles, I did not consult anyone; [17] and I did not go up to *Yerushalayim* to see those who were emissaries before me. Instead, I immediately went off to Arabia and afterwards returned to *Dammesek.* [18] Not until three years later did I go up to *Yerushalayim* to make *Kefa's* acquaintance, and I stayed with him for two weeks, [19] but I did not see any of the other emissaries except *Ya'akov* the Lord's brother. [20] (Concerning these matters, I am writing you about, I declare before God that I am not lying!)" [3 (page 1670)]

Galatians [2:2] "I went up in obedience to a revelation, and I explained to them the Good News as I proclaim it among the Gentiles – but privately, to the acknowledged leaders. I did this out of concern that my current or previous work might have been in vain. [3] But they didn't force my Gentile companion Titus to undergo *b'rit-milah.* [4] Indeed, the question came up only because some men who pretended to be brothers had been sneaked in – they came in surreptitiously to spy out the freedom we have in the Messiah *Yeshua*, so that they might enslave us." [3 (page 1670)]

Galatians [2:11] "Furthermore, when *Kefa* came to *Antioch*, I opposed him publicly, because he was clearly in the wrong. [12] For prior to the arrival of certain people from [the community headed by] *Ya'akov*, he had been eating with the Gentile believers; but when they came, he withdrew and separated himself, because he was afraid of the faction who favored circumcising Gentile believers. [13] And the other Jewish believers became hypocrites along with him, so that even *BarNabba* was led astray by their hypocrisy." [3 (page 1671)]

Galatians [3:8] "Also the *Tanakh* foreseeing that God would consider the Gentiles righteous when they live by trusting and being faithful, told the Good News to *Avraham* in advance by saying, '**In connection with you, all the nations will be blessed.**' [9] So then those who rely on trusting and being faithful are blessed along with *Avraham*, who trusted and was faithful." [3 (page 1672)]

Galatians [6:2] "Bear one another's burdens – in this way you will be fulfilling the *Torah's* true meaning which the Messiah upholds. [3] For if anyone thinks he is something when he is really nothing, he is fooling himself. [4] So let each of you scrutinize his owns actions. Then if you do find something to boast about, at least the boasting will be based on what you have actually done and not merely on a judgement that you are better than someone else; [5] for each person will carry his own load." [3 (page 1677)]

***B'resheet* (*Genesis*)** [9:5] "I will certainly demand an accounting for the blood of your lives: I will demand it from every animal and from every human being. I will demand from every human being an accounting for the life of his fellow human being. [6] Whoever sheds human blood, by a human being will his own blood be shed; for God made human beings in his image. [7] And you people, be fruitful, multiply, swarm on the earth and multiply on it." [3 (page 13)]

***B'resheet* (*Genesis*)** [12:7] "*ADONAI* appeared to *Avram* and said, 'To your descendants (Heb. *l'zer'akhal* 'to your seed') I will give this land.' So, he built an altar there to *ADONAI*, who had appeared to him." [3 (page 16)]

***B'resheet* (*Genesis*)** 13:15 "All the land you see I will give to you and your descendants (Heb. *'ul'zer'akhal* 'and to your seed') forever,"[3 (page 18)]

***B'resheet* (*Genesis*)** 15:6 "He believed in *ADONAI*, and he (God) credited it to him as righteousness."[3 (page 19)]

***B'resheet* (*Genesis*)** 17:7 "I am establishing my covenant between me and you, along with your descendants after you, generation after generation, as an everlasting covenant, to be God for you and for your descendants after you."[3 (page 22)]

***B'resheet* (*Genesis*)** 24:7 "*ADONAI*, the God of heaven – who took me away from my father's house and away from the land I was born in, who spoke to me and swore to me, 'I will give this land to your descendants' – he will send his angel ahead of you; and you are to bring a wife for my son from there.'"[3 (page 31)]

***Yesha'yahu* (*Isaiah*)** 29:13 "Then *Adonai* said: 'Because these people approach me with empty words, and the honor they bestow on me is mere lip-service; while in fact they have distanced their hearts from me, and their 'fear of me' is just a *mitzvah* of human origin – '"[3 (page 533)]

***Yesha'yahu* (*Isaiah*)** 41:8 "'But you, *Isra'el*, my servant; *Ya'akov*, whom I have chosen, descendants of *Avraham*, my friend, 9 I have taken you from the ends of the earth, summoned you from its most distant parts and said to you, 'You are my servant' – I have chosen you, not rejected you."[3 (page 554)]

***Yesha'yahu* (*Isaiah*)** 43:6 "I will say to the north, 'Give them up!' and to the south, 'Don't hold them back! Bring my sons from far away, and my daughters from the ends of the earth, 7 everyone who bears my name, whom I created for my glory – I formed him, yes, I made him.'"[3 (page 559)]

***Yesha'yahu* (*Isaiah*)** 45:23 "'In the name of myself I have sworn, from my mouth has rightly gone out, a word that will not return – that to me every knee will bow, and every tongue will swear 24 about me that only in *ADONAI* are justice and strength.'"[3 (page 566)]

***Yesha'yahu* (*Isaiah*)** 52:11 "Leave! Leave! Get out of there! Don't touch anything unclean! Get out from inside it, and be clean, you who carry *ADONAI'S* Temple equipment."[3 (page 578)]

***Yesha'yahu* (*Isaiah*)** 53:7 "Though mistreated, he was submissive – he did not open his mouth. Like a lamb led to be slaughtered, like a sheep silent before its shearers, he did not open his mouth. 8 After forcible arrest and sentencing, he was taken away; and none of his generation protested his being cut off from the land of the living."[3(page 580)]

***Yesha'yahu* (*Isaiah*)** 53:12 "Therefore I will assign him a share with the great, he will divide the spoil with the mighty, for having exposed himself to death and being counted among the sinners, while actually bearing the sin of many and interceding for the offenders."[3 (page 581)]

***Yesha'yahu* (*Isaiah*)** 63:10 "However, they rebelled, they grieved his Holy Spirit; so he became their enemy and himself fought against them."[3 (page 598)]

***Yesha'yahu* (*Isaiah*)** 66:1 "'Heaven is my throne,' says *ADONAI*, 'and the earth is my footstool. What kind of house could you build for me? What sort of place could you devise for my rest? 2 Didn't I myself make all these things? This is how they all came to be,'" 3 (page 603)

Ya'akov* (*James*)** 2:12 "Keep speaking and acting like people who will be judged by a *Torah* which gives freedom. 13 For judgement will be without mercy toward one who doesn't show mercy; but mercy wins out over judgement. 14 What good is it, my brothers, if someone claims to have faith but has no actions to prove it? Is such 'faith' able to save him? 15 Suppose a brother or sister is without clothes and daily food, 16 and someone says to him, 'Shalom! Keep warm and eat hearty!' without giving him what he needs, what good does it do? 17 Thus, faith by itself unaccompanied by actions, is dead. 18 But someone will say that you have faith and I have actions. Show me this faith of yours without actions, and I will show you my faith by my actions! 19 You believe that '**God is one**? [b] Good for you! The demons believe it too – the thought makes them shudder with fear! 20 But, foolish fellow, do you want to be shown that such 'faith' apart from actions is barren? 21 Wasn't *Avraham avinu* declared righteous because of actions when he offered up his son *Yitz'chak* on the altar? 22 You see that his faith was made complete; 23 and the passage of the *Tanakh* was fulfilled which says, 'Avraham*** **had faith in God, and it was credited to his account as righteousness.**' [c] He was even called **God's friend**. [d] 24 You see that a person is declared righteous because of actions and not because of faith alone. 25 Likewise, wasn't *Rachav* the prostitute also declared righteous because of actions when she welcomed the messengers and sent them out by another route? 26 Indeed, just as the body without a spirit is dead, so to faith without actions is dead." b Deuteronomy 6:4; c Genesis 15:6; d Isaiah 41:8; 2 Chronicles 20:7. 3 (page 1753)

***Yirmeyahu* (*Jeremiah*)** 6:10 *ADONAI-Tzva'ot* says, "'To whom should I speak? Whom should I warn? Who will still listen to me? Their ears are dull, they can't pay attention. For them the word of *ADONAI* has become unattractive, an object of scorn.'" 3 (page 621)

***Yirmeyahu* (*Jeremiah*)** 9:24(25) "'The days are coming,' says *ADONAI*, 'when I will punish all those who have been circumcised in their uncircumcision – 25(26) Egypt, *Y'hudah*, *Edom*, the people of *'Amon* and *Mo 'av*, and all those living in the desert who cut the edges [of their beard]: For although all the Gentiles are uncircumcised, all the house of *Isra'el* have uncircumcised hearts.'" 3 (page 629)

***Yirmeyahu* (*Jeremiah*)** 31:30(31) "'Here, the days are coming,' says *ADONAI*, 'when I will make a new covenant with the house of *Isra'el* and with the house of *Y'hudah*. 31(32) It will not be like the covenant I made with their fathers on the day I took them by their hand and brought them out of the land of Egypt; because they, for their part, violated my covenant, even though I, for my part, was a husband to them.' Says *ADONAI*. 32(33) 'For this is the covenant I will make with the house of *Isra'el* after those days,' says *ADONAI*: 'I will put my *Torah* within them and write it on their hearts; I will be their God, and they will be my people. 33(34) No longer will any of them teach his fellow community member or his brother, 'Know *ADONAI*'; for all will know me, from the least of them to the greatest; because I will forgive their wickedness and remember their sins no more.'" 3 (page 670-671)

***Yirmeyahu* (*Jeremiah*)** 32:38 "They will be my people, and I will be their God." 3 (page 673))

***Yo'el* (*Joel*)** [3:1(2:28)] "'After this, I will pour out my Spirit on all humanity. Your sons and
daughters will prophesy, your old men will dream dreams, your young men will see
visions; [2(2:29)] and also on male and female slaves in those days I will pour out my Spirit.
[3(2:30)] I will show wonders in the sky and on earth – blood, fire, and columns of smoke.
[4(2:31)] The sun will be turned into darkness and the moon into blood before the coming of
that great and terrible Day of *ADONAI*.' [5(2:32)] At that time, whoever calls on the name of
ADONAI will be saved. For in *Mount Tziyon* and *Yerushalayim* there will be those who
escape, as *ADONAI* has promised; among the survivors will be those whom *ADONAI* has
called." [3 (page 809-810)]

***Yochanan* (*John*)** [6:4] "Now the Judean festival of *Pesach* was coming up," [3 (page 1530)]

***Yochanan* (*John*)** [16:16] "In a little while, you will see me no more; then, a little while later,
you will see me." [3 (page 1548)]

***Yochanan* (*John*)** [17:1] "After *Yeshua* had said these things, he looked up toward heaven
and said, 'Father, the time has come. Glorify your Son, so that the Son may glorify you –
[2] just as you gave him authority over all mankind, so that he might give eternal life to all
those whom you have given him. [3] And eternal life is this: to know you, the one true
God, and him whom you sent, *Yeshua* the Messiah. [4] I glorified you on earth by finishing
the work you gave me to do. [5] Now, Father, glorify me alongside yourself. Give me the
same glory I had with you before the world existed. [6] I made your name known to the
people you gave me out of the world. They were yours, you gave them to me, and they
have kept your word. [7] Now they know that everything you have given me is from you, [8]
because the words you gave me, I have given to them, and they have received them.
They have really come to know that I came from you, and they have come to trust that
you sent me. [9] I am praying for them. I am not praying for the world, but for those you
have given to me, because they are yours. [10] Indeed, all I have is yours, and all you have
is mine, and in them I have been glorified. [11] Now I am no longer in the world. They are
in the world, but I am coming to you. Holy Father, guard them by the power of your
name, which you have given to me; so that they may be one, just as we are. [12] When I
was with them, I guarded them by the power of your name, which you have given to me;
yes, I kept watch over them; and not one of them was destroyed (except the one meant for
destruction, so that the *Tanakh* might be fulfilled). [13] But now, I am coming to you; and I
say these things while I am still in the world so that they may have my joy made
complete in themselves. [14] I have given them your word, and the world hated them,
because they do not belong to the world – just as I myself do not belong to the world. [15] I
don't ask you to take them out of the world, but to protect them from the Evil One. [16]
They do not belong to the world, just as I do not belong to the world. [17] Set them apart
for holiness by means of the truth – your word is truth. [18] Just as you sent me into the
world, I have sent them into the world. [19] On their behalf I am setting myself apart for
holiness, so that they too may be set apart for holiness by means of the truth. [20] I pray not
only for these, but also for those who trust in me because of their word, [21] that they may
all be one. Just as you, Father, are united with me and I with you, I pray that they may be
united with us, so that the world may believe that you sent me. [22] The glory which you
have given to me, I have given to them; so that they may be one, just as we are one – [23] I
united with them and you with me, so that they may be completely one, and the world
thus realize that you sent me, and that you have loved them just as you have loved me. [24]

Father, I want those you have given me to be with me where I am; so that they may see my glory, which you have given me because you loved me before the creation of the world. [25] Righteous Father, the world has not known you, but I have known you, and these people have known that you sent me. [28] I made your name known to them, and I will continue to make it known; so that the love with which you have loved me may be in them, and I myself may be united with them.'" [3 (page 1548-1549)]

***Yochanan* (*John*)** [20:22] "Having said this, he breathed on them and said to them, 'Receive the *Ruach HaKodesh*! [23] If you forgive someone's sins, their sins are forgiven; if you hold them, they are held.'" [3 (page 1554)]

***1 Yochanan* (*1 John*)** 2:3 "The way we can be sure we know him (*Yeshua*) is if we are obeying his commands. [4] Anyone who says, 'I know him,' but isn't obeying his commands is a liar – the truth is not in him. [5] But if someone keeps doing what he says, then truly love for God has been brought to its goal in him. This is how we are sure that we are united with him. [6] A person who claims to be continuing in union with him ought to conduct his life the way he did." [3 (page 1771)]

***1 Yochanan* (*1 John*)** [5:3] "For loving God means obeying his commands. Moreover, his commands are not burdensome, [4] because everything which has God as its Father overcomes the world. And this is what victoriously overcomes the world: our trust. [5] Who does overcome the world if not the person who believes that *Yeshua* is the Son of God?" [3 (page 1775)]

***Vayikra* (*Leviticus*)** [3:17] "It is to be a permanent regulation through all your generations wherever you live that you will eat neither fat nor blood." [3 (page 132)]

***Vayikra* (*Leviticus*)** [9:18] "He slaughtered the ox and the ram, the peoples sacrifice as peace offerings; *Aaron's* sons brought him the blood, which he splashed against all sides of the altar, [19] and the fat of the ox and of the ram – the fat tail, the fat which covers the inner organs, the kidneys and the covering of the liver." [3 (page 139)]

***Vayikra* (*Leviticus*)** [26:11] "I will put my tabernacle among you, and I will not reject you, [12] but I will walk among you and be your God, and you will be my people." [3 (page 167)]

***Vayikra* (*Leviticus*)** [26:41] "'At that time I will be going against them, bringing them into the lands of their enemies. But if their uncircumcised hearts will grow humble, and they are paid the punishment for their misdeeds; [42] then I will remember my covenant with *Ya'akov*, also my covenant with *Yitz'chak* and my covenant with *Avraham*; and I will remember the land.'" [3 (page 168)]

Luke [1:6] "Both of them (*Z'kharyah* and *Elisheva*) were righteous before God, observing all the *mitzvot* and the ordinances of *ADONAI* blamelessly." [3 (page 1469)]

Luke [22:7] "Then came the day of *matzah*, on which the Passover lamb had to be killed. [8] *Yeshua* sent *Kefa* and *Yochanan*, instructing them, 'Go and prepare our *Seder*, so we can eat.' [9] They asked him, 'Where do you want us to prepare it?' [10] He told them, 'As you're going into the city, a man carrying a jar of water will meet you. Follow him into the house he enters, [11] and say to its owner,' 'The Rabbi says to you, where is the guest room where I am to eat the *Pesach* meal with my *talmidim*?' [12] He will show you a large room upstairs already furnished; make the preparations there.' [13] They went and found things just as *Yeshua* had told them they would be, and they prepared for the *Seder*. [14] When the time came, *Yeshua* and the emissaries reclined at the table, [15] and he said to them, 'I have really wanted so much to celebrate this *Seder* with you before I die! [16] For I tell you, it is certain that I will not celebrate it again until it is given its full meaning in the Kingdom of God.' [17] Then, taking a cup of wine, he made the *b'rakhah* and said, 'Take this and share it among yourselves. [18] For I tell you that from now on, I will not drink the 'fruit of the vine' until the Kingdom of God comes." [19] Also, taking a piece of matzah, he made the *b'rakhah*, broke it, gave it to them and said, 'This is my body, which is being given for you; do this in memory of me.' [20] He did the same with the cup after the meal, saying 'This cup is the New Covenant, ratified by my blood, which is being poured out for you.'" [3 (page 1510-1511)]

Luke [24:28] "They (*Cleopas* and *Ya'akov*) approached the village where they were going. He (*Yeshua*) made as if he were going on farther; [29] but they held him back, saying, 'Stay with us, for it's almost evening, and it's getting dark.' So, he went in to stay with them. [30] As he was reclining with them at the table, he took the *matzah*, made the *b'rakhah*, broke it and handed it to them. [31] Then their eyes were opened, and they recognized him. But he became invisible to them. [32] They said to each other, 'Didn't our hearts burn inside us as he spoke to us on the road, opening up the *Tanakh* to us.'" [3 (page 1516)]

Mal'akhi **(*Malachi*)** [3:6] "But because I, *ADONAI*, do not change, you sons of *Ya'akov* will not be destroyed." [3 (page 895)]

Mark [10:18] "*Yeshua* said to him, 'Why are you calling me good? No one is good except God! [19] You know the *mitzvot* – **Don't murder, don't commit adultery, don't steal, don't give false testimony, don't defraud, honor your father and mother…**'" [3 (page 1455)]

Mattiyahu **(*Matthew*)** [5:17] "Don't think that I have come to abolish the *Torah* or the Prophets. I have come not to abolish but to complete. [18] Yes indeed! I tell you that until heaven and earth pass away, not so much as a *yud* or a stroke will pass from the *Torah* – not until everything that must happen has happened. [19] So, whoever disobeys the least of these *mitzvot* and teaches others to do so will be called least in the Kingdom of Heaven. But whoever obeys them and so teaches will be called great in the Kingdom of Heaven." [3 (page 1390)]

B'midbar **(*Numbers*)** [11:17] "I will come down and speak with you there, and I will take some of the Spirit which rests on you and put it on them. Then they will carry the burden of the people along with you, so that you won't carry it yourself alone." [3 (page 188)]

B'midbar **(*Numbers*)** [11:29] "But *Moshe* replied, 'Are you so zealous to protect me? I wish all of *ADONAI's* people were prophets! I wish *ADONAI* would put his Spirit on all of them!" [3 (page 188)]

Philippians [2:19] "But I hope in the Lord *Yeshua* to send Timothy to you shortly, so that I too may be cheered by knowing how you are doing. [20] I have no one who compares with him, who will care so sincerely for your welfare – [21] people all put their own interests ahead of the Messiah *Yeshua's*. [22] But you know his character, that like a child with his father he slaved with me to advance the Good News." [3 (page 1690)]

***Tehillim* (*Psalms*)** [16:8] "I always set *ADONAI* before me; with him at my right hand, I can never be moved; [9] so my heart is glad, my glory rejoices, and my body too rests in safety; [10] for you will not abandon me to *Sh'ol*, you will not let your faithful one see the *Abyss*. [11] You make me know the path of life; in your presence is unbounded joy, in your right-hand eternal delight." [3 (page 911-912)]

***Tehillim* (*Psalms*)** [24:1] "By David. A psalm: The earth is *ADONAI*'s, with all that is in it, the world and those who live there;" [3 (page 922)]

***Tehillim* (*Psalms*)** [41:10(9)] "Even my close friend, on whom I relied, who shared my table, has turned against me." [3 (page 942)]

***Tehillim* (*Psalms*)** [50:12] "If I (God) were hungry, I would not tell you; for the world is mine, and everything in it." [3 (page 951)]

***Tehillim* (*Psalms*)** [51:6(4)] "Against you, you only, have I sinned and done what is evil from your perspective; so that you are right in accusing me and justified in passing sentence." [3 (page 952))]

***Tehillim* (*Psalms*)** [69:26(25)] "Let the place where they live be desolate, with no one to live in their tents, [27(26)] for persecuting someone you had already stricken, for adding to the pain of those you wounded." [3 (page 971)]

***Tehillim* (*Psalms*)** [89:12(11)] "The heavens are yours, and the earth is yours; you founded the world and everything in it." [3 (page 994)]

***Tehillim* (*Psalms*)** [93:1] "*ADONAI* is king, robed in majesty; *ADONAI* is robed, girded with strength. The world is well established; it cannot be moved." [3 (page 1000)]

***Tehillim* (*Psalms*)** [109:8] "May his days be few, may someone else take his position." [3 (page 1019)]

***Tehillim* (*Psalms*)** [110:1] "*ADONAI* says to my Lord, 'Sit at my right hand, until I make your enemies your footstool.'" [3 (page 1021)]

***Tehillim* (*Psalms*)** [143:2] "Don't bring your servant to trial, since in your sight no one alive would be considered righteous." [3 (page 1054)]

Revelation [13:8] "Everyone living on earth will worship it except those whose names are written in the *Book of Life* belonging to the *Lamb* slaughtered before the world was founded." [3 (page 1797)]

Romans [1:16] "For I am not ashamed of the Good News, since it is God's powerful means of bringing salvation to everyone who keeps on trusting, to the Jew especially, but equally to the Gentile." [3 (page 1606)]

Romans [3:4] "Heaven forbid! God would be true even if everyone were a liar! – as the *Tanakh* says, '**so that you, God, may be proved right in your words and win the verdict when you are put on trial.**'" [a Psalm 51:6(4); 3 (page 1608)]

Romans [3:31] "Does it follow that we abolish *Torah* by this trusting? Heaven forbid! On the contrary, we confirm *Torah*." [3 (page 1610)]

Romans [6:23] "For what one earns from sin is death; but eternal life is what one receives as a free gift from God, in union with the Messiah *Yeshua*, our Lord."

Romans [7:12] "So the *Torah* is holy; that is, the commandment is holy, just and good." [3 (page 1615)]

Romans [8:2] "Why? Because the *Torah* of the Spirit, which produces this life in union with Messiah *Yeshua*, has set me free from the '*torah*' of sin and death. [3] For what the *Torah* could not do by itself, because it lacked the power to make the old nature cooperate, God did by sending his own Son as a human being with a nature like our own sinful one [but without sin]." [3 (page 1616)]

Romans [10:4] "For the goal at which the *Torah* aims is the Messiah, who offers righteousness to everyone who trusts." [3 (page 1620)]

Romans [10:12] "That means that there is no difference between Jew and Gentile – *ADONAI* is the same for everyone, rich toward everyone who calls on him, [13] since **everyone who calls on the name of *ADONAI* will be delivered**." [b (b Joel 3:5(2:32) 3 (page 810) 3 (page 1621)]

Romans [11:17] "But if some of the branches were broken off and you – a wild olive – were grafted in among them and have become equal sharers in the rich root of the olive tree, [18] then don't boast as if you were better than the branches! However, if you do boast, remember that you are not supporting the root, the root is supporting you." [3 (page 1623)]

***Sh'm'uel Alef* (*1 Samuel*)** [10:6] "Then the Spirit of *ADONAI* will fall on you; you will prophesy with them and be turned into another man!" [3 (page 346)]

***Sh'm'uel Bet* (*2 Samuel*)** [7:14] "'I (*ADONAI*) will be a father for him (David), and he will be a son for me. If he does something wrong, I will punish him with a rod and blows, just as everyone gets punished; [15] nevertheless, my grace will not leave him, as I took it away from *Sha'ul*, whom I removed from before you. [16] Thus your house and your kingdom will be made secure forever before you; your throne will be set up forever.'" [3 (page 382)]

Chapter Four: Scripture References

***B'resheet* (*Genesis*)** [3:4] "The serpent said to the woman, 'It is not true that you will surely die; [5] because God knows that on the day you eat from it, your eyes will be opened, and you will be like God, knowing good and evil.'" [1 (page 7)]

Sh'mot (*Exodus*) [12:46] "It is to be eaten in one house. You are not to take any of the meat outside the house, and you are not to break any of its bones." [1 (page 88)]

Galatians [4:1] "What I am saying is that as long as the heir is a minor, he is no different from a slave, even though he is the legal owner of the estate; [2] rather, he is subject to guardians and caretakers until the time previously set by his father. [3] So it is with us – when we were 'children' we were slaves to the elemental spirits of the universe; [4] but then the appointed time arrived, God sent forth his Son. He was born from a woman, born into a culture in which legalistic perversion of the *Torah* was the norm, [5] so that he might redeem those in subjection to this legalism and thus enable us to be made God's sons. [6] Now because you are sons, God has sent forth into our hearts the Spirit of his Son, the Spirit who cries out, 'Abba!' (that is, 'Dear Father!'). [7] So through God you are no longer a slave but a son and if you are a son, you are also an heir." [1 (page 1673-1674)]

***Yesha-Yahu* (*Isaiah*)** [65:1] "'I made myself accessible to those who didn't ask for me, I let myself be found by those who didn't seek me. I said, 'Here I am! Here I am!' to a nation not called by my name. [2] I spread out my hands all day long to a rebellious people who live in a way that is not good, who follow their own inclinations; [3] a people who provoke me to my face all the time, sacrificing in gardens and burning incense on bricks. [4] They sit among the graves and spend the night in caverns; they eat pig meat, and their pots hold soup made from disgusting things.'" [1 (page 600)]

***Mattityahu* (*Matthew*)** [8:28] "When *Yeshua* arrived at the other side of the lake, in the *Gadarenes*' territory, there came out of the burial caves two men controlled by demons, so violent that no one dared travel on that road. [29] They screamed, 'What do you want with us, Son of God? Have you come here to torture us before the appointed time?' [30] Now some distance from them a large herd of pigs was feeding. [31] The demons begged him, 'If you are going to drive us out, send us into the herd of pigs.' [32] 'All right, go!' he told them. So, they came out and went into the pigs, whereupon the entire herd rushed down the hillside into the lake and drowned. [33] The swineherds fled, went off to the town and told the whole story, including what happened to the demonized men. [34] At this, the whole town came out to meet *Yeshua*. When they saw him, they begged him to leave their district." [1 (page 1399)]

Note: [8:30] A large herd of pigs. The *Gadarenes* were not Jewish and had no compunctions about raising pigs. (cf. *Mark* 5:11-17). [1 (page 1399)]

Mark [5:11] "Now there was a large herd of pigs feeding near the hill, [12] and the unclean spirits begged him (*Yeshua*), 'Send us to the pigs, so we can go into them.' *Yeshua* gave them permission. They came out and entered the pigs; and the herd, numbering around two thousand, rushed down the hillside into the lake and were drowned. [14] The swineherds fled and told it in the town and in the surrounding country, and the people went to see what had happened. [15] They came to *Yeshua* and saw the man who had had the legion of demons, sitting there, dressed and in his right mind; and they were frightened. [16] Those who had seen it told what had happened to the man controlled by demons and to the pigs; [17] and the people began begging *Yeshua* to leave their district." [1 (page 1447)]

Chapter Five: Scripture References

'Amos [6:4] "You lie on beds of ivory and lounge sprawled out on your couches, dining on meat from lambs in the flock and from calves fattened in stalls." [1 (page 823)]

***M'Lakhim Alef* (*1 Kings*)** [4:22 (5:2)] "*Shlomo's* provisions for one day consisted of 150 bushels of fine flour, 310 bushels of meal, [23 (3)] ten fattened oxen, twenty pasture-fed oxen and one hundred sheep, in addition to deer, gazelles, roebucks and fattened poultry." [1 (page 417)]

***D'varim* (*Deuteronomy*)** [23:13(12)] "Also you are to have an area outside the camp to use as a latrine. [14(12)] You must include a trowel with your equipment, and when you relieve yourself, you are to dig a hole first and afterwards cover your excrement." [1 (page 256)]

Chapter Seven: Scripture References

***B'resheet* (*Genesis*)** [1:29] "Then God said, 'Here! Throughout the whole earth I am giving you as food every seed-bearing plant and every tree with seed-bearing fruit." [1 (page 4)]

***B'resheet* (*Genesis*)** [2:16] "*ADONAI*, God, gave the person this order: 'You may freely eat from every tree in the garden [17] except the tree of the knowledge of good and evil. You are not to eat from it because on the day that you eat from it, it will become certain that you will die.'" [1 (page 6)]

***B'resheet* (*Genesis*)** [3:18] "It will produce thorns and thistles for you, and you will eat field plants." [1 (page 7)]

***B'resheet* (*Genesis*)** [9:20] "*Noach*, a farmer, was the first to plant a vineyard. [21] He drank so much of the wine that he got drunk and lay uncovered in his tent." [1 (page 14)]

***D'Varim* (*Deuteronomy*)** [8:1] "All the *mitzvot* I am giving you today you are to take care to obey, so that you will live, increase your numbers, enter, and take possession of the land *ADONAI* swore about to your ancestors. [2] You are to remember everything of the way in which *ADONAI* led you these forty years in the desert. Humbling and testing you in order to know what was in your heart – whether you would obey His *mitzvot* or not. [3] He humbled you, allowing you to be known, to make you understand that a person does not live on food alone but on everything that comes from the mouth of *ADONAI*. [4] During these forty years the clothing you were wearing didn't grow old, and your feet didn't swell up. [5] Think deeply about it: *ADONAI* Was disciplining you, just as a man disciplines his child. [6] So obey the *mitzvot* of *ADONAI* your God, living as he directs and fearing him. [7] For *ADONAI* your God is bringing you into a good land, a land with streams, springs and water welling up from the depths in valleys and on hillsides. [8] It is a land of wheat and barley, grapevines, fig trees and pomegranates; a land of olive oil and honey, [9] a land where you will eat food in abundance and lack nothing in it; a land where stones contain iron, and the hills can be mined for copper. [10] So you will eat and be satisfied, and you will bless *ADONAI* your God for the good land he has given you. [11] Be careful not to forget *ADONAI* your God by not obeying his *mitzvot*, rulings, and regulations that I am giving you today. [12] Otherwise, after you have eaten and are satisfied, built fine houses, and lived in them, [13] and increased your herds, flocks, silver, gold, and everything else you own, [14] you will become proud-hearted. Forgetting *ADONAI* your God…" [1 (page 237-238)]

***Sh'mot* (*Exodus*)** [12:8] "That night, they are to eat meat, roasted in the fire; they are to eat it with *matzah* and *maror* (bitter herbs)." [1 (page 85)]

***M'lakhim Alef* (*1 Kings*)** [19:16] "Turn your ear, *ADONAI*, and hear! Open your eyes, *ADONAI*, and see! Hear the words that *Sancheriv* sent to taunt the living God." [1 (page 472)]

Vayikra (***Leviticus***) 7:22 "*ADONAI* said to *Moshe*, [23] Say to the people of *Is'rael*, 'You are not to eat the fat of bulls, sheep, or goats. [24] The fat of animals that die of themselves or are killed by wild animals may be used for any other purpose, but under no circumstances are you to eat it. [25] For whoever eats the fat of animals of the kind used in presenting an offering made by fire to *ADONAI* will be cut off from his people. [26] You are not to eat any kind of blood, whether from birds or animals, in any of your homes. [27] Whoever eats any blood will be cut off from his people.'" [1 (page 137)]

Vayikra (***Leviticus***) 11:9 "'Of all the things that live in the water, you may eat these: anything in the water that has fins and scales, whether in the seas or in rivers – these you may eat. [10] But everything in the seas and rivers without both fins and scales, of all the small water-creatures and of all the living creatures in the water, is a detestable thing for you. [11] Yes these will be detestable for you – you are not to eat their meat, and you are to detest their carcasses. [12] Whatever lacks fins and scales in the water is a detestable thing for you." [1 (page 141)]

Vayikra (Leviticus) 23:17 "You must bring bread from your homes for waving - two loaves made with one gallon of fine flour, baked with leaven - as firstfruits for *ADONAI*." [1 (page 160)]

B'midbar (***Numbers***) 9:11 "But he will observe it in the second month on the fourteenth day at dusk. They are to eat it with *matzah* and *maror*," [1 (page 185)]

B'midbar (Numbers) 15:20 "Set aside from your first dough a cake as a gift; set it aside as you would set aside a portion of the grain from the threshing-floor. [21] From your first dough you will give *ADONAI* a portion as a gift through all your generations." [1 (page 193)]

D'varim (***Deuteronomy***) 8:7 "For *ADONAI* your God is bringing you into a good land, a land with streams, springs, and water welling up from the depths in valleys and on hillsides. [8] It is a land of wheat and barley, grapevines, fig trees and pomegranates, a land of olive oil and honey; [9] a land where you will eat food in abundance and lack nothing in it; a land where stones contain iron, and the hills can be mined for copper. [10] So you will eat and be satisfied, and you will bless *ADONAI* your God for the good land he has given you." [1 (page 237-238)]

D'varim (***Deuteronomy***) 12:21 If the place which *ADONAI* your God chooses to place his name is too far away from you; then you are to slaughter animals from your cattle or sheep, which *ADONAI* has given you; and eat on your own property, as much as you want." [1 (page 244)]

D'varim (***Deuteronomy***) 14:19 "All winged swarming creatures are unclean for you; they are not to be eaten; [20] but all clean flying creatures you may eat." [1 (page 246)]

D'varim (***Deuteronomy***) 30:15 "Look! I am presenting you today with, on the one hand, life and good; and on the other, death and evil – [16] in that I am ordering you today to love *ADONAI* your God, to follow his ways, and to obey his *mitzvot*, regulations and rulings; for if you do, you will live and increase your numbers; and *ADONAI*, your God will bless you in the land you are entering in order to take possession of it. [17] But if your heart turns away, if you refuse to listen, if you are drawn away to prostrate yourselves before other gods and serve them; [18] I am announcing to you today that you will certainly perish; you will not live long in the land you are crossing the *Yarden* to enter and possess. [19] I call on heaven and earth to witness against you today that I have presented you with life and death, the blessing, and the curse. Therefore, choose life, so that you will live, you and your descendants, [20] loving *ADONAI* your God, paying attention to what he says and clinging to him – for that is the purpose of your life! On this depends the length of time you will live in the land *ADONAI* swore he would give to your ancestors *Avraham, Yitz'chak* and *Ya'akov*." [1 (page 265)]

***D'varim* (*Deuteronomy*)** [32:13] "He made them ride on the heights of the earth. They ate the produce of the fields. He had them suck honey from the rocks and olive oil from the crags, [14] curds from the cows and milk from the sheep, with lamb fat, rams from *Bashan* and goats, with the finest wheat flour; and you drank sparkling wine from the blood of grapes." [1 (page 268)]

***Sh'mu'el Alef* (*1 Samuel*)** [17:18] "Also bring these ten cheeses to their field officer. Find out if your brothers are well and bring back some token from them." [1 (page 356)]

***Sh'mu'el Alef* (*1 Samuel*)** [25:18] "*Avigayil* wasted no time in taking 200 loaves of bread, two skins of wine, five sheep already prepared, six quarts of roasted grain, a hundred clusters of raisins and 200 fig cakes, and having them loaded on donkeys." [1 (page 266)]

***Sh'mu'el Bet* (*2 Samuel*)** [5:23] "When David consulted *ADONAI*, he said, 'Don't attack! Circle behind them and engage them opposite the balsam trees. [24] When you hear the sound of marching in the tops of the balsam trees, advance, because then *ADONAI* has gone out ahead of you to defeat the army of the *P'lishtim*.'" [1 (page 381)]

***Sh'mu'el Bet* (*2 Samuel*)** [16:1] "When David had gone a little past the summit, there was *Tziva*, the servant of *M'fivoshet*, who met him with a pair of donkeys saddled and on them 200 loaves of bread, 100 bunches of raisins, 100 pieces of summer fruit and a skin of wine." [1 (page 394)]

***M'laakhim Alef* (*1 Kings*)** [19:16] "Also anoint *Yehu* the son of *Nimshi* to be king over *Isra'el* and anoint *Elisha* the son of *Shafat* of *Avel-M'cholah* to be prophet after you." [1 (page 440)]

***Divrei- HaYamin Alef* (*1 Chronicles*)** [14:14] "David consulted God again, but God told him, 'Don't attack them! Turn away from them and engage them opposite the balsam trees. [15] When you hear the sound of marching in the tops of the balsam trees, move out, and attack; because God has gone out ahead of you to defeat the army of the *P'lishtim*." [1 (page 1318)]

***Yesha'Yahu* (*Isaiah*)** [1:8] "The daughter of *Tziyon* is left like a shack in a vineyard, like a shed in a cucumber field, like a city under siege." [1 (page 484)]

***Yesha'Yahu* (*Isaiah*)** [38:21] "Then *Yesha'yahu* said, 'Have them take a fig plaster and apply it to the inflammation, and he will recover.'" [1 (page 548)]

***Yechezk'el* (*Ezekiel*)** [4:9] "Take wheat, barley, beans, lentils, millet and buckwheat; put them together in one bowl; and make bread from it. For as long as you lie on your side, 390 days, this is what you are to eat. [10] Each day the food you eat must weigh only three-quarters of a pound; you may eat it from time to time [during the day]. [11] You are to drink a limited amount of water, two-thirds of a quart; you may drink it from time to time [during the day]. [12] [The bread] you eat is to be baked like barley cakes; you are to bake it before their eyes, using human dung as fuel." [1 (page 717)]

***Tehillim* (*Psalm*)** [92:13 (12)] "The righteous will flourish like a palm tree; they will grow like a cedar in the *L'vanan*." [1 (page 999)]

***Mishlei* (*Proverbs*)** [18:21] "The tongue has power over life and death; those who indulge it must eat its fruit." [1 (page 1092)]

***Mishlei* (*Proverbs*)** [30:32] "If you have been boorish, exalting yourself, or if you have been scheming, lay your hand on your mouth." [1 (page 1115)]

***Shir-Hashirim* (*Song of Songs*)** [2:5] "Sustain me with raisins, refresh me with apples, for I am sick with love." [1 (page 1180)]

***Shir-Hashirim* (*Song of Songs*)** [5:13] "His cheeks are like a bed of spices, like banks of fragrant herbs. His lips are like lilies dripping with sweet myrrh." [1 (page 1184)]

***Shir-Hashirim* (*Song of Songs*)** [8:5] "Who is this coming up from the desert, leaning on her darling? I awakened you under the apple tree. It was there that your mother conceived you; there she who bore you conceived." [1 (page 1187)]

***Mattityahu* (*Matthew*)** [14:13] "On hearing about this, *Yeshua* left in a boat to be by himself in the wilderness. But the people learned of it and followed him from the towns by land.
[14] So when he came ashore, he saw a huge crowd; and, filled with compassion for them, he healed those of them who were sick. As evening approached, the *talmidim* came to him and said, 'This is a remote place and it's getting late. Send the crowds away, so that they can go and buy food for themselves in the villages!' [17] 'All we have with us,' they said, 'is five loaves of bread and two fish.' [18] He said, 'Bring them here to me.' [19] After instructing the crowds to sit down on the grass, he took the five loaves and the two fish and, looking up toward heaven, made a *b'rakhah*. Then he broke the loaves and gave them to the *talmidim*, who gave them to the crowds. [20] They all ate as much as they wanted, and they took up twelve baskets full of the pieces left over. [21] Those eating numbered about five thousand men, plus women and children." [1 (page 1413-1414)]

***Mattityahu* (*Matthew*)** [23:37] "Woe to you hypocritical *Torah*-teachers and *P'rushim*! You clean the outside of the cup and the dish, but inside they are full of robbery and self-indulgence." [1 (page 1426)]

Luke [6:1] "One Shabbat, while *Yeshua* was passing through some wheat fields, his *talmidim* began plucking the heads of grain, rubbing them between their hands and eating the seeds." [1 (page 1482)]

***Yochanan* (*John*)** [19:28] "After this, knowing that all things had accomplished their purpose, *Yeshua*, in order to fulfill the words of the *Tanakh*, said, 'I'm thirsty.' [29] A jar full of cheap sour wine was there, so they soaked a sponge in the wine, coated it with oregano leaves and held it up to his mouth. [30] After *Yeshua* had taken the wine, he said, 'It is accomplished!' And, letting his head droop, he delivered up his spirit." [1 (page 1553)]

1 Timothy [5:23] "Stop drinking water; instead, use a little wine for the sake of your digestion and because of your frequent illnesses." [1 (page 1714]

END NOTES

ABSTRACT – END NOTES

1 Stern, David H. *The Complete Jewish Study Bible, Insights for Jews and Christians, Illuminating the Jewishness of God's Word.* Hendrickson Publishers, Peabody, MA 2016

2 Sharps, Jim. *Concepts of Ordiginal Medicine*, Copyright IIOM, Revised November 2006

3 DeHaan, Roger L. *Restoring the Creation Mandate*, Huntsville, AL: Milestone International Publishers, 2007

CHAPTER ONE – END NOTES

1 Joseph Lumpkin, *Book of Jubilees, The Apocrypha: Including Books from the Ethiopic Bible,* Fifth Estate Publishers, PO Box 116, Blountsville, AL 35031, copyright 2009

2 David H Stern. *The Complete Jewish Study Bible, Insights for Jews and Christians, Illuminaing the Jewishness of God's Word.* Hendrickson Publishers, Peabody, MA 2016

3 *Life Application Study Bible, NIV.* Tyndale House Publishers, Inc. 1820 Jet Stream Drive, Colorado Springs, CO 80921-3696. Revised August 1983

4 *The System Bible Study or The Busy People's Bible.* The System Bible Company, Chicago, IL, 1922

5 Jim Sharps. *Concepts of Original Medicine*, Copyright IIOM, Revised November 2006

6 S. I. McMillen. *None of These Diseases.* Fleming H. Revell Company, in Westwood, NJ., MCMLXIII

Prothrombin: "a protein made by the liver – helps blood to clot." (Page 22)

7 "So Will I (100 Billion X), Word and Music by Joel Houston, Benjamin Hastings, & Michael Fatkin, 2017 Hillsong Music Publishing CCLL: 7084123

https://www.youtube.com/watch?v=GfVd5x9W1Xc

8 J. Jasher *The Book of Jasher*, AncientWisdomBooks.com, 2020

9 Michelle M. Karten, MD. *Kids Health from Nemours – Why Do Newborns Need a Vitamin K Shot?* April 2018, https://kidshealth.org/en/parents/vitamin-k-shot.prt-en-html

CHAPTER TWO – END NOTES

[1] Michael J. Rood, *The Chronological Gospels, The Acceptable Year of the LORD. The Life and Seventy Week Ministry of the Messiah.* Aviv Moon Publishing, Fort Mill, SC 2013

[2] David H. Stern. *The Complete Jewish Study Bible, Insights for Jews and Christians, Illuminating the Jewishness of God's Word.* Hendrickson Publishers, Peabody, MA 2016

Note: *Matthew* 11:13,14 "This does not suggest that *Yochanan* was *Eliyahu* (*Elijah*) reincarnated. On the contrary, *Hebrews* 9:27 specifically teaches that reincarnation does not occur; and when asked, *Yochanan* himself denies that he is *Eliyahu* (*John* 1:21). Rather, he comes in the spirit of *Eliyahu* and precedes the Messiah's first coming in the same way that another *Eliyahu*-like figure is to precede his second coming. *Yeshua* affirms this understanding in *Matthew* 17:11-12." [2 (page 1405)]

[3] Shawn Brasseaux. *Why Is Jesus Christ Called "The Word of God?",* https://forwhatsaiththescriptures.org' 4/23/2018 Christian Ambassador (Shawn Brasseaux)

[4] Nehemia Gordon. *The Hebrew Yeshua vs. The Greek Jesus*, Hilkiah Press, 2006. www.NehemiasWall.com.

[5] R.C. Sproul, "*What Does the Word "Gospel" Mean in the New Testament*?" November 30, 2020. (Blog/Teacher/Rc-Sproul)

CHAPTER THREE – END NOTES

1 Brad H. Young. *Jesus the Jewish Theologian.* Baker Academic, a division of Baker Publishing Group, Grand Rapids, MI

2 Michael J. Rood. *The Chronological Gospel, The Acceptable Year of the LORD. The Life and Seventy Week Ministry of the Messiah.* Aviv Moon Publishing, Fort Mill, SC, 2013

3 David H. Stern, *The Complete Jewish Study Bible, Insights for Jews and Christians.* Messianic Jewish Publishers and Resources. 2016 by Hendrickson Publishers Marketing, LLC, P.O. Box 3473, Peabody, MA 01961-3473

[4] *Chronology – From the Crucifixion in 30 AD to the Destruction of Jerusalem in 70 AD* (all years are reckoned AD). www.churchathome.org/day-jesus-died/pdf/chronology%20v.pdf

[5] Perry Stone. *The Meal That Heals.* Charisma House – A Strang Company, 600 Rinehart Road, Lake Mary, FL 32746. www.charismaHouse.com, copyright 2008

[6] Dr. Miles R. Jones, *The Epistle of James (Ya'akov) – A Translation from the Hebrew.* Little Team Jones Report, 18, July 2021. Copyright 2021. Published by B'nai Emunah Institute for Accelerated Learning. www.writingofgod.com; administrator@jonesgeniuses.com

[7] Brad H. Young. *Paul the Jewish Theologian.* Baker Publishing Group, P.O. Box 6287, Grand Rapids, MI 49516-6287, Copyright 1997, ISBN. 978-0-8010-4821-0

[8] Bishop J.L Payne, BS. DD. PhD. *God's Health and Natural Healing, Biblical and Dietary Laws, Volume One and Two*, http://churchhousepublisher.com; 426 West Silas Brown Street, Jackson, MI 39204. Copyright 2007. ISBN 978-0-9800202-0-5

[9] Mike Gascoigne. *Chronology of the Early Church.* Anno Mundl Books. www.annomundl.com/bible/chronology-of-the-early-church. Copyright 1997

[10] Rabbi Gavriel. Messiahyeshua.blogspot

[11] Daniel Leonard Harris. *God Cares What You Eat – Dietary Laws of the Bible.* Columbia, SC. Made in USA, Copyright 2019. 22, April 2020. ISBN 93652979R00045

CHAPTER FOUR – END NOTES

1 David H. Stern, *The Complete Jewish Study Bible, Insights for Jews and Christians.* Peabody, MA. (Hendrickson Publishers Marketing, LLC, Copyright 2016)

2 Daniel Leonard Harris. *God Cares What You Eat – Dietary Laws of the Bible.* Columbia, SC (Daniel Leonard Harris, Copyright 2019. ISBN 13:978 1792 169175)

3 Bishop J. L. Payne, *God's Health, Natural Healing, Biblical and Dietary Law. Perspective on Health, Healing Living Volume One and Two.*
Jackson Mississippi, 2007. (God's Health and Natural Healing, Copyright 2007).

4 "What the Bible Says About Boiling a Kid in its Mother's Milk", (Church of the Great God, Copyright 1992-2022).
www.bibletools.org/index.cfm/fuseaction/topical.show/RTD/CGG/ID/9313/Boiling-Kid-its-mothers-milk.htm.

5 Rex Russell, M.D. *What the Bible Says About Healthy Living.* Grand Rapids, MI, (Baker Publishing, Copyright 2014)

6 "Do Not Boil a Young Goat in its Mother's Milk. Another Possibility". Christy Jordan.
(https://seekingscripture.com/do-not-boil-a-young-goat-in-its-mothers-milk-another-possibility , Copyright 2022)

7 Betty Reams Hernandez. *RBTI and Foods-Eating By the Numbers – The Bible on Foods, Module 6.* (IIOM/RBTI)

CHAPTER FIVE – END NOTES

1 David H. Stern, *The Complete Jewish Study Bible, Insights for Jews and Christians.* (Peabody, MA. Hendrickson Publishers Marketing, LLC, Copyright 2016)

2 "*Diet, Hygiene, Quarantine, and Hell to Pay*" Topic #01004. www.GodSaidManSaid.com

3 "*Revelation 18:23-Discover Babylon's Deception by Pharmakeia/Sorcery.*" https://revelationscriptures/revelation-18-23-babylons-pharmakeia

4 *What Is a Retrovirus?* Healthline, medically reviewed by Vincent J. Tavelle et al. March 1, 2019. https://www.healthline.com/health/what-is-a-retrovirus
5 "*The Coronavirus: You Won't Believe It!*" Topic 00991. www.GodSaidManSaid.com
6 Michael Rood. "*These Things Are Unclean to You.*". DVD (Fort Mill, SC 29716 copyright 2020). www.aroodawakening.tv. 1- 866-766-3610
7 Rex Russell, *What the Bible Says About Healthy Living.* (Grand Rapids, MI. Revell a division of Baker Publishing Group. Copyright 2006).
8 Judy Mikovits, Kent Heckenlively. *Plague of Corruption.* (New York, NY. Skyhorse Publishing, copyright 2020)
9 "*Petroleum in Real Life: Pills*". Agnes Zalewski http://context.capp.ca/article/2019/feature-petroleum-in-real-life-pills
10 Francisco Contreras, *Health in the 21st Century – Will Doctors Survive?.* (Chula Vista, CA. Interpacific Press, copyright February 1997)
11 Susan M. Turley. Understanding Pharmacology for Health Professionals. Third Edition. (Upper Saddle River, New Jersey. Pearson Education, Inc., copyright 2003)
12 Julie Von Vett and Bruce Malone. *Inspired Evidence Only One Reality.* (Midland, MI., Search for the Truth Publications. Copyright 2011.)
13 Richard Brouse. Build a Better You. (Portland, OR. Dr. Richard Brouse, copyright 2011)
14 *Merck Manual of Medical Information.* Robert Berkow, M.D. et al. Whitehouse Station, NJ, Merck Research Laboratories, copyright 1997)

CHAPTER SIX: END NOTES

1 Stern, David H. *The Complete Jewish Study Bible, Insights for Jews and Christians, Illuminating the Jewishness of God's Word.* Hendrickson Publishers, Peabody, MA 2016
2 Brennan, Barbara Ann. *Hands of Light-A Guide to Healing Through the Human Energy Field.* Bantam Books, a division of Random House, Inc. New York, NY. Copyright 1987.
3 Reams Hernandez, Betty. *Book One: In His Footsteps: My Life with Carey Reams.* Third Printing, Published by Daily Manufacturing, Inc. 4920 Pless Rd., Rockwell, NC 28138, Copyright 2017, www.dailymfg.com.
4 Reams, Carey A., Dudley, Cliff. *Choose Life or Death.* Self-Published
5 Tennant, Jerry *Healing is Voltage-Healing Eye Disease*, Jerry Tennant, Middleton, DE., copyright 2011.
6 Beddoe, Alexander F., *Biological Ionization as Applied to Human Nutrition.* Advanced Ideals Institute, eBook, c/o P.O. Box 23709, Santa Barbara, CA 93121. Copyright 1984-2008. ISBN 978-0-9763669-7-3.
7 Guralnik, David B., General Editor. *Webster's New World Dictionary of the American Language*. The World Publishing Co., The South Western Company, Nashville, TB. Copyright 1963.

8 *The Winston Dictionary College Edition.* The John C. Winston Company. Copyright 1946.
9 Whitney, Eleanor Noss; Hamilton, Eva May Nunnelley; Rolfes, Sharon Rady. *Understanding Nutrition: Fifth Edition.* West Publishing Company, 50 W. Kellogg Blvd., St. Paul, MN 55164-1003, Copyright 1990. ISBN 0-314-57831-5

10 Julie Von Vett and Bruce Malone. *Inspired Evidence Only One Reality.* (Midland, MI., Search for the Truth Publications. Copyright 2011.)

CHAPTER SEVEN - END NOTES

1 David H. Stern, *The Complete Jewish Study Bible, Insights for Jews and Christians*. (Peabody, MA. Hendrickson Publishers Marketing, LLC, Copyright 2016)
2 Ellen G. White, *Counsels on Diet and Food.* (Herald Publishing Association. The Ellen G. White Publications, USA. Copyright 1938, 1946, 1976, 2001)
3 Don Colbert, M.D., *What Would Jesus Eat?* (Thomas Nelson, Inc. Copyright 2002)
4 Sue Becker, *The Essential Home – Ground Flour Book.* Robert Rose, Inc., Copyright 2016)

5 D. C. Jarvis, M.D., *Folk Medicine*. (Fawcett Crest Books. Copyright 1958.)

CONCLUSION AND SUMMARY - END NOTES:

1 Burgess, Stuart. *The Design and Origin of Man.* Day One Publications. Ryelands Road, Leominster, HR6 8NZ. 2004. www.dayone.co.uk
2 Sharps, Jim. *Concepts of Original Medicine*, Copyright IIOM, Revised November 2006.

GLOSSARY OF HEBREW TERMS AND WORDS - END NOTES:

1 David Stern. *The Complete Jewish Study Bible, Insight for Jews and Christians Illuminating the Jewishness of God's Word.* Hendrickson Publishers, Peabody, MA. Copyright © 2016

2 Nehemia Gordon. *The Hebrew Yeshua vs The Greek Jesus*. Hilkiah Press, Copyright © 2006, (www.HilkiahPress.com)

3 Nehemia Gordon. "The Hebrew Yeshua vs The Greek Jesus, Live Video Teaching". DVD 8907638452, Hilkiah Press, (www.HilkiahPress.com)

4 Roger L. DeHaan. *Restoring the Creation Mandate*, Huntsville, AL: Milestone International Publishers. Copyright © 2007

[5] Daniel Leonard Harris. *God Cares What You Eat – Dietary Laws of the Bible*. Daniel Leonard Harris, Columbia, SC. Copyright © 2019

[6] Nehemia Gordon, *The Naming of Jesus in Hebrew Matthew*, Makor Hebrew Foundation, 2008 (www.HilkiahPress.com)

[7] Sharonne Cohen. *What Is An Eruv?* My Jewish Learning. https://www.myjewishlearning.com/article/eruv/. January 9, 2022.

[8] Bob Dodson. *Jewish Dress and Custom – A Study of Haluk, Tallit, Kanaf, Tzitzit, and Tefillin.* Acts 242 Study, February 8, 2013. https://acts242study.com/jewosh-dress-and- custom-a-study-of-haluk-tallit-kanaf-tzitzit-and-tfillin/

[9] Michael Rood. *The Chronological Gospels-The Acceptable Year of the Lord.* Aviv Moon Publishing, P.O. Box 1559, Fort Mill, SC 29716. Copyright © 2013.

RESOURCES

Websites:

Kosher approved food supplements, personal care products, cleaning products, etc. – Shaklee Corporation. www.shaklee.com; www.sutterbysolutions.com.

Education: International Institute of Original Medicine. Various certifications and degrees in RBTI, Original Medicine, Nutrition and Medical Ministry available. www.iiomonline.org.

Azure Standard: Family-owned source for organic and non-GMO foods and products. www.azurestandard.com.

Bread Beckers: Whole grains, cooking and baking supplies, and equipment. www.breadkbeackers.com

Cookbooks:

The Essential Home-Ground Flour Book by Sue Becker, copyright © 2016, ISBN 978-0-7788-0534-2

The What Would Jesus Eat Cook Book by Don Colbert, M.D., copyright © 2002, ISBN 0-7852-6519-8

What The Bible Says About Healthy Living Cookbook by Hope Egan & Amy Cataldo, copyright © 2009, ISBN 979-8-9902299-3-8

Healthcare Providers Mentioned (alphabetical order):

Dr. Don Colbert (Integrative & Holistic Medicine)
Divine Health
Divinehealth.com

Oasis of Hope Hospital (Holistic & Alternative Cancer Treatment)
Dr. Francisco Contreras
OasisofHope.com

Dr.s Jim and Elisa Sharps. IIOM
International Institute of Original Medicine (Biblically based Integrative Health)
iiomonline.org

Cheryl Sutterby, DNOM, Original Medicine Health Professional, RBTI, Kosher approved supplements and products. www.cherylsutterbydnom.com , BetterHealthin31Days.com/sunnysideup;

Tennant Institute (Integrative and Functional Medicine)
Dr. Jerry Tennant
www.tennantinstitute.com

BIBLIOGRAPHY

Becker, Sue. *The Essential Home – Ground Flour Book.* Toronto, Canada. Robert Rose, Inc., Copyright © 2016

Beddoe, Alexander F., *Biological Ionization as Applied to Human Nutrition.* Advanced Ideals Institute, eBook, c/o P.O. Box 23709, Santa Barbara, CA 93121. Copyright © 1984-2008. ISBN 978-0-9763669-7-3.

Berkow, Robert., et al., *Merck Manual of Medical Information.* Whitehouse Station, NJ, Merck Research Laboratories, copyright © 1997

Brennan, Barbara Ann. *Hands of Light-A Guide to Healing Through the Human Energy Field.* Bantam Books, a division of Random House, Inc. New York, NY. Copyright © 1987.

Brasseaux, Shawn. *Why Is Jesus Christ Called "The Word of God?",* https://forwhatsaiththescriptures.org' 4/23/2018 Christian Ambassador (Shawn Brasseaux)

Brouse, Richard. *Build a Better You.* (Portland, OR. Dr. Richard Brouse, copyright © 2011)

Burgess, Stuart. *The Design and Origin of Man.* Day One Publications. Ryelands Road, Leominster, HR6 8NZ. Copyright © 2004. www.dayone.co.uk

Cavanaugh, Madison. *The One-Minute Cure-The Secret to Healing Virtually All Diseases.* Second Edition. Think Outside the Book, Inc. Publisher. Summerlin, Nevada. Copyright© 2021

Chronology – From the Crucifixion in 30 AD to the Destruction of Jerusalem in 70 AD (all years are reckoned AD). www.churchathome.org/day-jesus-died/pdf/chronology%20v.pdf

Cohen, Sharonne. *What Is an Eruv?* My Jewish Learning. https://www.myjewishlearning.com/article/eruv. January 9, 2022.

Colbert, Don. *What Would Jesus Eat?* (Thomas Nelson, Inc. Copyright © 2002)

Contreras, Francisco, *Health in the 21st Century – Will Doctors Survive?* (Chula Vista, CA. Interpacific Press, copyright © February 1997)

DeHaan, Roger L., *Restoring the Creation Mandate*, Huntsville, AL: Milestone International Publishers, copyright © 2007

Dodson, Bob. *Jewish Dress and Custom – A Study of Haluk, Tallit, Kanaf, Tzitzit, and Tefillin.* Acts 242 Study, February 8, 2013. https://acts242study.com/jewosh-dress-and-custom-a-study-of-haluk-tallit-kanaf-tzitzit-and-tfillin/cts 242 Study, February 8, 2013.

Gascoigne, Mike. *Chronology of the Early Church.* Anno Mundl Books. Copyright 1997 www.annomundl.com/bible/chronology-of-the-early-church.

Gavriel, Rabbi. Messiahyeshua.blogspot

God Said Man Said. "Black Plague Leveled by Leviticus—And Here It Is Again." Topic #: 00715, Retrieved May 4, 2021 (http://www.godsaidmansaid.org)

God Said Man Said. "Corona Virus: You Won't Believe It!" Topic #: 00991, Retrieved May 4, 2021 (http://www.godsaidmansaid.org)

God Said Man Said. "Diet, Hygiene, Quarantine, and Hell to Pay." Topic #: 01004 (http://www.godsaidmansaid.org) Retrieved May 4, 2021

God Said Man Said. "The Coronavirus: You Won't Believe It!" Topic 00991. www.GodSaidManSaid.com

Gordon, Nehemia. *The Hebrew Yeshua vs. The Greek Jesus*, Hilkiah Press, copyright © 2006 (www.HilkiahPress.com) (www.NehemiasWall.com)

Gordon, Nehemia. "The Hebrew Yeshua vs. The Greek Jesus, Live Video Teaching". DVD 8907638452, Hilkiah Press, (www.HilkiahPress.com) (www.NehemiasWall.com)

Gordon, Nehemia. *The Naming of Jesus in Hebrew Matthew.* Makor Hebrew Foundation, copyright © 2008 (www.makorhebrew.org) (NehemiasWall.com)

Gordon, Nehemia. *Torah* Pearls #47 – Re'eh (*Deuteronomy* 11:26-16:17),

Guralnik, David B., General Editor. *Websters New World Dictionary of the American Language*. The World Publishing Co., The South Western Company, Nashville, TB. Copyright © 1963.

Harris, Daniel Leonard. *God Cares What You Eat – Dietary Laws of the Bible.* Daniel Leonard Harris, Columbia, SC, copyright © 2019

Hillsong Music Publishing, "So Will I (100 Billion X)", Words and Music by Joel Houston, Benjamin Hastings, & Michael Fatkin, copyright © 2017 Hillsong Music Publishing CCLL: 7084123, https://www.youtube.com/watch?v=GfVd5x9W1Xc

Jarvis, D. C., *Folk Medicine*, Fawcett Crest Books, Greenwich, Connecticut. Copyright 1958.

Jasher, J., "*The Book of Jasher, From the Original Hebrew Into English*", www.ancientwisdombooks.com, 2020

Jones, Dr. Miles R., *The Epistle of James (Ya'akov) – A Translation from the Hebrew*.

Jones Report. 18, July 2021. copyright © 2021. Published by B'nai Emunah Institute from Accelerated Learning. www.writingofgod.com ; administrator@jonesgeniuses.com

Jordan, Christy. "Do Not Boil a Young Goat in its Mother's Milk. Another Possibility". (https://seekingscripture.com/do-not-boil-a-young-goat-in-its-mothers-milk-another-possibility , copyright © 2022)

Karten, Michelle M. Kids Health from Nemours – *Why Do Newborns Need a Vitamin K Shot?* Date Reviewed: April 2018, https://kidshealth.org/en/parents/vitamin-k-shot.prt-en.html

Life Application Study Bible, NIV. Tyndale House Publishers, Inc. 1820 Jet Stream Drive, Colorado Springs, CO 80921-3696. copyright Revised August 1983

Lumpkin, Joseph, "*The Apocrypha: Including Books from the Ethiopic Bible*", Fifth Estate Publishers, PO Box 116, Blountsville, AL 35031, copyright © 2009

Malkus, George H. *Why Christians Get Sick*. Hallelujah Acres Publishing, Eidson, Tennessee, copyright ©1989

McMillen, S. I. *None of These Diseases*. Fleming H. Revell Company, Westwood, NJ, copyright © 1963, 1984, 2000

Mikovits, Judy. Kent Heckenlively. *Plague of Corruption*. (New York, NY. Skyhorse Publishing, copyright © 2020)

Ott, John N. *Health and Light, The Extraordinary Study That Shows How Light Affects Your Health and Emotional Well-Being*. Ariel Press, Mar le Hill, GA, copyright © 1973

Payne, Bishop J.L. *God's Health, Natural Healing, Biblical Dietary Laws, Perspective on Health, Healing, Living, Volumes 1 and 2.* Church House Publisher, Jackson, Mississippi, copyright © 2007

Reams, Betty. "RBTI & Foods, Eating by the Numbers-Module Six", IIOM RBTI January 2021

Reams Hernandez, Betty. *Book One: In His Footsteps: My Life with Carey Reams*. Third Printing, Published by Daily Manufacturing, Inc. 4920 Pless Rd., Rockwell, NC 28138, copyright © 2017, www.dailymfg.com.

Reams, Carey. *Choose Life or Death.* New Leaf Press, Harrison, Arkansas, copyright © 1978

Reams, Carey A., Dudley, Cliff. *Choose Life or Death*. Self-Published

"*Revelation 18:23-Discover Babylon's Deception by Pharmakeia/Sorcery*." https://revelationscriptures/revelation-18-23-babylons-pharmakeia

Robinson, Lucinda Gibbs. *Natural Herbal Therapy, A Scriptural/Torah Based Plan to Reclaim Your Health*. Lucinda Gibbs Robinson, copyright © 2011, 2020, 2024, 2026. www.naturalherbaltherapy.info

Rood, Michael J. *The Chronological Gospel, The Acceptable Year of the LORD. The Life and Seventy Week Ministry of the Messiah."* Aviv Moon Publishing, Fort Mill, SC, copyright © 2013

Rood, Michael J. "These Are Unclean to You. Five Episode Teaching." Michael Rood Presents, Fort Mill, SC, copyright © 2020

Rood, Michael. "*These Things Are Unclean to You.*". DVD (Fort Mill, SC 29716, copyright © 2020). www.aroodawakening.tv. 1- 866-766-3610

Russell, Rex M.D. *What the Bible Says About Healthy Living.* Grand Rapids, MI, (Baker Publishing, Copyright © 2014) ISBN 978-0-8007-2569-3

Sharps, Jim. *Concepts of Original Medicine.* IIOM, Smithfield, VA, copyright © 2006

Sproul, R.C., (Blog/Teacher/Rc-Sproul). November 30, 2020. Excerpt adapted from *Romans: An Expositional Commentary* (https://www.ligonier.org/store/romans-an-expositional-commentary-hardcover/) by R.C. Sproul

Stern, David H. *The Complete Jewish Study Bible, Insights for Jews and Christians, Illuminating the Jewishness of God's Word.* Hendrickson Publishers, Peabody, MA, copyright © 2016

Stone, Perry. *The Meal That Heals.* Charisma House – A Strang Company,

600 Rinehart Road, Lake Mary, FL 32746. www.charismaHouse.com, copyright © 2008

The Holy Bible Revised Standard Version. Revised A.D. 1952; Thomas Nelson & Sons, USA copyright © 1952

"*The Dead Sea Scrolls: History and Overview*;" Original article by Ayala Sussman and Ruth Peled. Jewish Virtual Library. www.jewishvirtuallibrary.org

The Israel Bible. Edited by Rabbi Tuly Weisz. Jewish Publication Society, Menorah Books, Milford, CT, 1985, First Edition copyright © 2018

The System Bible Study or The Busy People's Bible. Authors: By Many of the World's Greatest Bible Scholars. The System Bible Company, Chicago, IL, copyright © 1922

Tennant, Jerry *Healing is Voltage-Healing Eye Disease*, Jerry Tennant, Middleton, DE., copyright © 2011.

The Winston Dictionary College Edition. The John C. Winston Company. Copyright © 1946.

Turley Susan M., *Understanding Pharmacology for Health Professionals.* Third Edition. (Upper Saddle River, New Jersey. Pearson Education, Inc., copyright © 2003)

Von Vett, Julie and Malone, Bruce. *Inspired Evidence Only One Reality.* (Midland, MI., Search for the Truth Publications. Copyright © 2011.)

What Is a Retrovirus? Healthline, medically reviewed by Vincent J. Tavelle et al. March 1, 2019. https://www.healthline.com/health/what-is-a-retrovirus

"What the Bible Says About Boiling a Kid in its Mother's Milk", (Church of the Great God, Copyright © 1992-2022).

www.bibletools.org/index.cfm/fuseaction/topical.show/RTD/CGG/ID/9313/Boiling-Kid-its-mothers-milk.htm

White, Ellen G. *Counsels on Diet and Food.* (Herald Publishing Association. The Ellen G. White Publications, USA. Copyright © 1938, 1946, 1976, 2001)

White, Ellen G. *Healthful Living.* Premium Classic Books, Columbia, SC, copyright © 2018

Whitney, Eleanor Noss; Hamilton, Eva May Nunnelley; Rolfes, Sharon Rady. *Understanding Nutrition: Fifth Edition.* West Publishing Company, 50 W. Kellog Blvd., St. Paul, MN 55164-1003, Copyright © 1990. ISBN 0-314-57831-5

Young, Brad H., *Jesus The Jewish Theologian*, Baker Academic, a division of Baker Publishing Group, Grand Rapids, Michigan, PO Box 6287, Grand Rapids, MI 49516-6287; copyright © 1995. Published 2011. www.bakeracademic.com ISBN 978-0-8010-4817-3

Young, Brad H., *Paul the Jewish Theologian*, Baker Academic, a division of Baker Publishing Group, Grand Rapids, Michigan, PO Box 6287, Grand Rapids, MI 49516-6287; copyright © 1997. www.bakeracademic.com ISBN 978-0-8010-4821-0

Zalewski, Agnes. "*Petroleum in Real Life: Pills*". http://context.capp.ca/article/2019/feature-petroleum-in-real-life-pills

www.ingramcontent.com/pod-product-compliance
Lightning Source LLC
LaVergne TN
LVHW070852210926
848482LV00016B/918